T0137195

Voice Disorders in Athletes, Coaches and other Sports Professionals

Abdul-Latif Hamdan • Robert Thayer Sataloff
Mary J. Hawkshaw

Voice Disorders in Athletes, Coaches and other Sports Professionals

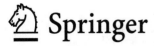

Springer

Abdul-Latif Hamdan
Department of Otolaryngology – Head and
Neck Surgery
American University of Beirut
Medical Center
Beirut
Lebanon

Adjunct Professor, Department of
Otolaryngology – Head and
Neck Surgery
Drexel University College of Medicine
Philadelphia, PA
USA

Mary J. Hawkshaw
Department of Otolaryngology – Head and
Neck Surgery
Drexel University College of Medicine
Philadelphia, PA
USA

Robert Thayer Sataloff
Department of Otolaryngology – Head and
Neck Surgery
Drexel University College of Medicine
Philadelphia, PA
USA

Lankenau Institute for Medical Research
Wynnewood, PA
USA

ISBN 978-3-030-69833-1   ISBN 978-3-030-69831-7   (eBook)
https://doi.org/10.1007/978-3-030-69831-7

This Springer imprint is published by the registered company Springer Nature Switzerland AG
The registered company address is: Gewerbestrasse 11, 6330 Cham, Switzerland

To our families.

Preface

The last few decades have witnessed an increase in sports activities in a growing percentage of the population. It is estimated that one out of four adults in the United States plays at least one type of sport, with younger individuals being more attracted to high-velocity sports while elderly people tend to pursue less volatile, non-competitive sports. The fitness and sports industry, like other occupational industries that require extensive voice use, has a high prevalence of voice disorders among its occupational voice users. Athletes, fitness instructors, and coaches often engage in abusive voice behavior because of the need to project their voices while performing strenuous exercise. This vocal loading is compounded by environmental factors such as background noise, poor environment acoustics, and environmental allergies. Additional individual-related voice risk factors include dehydration, exercise-induced asthma, laryngopharyngeal reflux disease, and the intake of supplements such as anabolic steroids, and other factors. Moreover, athletes are prone to laryngeal trauma, with sports-related laryngeal trauma being common causes of laryngeal injury, in addition to motor vehicle accidents and strangulation. Musculoskeletal injuries may also jeopardize voice given the strong interplay between the phonatory apparatus and musculoskeletal structures. Exercise-induced laryngeal dysfunction, also called paradoxical vocal fold motion, is a significant threat to athletes that warrants consideration given its dramatic impact on quality of life, and that also may result in dysphonia.

Sports lead to numerous voice symptoms and laryngeal pathologies that affect athletes, coaches, and fitness instructors, often leading to absenteeism, abstention from sports, and interference with other normal activities. This book reviews the literature on voice health risk factors in the sports industry. The first four chapters provide core knowledge helpful in understanding voice disorders. This information is included in this book for the convenience of readers who are not otolaryngologists or speech-language pathologists. A fundamental understanding of voice helps readers comprehend sports-related voice dysfunction. These four chapters provide basic information that is common knowledge among laryngologists, and they are modified from prior publications by the author (RTS), with permission. Chapter 1 presents a focused, brief review of anatomy and physiology of phonation. Chapters 2 and 3 explain the medical evaluation (history and physical examination) performed for patients with voice complaints. Many athletes, coaches, and instructors should be considered professional voice users. If a coach cannot be heard from the sidelines, or athletes cannot be heard calling signals to their teammates, their professional performance is impaired. Many voice disorders result in not only alterations in voice quality, but also in loudness and projection. Chapter 4, written in collaboration with Johnathan Sataloff, MD, offers an overview of many medical conditions that may afflict the voice, and of their treatments. These conditions may be seen in any population, including athletes. Chapter 5 provides a comprehensive review of voice health risk factors in sports-occupational voice users, highlighting individual and environmental factors. This review serves as a basis for development of strategies to prevent voice injuries and reduce the risks of laryngeal trauma in athletes and coaches. Chapter 6 discusses voice disorders associated with specific sports activities and highlights behaviors that lead commonly to dysphonia among athletes and coaches participating in specific sports. It also provides understanding of the pathophysiology of dysphonia and the measures that might decrease the prevalence of dysphonia in participants of these athletic endeavors. Chapter 7 provides a concise description of the interplay between musculoskeletal injuries, hyperkinetic body behavior, laryngeal hyperfunction, and voice disorders in athletes and coaches. Chapter 8 summarizes external laryngeal trauma in athletes. Such trauma can lead not only to voice, swallowing, and breathing disturbances, but also to death. The chapter also discusses team- and field-related collisions as causes of sports-related laryngeal trauma and highlights the development of sports-specific rules and equipment that help to minimize the occurrence of such injuries. Chapter 9 offers a comprehensive discussion of exercise-induced laryngeal obstruction in athletes. Also known as paradoxical vocal fold motion (PVFM) and by several other names, this condition is characterized by vocal fold adduction (closing) when the vocal folds should be adducting (opening). This condition can disable athletes, and differential diagnosis and treatment are discussed in detail in this chapter. Chapter 10 summaries sex hormone disturbances in athletes and their effects upon the voice. Related issues have been recognized among young female gymnasts and ballet dancers for many decades, but the implications go far beyond that demographic. Athletes of all ages and genders may be affected by sports-related sex hormone changes and use of related substances such as testosterone to enhance performance. Chapter 11 provides a summary/overview of management of voice health among sports professionals. It considers the information provided in previous chapters, as well as other factors, and offers guidance and strategies for preserving healthy voice while competing in sports at any level, coaching, or participating in any other activity in the sports industry. This chapter stresses the importance of increased awareness of voice hygiene and education, improvement in working environment acoustics when possible, and strategies to minimize the risk of laryngeal fractures.

This book has been written entirely by the three authors in order to optimize consistency and prevent duplication, with a contribution to Chapter 4 by Johnathan B. Sataloff, MD. This is the first book that addresses specifically the interactions between the sports industry and voice health. Dysphonia is extremely common among athletes, coaches, fitness instructors, and other sports professionals. However, it is preventable in most cases and treatable in virtually all cases. The authors hope that this book will provide insights not only for medical voice care professionals, but also for participants in the sports industry that may help them preserve healthy voice for everyone involved in sports.

Beirut, Lebanon   Abdul-Latif Hamdan
Philadelphia, PA, USA   Robert Thayer Sataloff
Philadelphia, PA, USA   Mary J. Hawkshaw

Acknowledgments

The authors are indebted to Deborah Westergon, Executive Assistant to Dr. Robert Sataloff, for her invaluable efforts in preparing and formatting this manuscript, identifying and correcting errors as the text was being written, and assuring accuracy of the references.

Contents

Contributor

Johnathan B. Sataloff, MD Department of Psychiatry, Beth Israel Deaconess Medical Center, Harvard Medical School, Boston, MA, USA

Chapter 1
Anatomy and Physiology of the Voice

To treat voice patients knowledgeably and responsibly, healthcare providers must understand the medical aspects of voice disorders and their treatment. This requires core knowledge of the anatomy and physiology of phonation. The human voice consists of much more than simply the vocal folds, popularly known as the vocal cords. State-of-the-art voice diagnosis, nonsurgical therapy, and voice surgery depend on understanding the complex workings of the vocal tract. Physicians and other healthcare professionals specializing in the care of voice patients, especially voice professionals, should be familiar with at least the basics of the latest concepts in voice function. The physiology of phonation is much more complex than this brief chapter might suggest, and readers interested in acquiring more than a clinically essential introduction are encouraged to consult other literature [1].

1.1 Anatomy

The larynx is essential to normal voice production, but the anatomy of the voice is not limited to the larynx. The vocal mechanism includes the abdominal and back musculature, rib cage, lungs, pharynx, oral cavity, and nose, among other structures. Each component performs an important function in voice production, although it is possible to produce voice even without a larynx—for example, in patients who have undergone laryngectomy. In addition, virtually all parts of the body play some role in voice production and may be responsible for voice dysfunction. Even something as remote as a sprained ankle may alter posture, thereby impairing abdominal, back, and thoracic muscle function and resulting in vocal inefficiency, weakness, and hoarseness.

The larynx is composed of four basic anatomic units: skeleton, intrinsic muscles, extrinsic muscles, and mucosa. The most important components of the laryngeal skeleton are the thyroid cartilage, cricoid cartilage, and two arytenoid cartilages

A.-L. Hamdan et al., *Voice Disorders in Athletes, Coaches and other Sports Professionals*, https://doi.org/10.1007/978-3-030-69831-7_1

(Fig. 1.1). Intrinsic muscles of the larynx are connected to these cartilages (Fig. 1.2). One of the intrinsic muscles, the *thyroarytenoid muscle* (its medial belly is also known as the vocalis muscle), extends on each side from the vocal process of the arytenoid cartilage to the inside of the thyroid cartilage just below and behind the

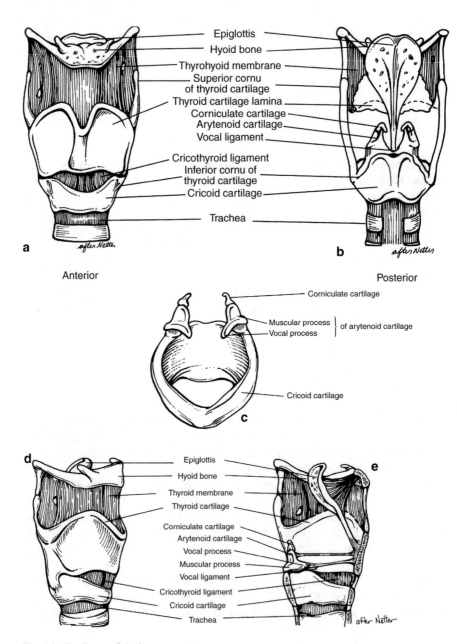

Fig. 1.1 Cartilages of the larynx

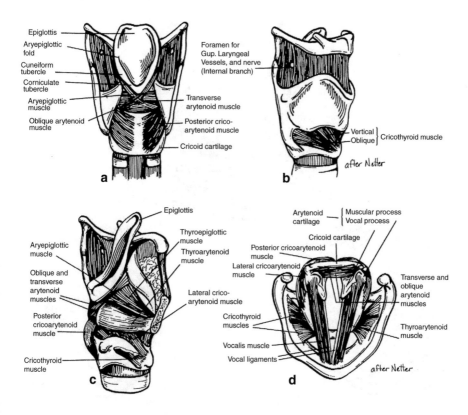

Intrinsic muscles of the larynx.

Fig. 1.2   Intrinsic muscles of the larynx

thyroid prominence ("Adam's apple"), forming the body of the vocal folds. The vocal folds act as the *oscillator* or *voice source* of the vocal tract. The space between the vocal folds is called the *glottis* and is used as an anatomic reference point. The intrinsic muscles alter the position, shape, and tension of the vocal folds, bringing them together (adduction), moving them apart (abduction), or stretching them by increasing longitudinal tension (Fig. 1.3). They are able to do so because the laryngeal cartilages are connected by soft attachments that allow changes in their relative angles and distances, thereby permitting alteration in the shape and tension of the tissues suspended between them. The arytenoid cartilages on their eliptoid cricoarytenoid joints are capable of motion in multiple planes, permitting complex vocal fold motion and alteration in the shape of the vocal fold edge associated with intrinsic muscle action (Fig. 1.4). All but one of the muscles on each side of the larynx are innervated by one of the two *recurrent laryngeal nerves*. Because this nerve runs in a long course (especially on the left) from the neck down into the chest and then back up to the larynx (hence, the name "recurrent"), it is injured easily by trauma, neck surgery, and chest surgery. Injury may result in vocal fold paresis or paralysis.

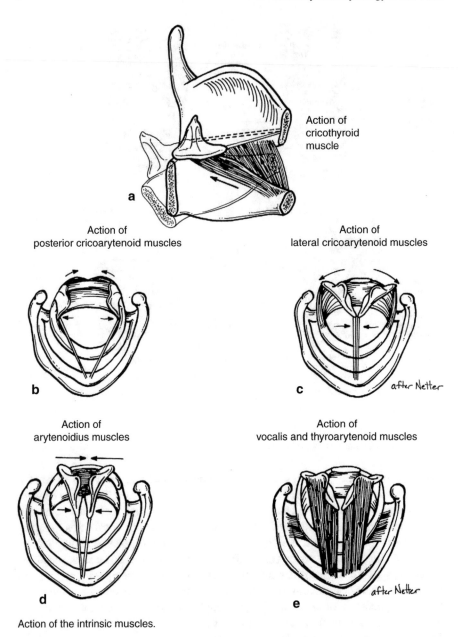

Action of
cricothyroid
muscle

Action of
posterior cricoarytenoid muscles

Action of
lateral cricoarytenoid muscles

after Netter

Action of
arytenoidius muscles

Action of
vocalis and thyroarytenoid muscles

after Netter

Action of the intrinsic muscles.

Fig. 1.3 Action of the intrinsic muscle

The remaining muscle (*cricothyroid muscle*) is innervated by the superior laryngeal nerve on each side, which is especially susceptible to viral and traumatic injury. It causes changes in longitudinal tension that are important in voice projection and pitch control. The "false vocal folds" are located above the vocal folds and, unlike

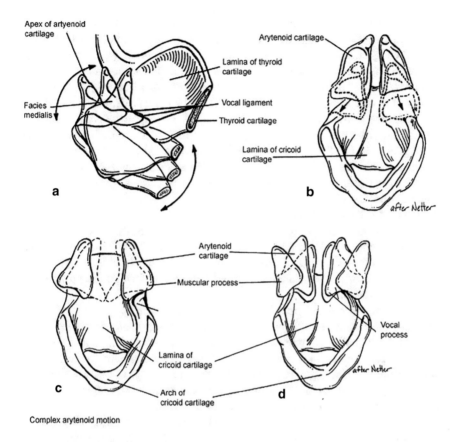

Complex arytenoid motion

Fig. 1.4 Complex arytenoid motion

the true vocal folds, usually do not make contact during normal speaking or singing [1]. The neuroanatomy and neurophysiology of phonation are extremely compli- cated and only partially understood. As the new field of neurolaryngology advances, a more thorough understanding of the subject is becoming increasingly important to clinicians. Readers interested in acquiring a deeper, scientific understanding of neu- rolaryngology are encouraged to consult other literature [2] and the publications cited therein.

Because the attachments of the laryngeal cartilages are flexible, the positions of the cartilages with respect to each other change when the laryngeal skeleton is ele- vated or lowered. Such changes in vertical height are controlled by the extrinsic laryngeal muscles, the strap muscles of the neck. When the angles and distances between cartilages change because of this accordion-like effect, the resting length of the intrinsic muscle changes. Such large adjustments in intrinsic muscle condi- tion interfere with fine control of smooth vocal quality. Classically trained singers generally are taught to use the extrinsic muscles to maintain the laryngeal skeleton at a relatively constant height regardless of pitch. That is, they learn to avoid the natural tendency of the larynx to rise with ascending pitch and fall with descending pitch, thereby enhancing unity of sound quality throughout the vocal range through effects on both resting muscle condition and supraglottic vocal tract posture.

The soft tissues lining the larynx are much more complex than originally thought. The mucosa forms the thin, lubricated surface of the vocal folds, which makes contact when the two vocal folds are approximated. Laryngeal mucosa might look superficially like the mucosa which lines the inside of the mouth, but it is not. Throughout most of the larynx, there are goblet cells and pseudostratified ciliated columnar epithelial cells designed for producing and handling mucous secretions, similar to mucosal surfaces found throughout the respiratory tract. However, the mucosa overlying the vocal folds is different. First, it is stratified squamous epithelium, which is better suited to withstand the trauma of vocal fold contact. Second, the vocal fold is not simply muscle covered with mucosa. Rather, it consists of five layers as described by Hirano [3]. Mechanically, the vocal fold structures act more like three layers consisting of the *cover* (epithelium and superficial layer of the lamina propria), *transition* (intermediate and deep layers of the lamina propria), and *body* (the vocalis muscle).

The *supraglottic vocal tract* includes the pharynx, tongue, palate, oral cavity, nose, and other structures. Together, they act as a *resonator* and are largely responsible for vocal quality or timbre and the perceived character of all phonated sounds. The vocal folds themselves produce only a "buzzing" sound. During the course of vocal training for singing, acting, or healthy speaking, changes occur not only in the larynx but also in the muscle motion, control, and shape of the supraglottic vocal tract and in aerobic, pulmonary, and bodily muscle function.

The *infraglottic vocal tract* (all anatomical structures below the glottis) serves as the *power source* for the voice. Singers and actors often refer to the entire power source complex as their "support" or "diaphragm." The anatomy of support for phonation is especially complicated and not completely understood. Yet, it is quite important because deficiencies in support frequently are responsible for voice dysfunction.

The purpose of the support mechanism is to generate a force that directs a controlled airstream between the vocal folds. Active respiratory muscles work in concert with passive forces. The principal muscles of inspiration are the diaphragm (a dome-shaped muscle that extends along the bottom of the rib cage) and the external intercostal muscles (located between the ribs). During quiet respiration, expiration is largely passive. The lungs and rib cage generate passive expiratory forces under many common circumstances such as after a full breath.

Many of the muscles used for active expiration also are employed in "support" for phonation. Muscles of active expiration either raise the intra-abdominal pressure, forcing the diaphragm upward, or lower the ribs or sternum to decrease the dimensions of the thorax, or both, thereby compressing air in the chest. The primary muscles of expiration are "the abdominal muscles," but internal intercostals and other chest and back muscles also are involved. Trauma or surgery that alters the structure or function of these muscles or ribs undermines the power source of the voice, as do diseases, such as asthma, that impair expiration. Deficiencies in the support mechanism often result in compensatory efforts that utilize the laryngeal muscles, which are not designed for power functions. Such behavior can result in impaired voice quality, rapid fatigue, pain, and even structural pathology such as vocal fold nodules. Current expert treatment for such vocal problems focuses on the correction of the underlying malfunction rather than surgery whenever possible.

1.2 Physiology

The physiology of voice production is extremely complex. The volitional production of voice begins in the cerebral cortex (Fig. 1.5).

The command for vocalization involves complex interactions among brain centers for speech, as well as other areas. For singing, speech directives must be integrated with information from the centers for musical and artistic expression, which are discussed elsewhere [1]. The "idea" of the planned vocalization is conveyed to the precentral gyrus in the motor cortex, which transmits another set of instructions to the motor nuclei in the brainstem and spinal cord. These areas send out the complicated messages necessary for coordinated activity of the larynx, thoracic and abdominal musculature lungs, and vocal tract articulators, among other structures. Additional refinement of motor activity is provided by the extrapyramidal and autonomic nervous systems. These impulses combine to produce a sound that is transmitted not only to the ears of the listener but also to those of the speaker or singer. Auditory feedback is transmitted from the ear through the brainstem to the cerebral cortex, and adjustments are made within milliseconds that permit the vocalist to match the sound produced with the sound intended, integrating the acoustic properties of the performance environment. Tactile feedback from the throat and other muscles involved in phonation also is believed to help in fine tuning vocal output, although the mechanism and role of tactile feedback are not understood fully. Many trained singers and speakers cultivate the ability to use tactile feedback effectively because of expected interference with auditory feedback data from ancillary sound such as an orchestra or band.

Phonation, the production of sound, requires interaction among the power source, oscillator, and resonator. The voice may be compared to a brass instrument such as a trumpet. Power is generated by the chest, abdominal, and back musculature, and a high-pressure air stream is produced. The trumpeter's lips open and close against the mouthpiece producing a "buzz" similar to the sound produced by vocal folds when they come together and move apart (oscillate) during phonation. This sound then passes through the trumpet, which has acoustic resonance characteristics that shape the sound we associate with trumpet music. If a trumpet mouthpiece is placed on a French horn, the sound we hear will sound like a French horn, not a trumpet. Quality characteristics are dependent upon the resonator more than on the oscillatory source. The non-mouthpiece portions of a brass instrument are analogous to the supraglottic vocal tract.

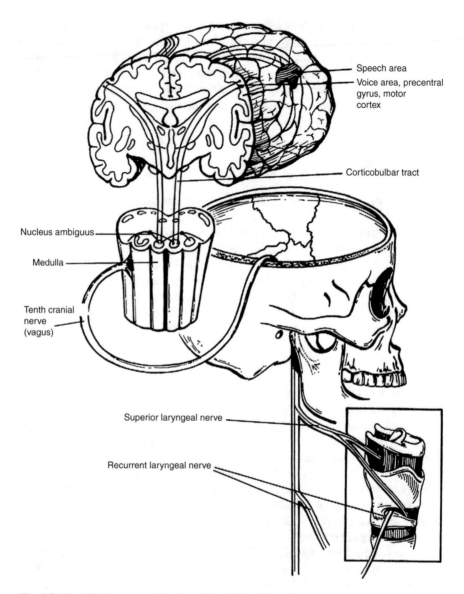

Fig. 1.5 Simplified summary of pathway for volitional phonation

During phonation, the infraglottic musculature must make rapid, complex adjustments because the resistance changes almost continuously as the glottis closes, opens, and changes shape. At the beginning of each phonatory cycle, the vocal folds are approximated, and the glottis is obliterated. This permits infraglottic air pressure to build, typically to a level of about 7 cm of water for conversational speech. At that point, the vocal folds are convergent (Fig. 1.6a). Because the vocal folds are closed, there is no airflow. The subglottic pressure then pushes the vocal folds progressively

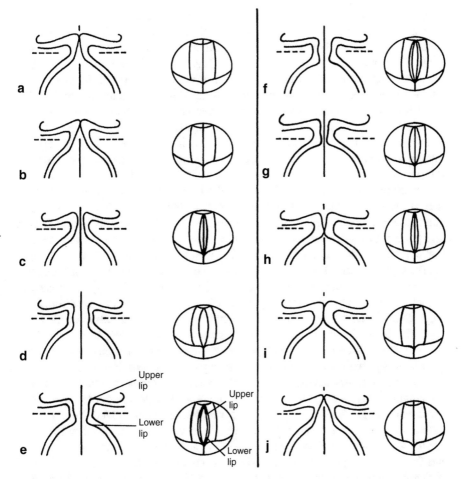

Fig. 1.6 Frontal view (left) and view from above (right) illustrating the normal pattern of vocal fold vibration. The vocal folds close and open from the inferior aspect of the vibratory margin upward and from posterior to anterior

farther apart from the bottom up and from the back forward (Fig. 1.6b) until a space develops (Fig. 1.6c, d) and air begins to flow. The Bernoulli force created by the air passing between the vocal folds combines with the mechanical properties of the folds to begin closing the lower portion of the vocal folds almost immediately (Fig. 1.6e–h) even while the upper edges are still separating. The principles and mathematics of the Bernoulli force are complex. It is a flow effect more easily understood by familiar examples such as the sensation of pull exerted on a vehicle when passed by a truck at high speed or the inward motion of a shower curtain when the water flows past it.

The upper portion of the vocal folds has elastic properties that also tend to make the vocal folds snap back to the midline. This force becomes more dominant as the upper edges are stretched and the opposing force of the air stream diminishes because of approximation of the lower edges of the vocal folds. The upper portions of the vocal folds are then returned to the midline (Fig. 1.6i), completing the glottic cycle. Subglottal pressure then builds again (Fig. 1.6j), and the events repeat. Thus, there is a vertical phase difference. That is, the lower portion of the vocal folds begins to open and close before the upper portion. The rippling displacement of the vocal fold cover produces a mucosal wave that can be examined clinically under stroboscopic light. If this complex motion is impaired, hoarseness or other changes in voice quality may cause the patient to seek medical evaluation. The frequency of vibration (number of cycles of openings and closings per second, measured in hertz [Hz]) is dependent on the air pressure and mechanical properties of the vocal folds, which are regulated in part by the laryngeal muscles. Pitch is the perceptual correlate of frequency. Under most circumstances, as the vocal folds are thinned and stretched and air pressure is increased, the frequency of air pulse emissions increases, and pitch goes up. The myoelastic-aerodynamic mechanism of phonation reveals that the vocal folds emit pulses of air, rather than vibrating like strings.

The sound produced by the oscillating vocal folds, called the voice source signal, is a complex tone containing a fundamental frequency and many overtones, or higher harmonic partials. The amplitude of the partials decreases uniformly at approximately 12 dB per octave. Interestingly, the acoustic spectrum of the voice source is about the same in ordinary speakers as it is in trained singers and speakers. Voice quality differences in voice professionals occur as the voice source signal passes through their supraglottic vocal tract resonator system (Fig. 1.7).

The pharynx, oral cavity, and nasal cavity act as a series of infinitely variable interconnected resonators, which are more complex than that in our trumpet example or other single resonators. As with other resonators, some frequencies are attenuated, and others are enhanced. Enhanced frequencies are radiated with higher relative amplitudes or intensities. Sundberg [4] showed long ago that the vocal tract has four or five important resonance frequencies called *formants* and summarized his early findings in a book that has become a classic. The presence of formants alters the uniformly sloping voice source spectrum and creates peaks at formant frequencies. These alterations of the voice source spectral envelope are responsible for distinguishable sounds of speech and song. Formant frequencies are determined by vocal tract shape, which can be altered by the laryngeal, pharyngeal, and oral cavity musculature. Overall, the vocal tract length and shape are individually fixed and determined by age and sex (females and children have shorter vocal tracts and formant frequencies that are higher than males). Voice training includes conscious physical mastery of the adjustment of vocal tract shape.

Although the formants differ for different vowels, one resonant frequency has received particular attention and is known as the "singer's formant." This formant occurs in the vicinity of 2300–3200 Hz for all vowel spectra and appears to be responsible for the "ring" in a singer's or trained speaker's ("speaker's formant") voice. The ability to hear a trained voice clearly even over a loud choir or orchestra is dependent primarily on the presence of the singer's formant [1]. Interestingly, there is little or no significant difference in maximum vocal intensity between

Generation of Vocal Sound

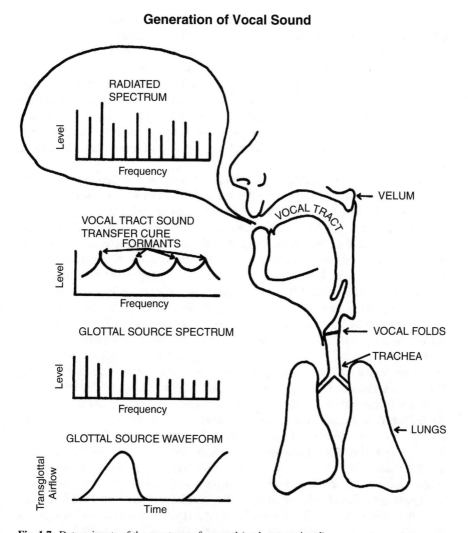

Fig. 1.7 Determinants of the spectrum of a vowel (oral-output signal)

trained and untrained singers. The singer's formant also contributes substantially to the differences in fach (voice classification) among voice categories, occurring in basses at about 2400 Hz, baritones at 2600 Hz, tenors at 2800 Hz, mezzo-sopranos at 2900 Hz, and sopranos at 3200 Hz. It is frequently much less prominent in high soprano singing [1].

The mechanisms that control two vocal characteristics are particularly important: fundamental frequency and intensity. Fundamental frequency, which corresponds to pitch, can be altered by changing either air pressure or the mechanical properties of the vocal folds, although the latter is more efficient under most conditions. When the cricothyroid muscle contracts, it makes the thyroid cartilage pivot on the cricothyroid joint and increases the distance between the thyroid and arytenoid cartilages, thus stretching the vocal folds. This increases the surface area exposed to subglottal pressure and makes the air pressure more effective in opening the glottis. In addition, stretching of elastic fibers of the vocal fold makes them more efficient at snapping back together. Hence, the cycles shorten and repeat more frequently, and the fundamental frequency (and pitch) rises. Other muscles, including the thyroarytenoid, also contribute [1]. Raising the pressure of the air stream also tends to increase fundamental frequency, a phenomenon for which singers must learn to compensate. Otherwise, their pitch would go up whenever they tried to sing more loudly.

Voice intensity corresponds to loudness and depends on the degree to which the glottal wave motion excites the air molecules in the vocal tract. Raising the air pressure creates greater amplitude of vocal fold oscillation and therefore increases vocal intensity. However, actually, it is not the oscillation of the vocal fold but rather the sudden cessation of airflow that is responsible for initiating an acoustic signal in the vocal tract and controlling intensity. This is similar to the mechanism of acoustic signal that results from buzzing lips. In the larynx, the sharper the cutoff of air flow, the more intense the sound [1]. In the evaluation of voice disorders, an individual's ability to optimize adjustments of air pressure and glottal resistance is assessed. When high subglottic pressure is combined with high adductory (closing) vocal fold force, glottal airflow and the amplitude of the voice source fundamental frequency are low. This is called *pressed phonation* and can be measured clinically through a technique known as flow glottography. Flow glottogram wave amplitude indicates the type of phonation being used, and the slope (closing rate) provides information about the sound pressure level or loudness. If adductory forces are so weak that the vocal folds do not make contact, the vocal folds become inefficient at resisting air leakage, and the voice source fundamental frequency is low. This is known as *breathy phonation. Flow phonation* is characterized by lower subglottic pressure and lower adductory force. These conditions increase the dominance of the fundamental frequency of the voice source in the perceived sound. Sundberg showed that the amplitude of the fundamental frequency can be increased by 15 dB or more when the subject changes from pressed phonation to flow phonation [4]. If a patient habitually uses pressed phonation, considerable effort will be required to achieve loud voicing. The muscle patterns and force that are used to compensate for this laryngeal inefficiency may cause vocal fold damage. Such voice behavior (i.e., pressed voice) can result from laryngeal structural problems, voice technique, psychological abnormalities, and other causes.

Acknowledgments Modified in part from Sataloff RT. *Professional Voice: The Science and Art of Clinical Care, 4th Edition.* San Diego, CA: Plural Publishing; 2017, with permission.

References

1. Sataloff RT. Professional voice: the science and art of clinical care. 4th ed. San Diego, CA: Plural Publishing; 2017.
2. Sataloff RT. Neurolaryngology. San Diego, CA: Plural Publishing; 2017.
3. Hirano M. Phonosurgery: basic and clinical investigations. Otologia (Fukuoka). 1975;21:239–442.
4. Sundberg J. The science of the singing voice. DeKalb, IL: Northern Illinois University Press; 1987.

Chapter 2
Patient History

2.1 Introduction

A comprehensive history and physical examination usually reveal the cause of voice dysfunction. Effective history taking and physical examination depend on a practical understanding of the anatomy and physiology of voice production [1–3]. Because dysfunction in virtually any body system may affect phonation, medical inquiry must be comprehensive. The current standard of care for all voice patients evolved from advances inspired by medical problems of voice professionals such as singers and actors. Even minor problems may be particularly symptomatic in singers and actors, because of the extreme demands they place on their voices. However, a great many other patients are voice professionals. They include teachers, salespeople, attorneys, clergy, physicians, politicians, telephone receptionists, and anyone else whose ability to earn a living is impaired in the presence of voice dysfunction. Because good voice quality is so important in our society, the majority of our patients are voice professionals, and all patients should be treated as such.

The scope of inquiry and examination for most patients is similar to that required for singers and actors, except that performing voice professionals have unique needs, which require additional history and examination. Questions must be added regarding performance commitments, professional status and voice goals, the amount and nature of voice training, the performance environment, rehearsal practices, abusive habits during speech and singing, and many other matters. Such supplementary information is essential to proper treatment selection and patient counseling in singers and actors. However, analogous factors must also be taken into account for stockbrokers, factory shop foremen, elementary school teachers, homemakers with several noisy children, and many others. Physicians familiar with the management of these challenging patients are well equipped to evaluate all patients with voice complaints.

Obtaining extensive historical background information is necessary for thorough evaluation of the voice patient, and the otolaryngologist who sees voice patients (especially singers) only occasionally cannot reasonably be expected to remember all the pertinent questions. Although some laryngologists consider a lengthy inquisition helpful in establishing rapport, many of us who see a substantial number of voice patients each day within a busy practice need a thorough but less time-consuming alternative. A history questionnaire can be extremely helpful in documenting all the necessary information, helping the patient sort out and articulate his or her problems, and saving the clinician time recording information. The author has developed a questionnaire [4] that has proven helpful. The patient is asked to complete the relevant portions of the form at home prior to his or her office visit or in the waiting room before seeing the doctor. A similar form has been developed for voice patients who are not singers.

No history questionnaire is a substitute for direct, penetrating questioning by the physician. However, the direction of most useful inquiry can be determined from a glance at the questionnaire, obviating the need for extensive writing, which permits the physician greater eye contact with the patient and facilitates rapid establishment of the close rapport and confidence that are so important in treating voice patients. The physician is also able to supplement initial impressions and historical information from the questionnaire with seemingly leisurely conversation during the physical examination. The use of the history questionnaire has added substantially to the efficiency, consistent thoroughness, and ease of managing these delightful, but often complex, patients. A similar set of questions is used by the speech-language pathologist with new patients and by many enlightened singing teachers when assessing new students. The following questions help identify the cause(s) of the voice complaint.

2.1.1 How Old Are You?

Serious vocal endeavor may start in childhood and continue throughout a lifetime. As the vocal mechanism undergoes normal maturation, the voice changes. The optimal time to begin serious vocal training is controversial. For many years, most singing teachers advocated delay of vocal training and serious singing until near puberty in the female and after puberty and voice stabilization in the male. However, in a child with earnest vocal aspirations and potential, starting specialized training early in childhood is reasonable. Initial instruction should teach the child to vocalize without straining and to avoid all forms of voice abuse. It should not permit premature indulgence in operatic bravado. Most experts agree that taxing voice use and singing during puberty should be minimized or avoided altogether, particularly by the male. Voice maturation (attainment of stable adult vocal quality) may occur at any age from the early teenage years to the fourth decade of life. The dangerous tendency for young singers to attempt to sound older than their vocal years frequently causes vocal dysfunction.

All components of voice production are subject to normal aging. Abdominal and general muscular tone frequently decrease, the lungs lose elasticity, the thorax loses its distensibility, the mucosa of the vocal tract atrophies, mucous secretions change character and quantity, nerve endings are reduced in number, and psychoneurologic functions change. Moreover, the larynx itself loses muscle tone and bulk and may show depletion of submucosal ground substance in the vocal folds. The laryngeal cartilages ossify, and the joints may become arthritic and stiff. Hormonal influence is altered. Vocal range, intensity, and quality all may be modified. Vocal fold atrophy may be the most striking alteration. The clinical effects of aging seem more pronounced in female singers, although vocal fold histologic changes may be more prominent in males. Excellent male singers occasionally extend their careers into their 70s or beyond [5, 6]. However, some degree of breathiness, decreased range, and other evidence of aging should be expected in elderly voices. Nevertheless, many of the changes we typically associate with elderly singers (wobble, flat pitch) are due to lack of conditioning, rather than inevitable changes of biological aging. These aesthetically undesirable concomitants of aging can often be reversed.

2.1.2   What Is Your Voice Problem?

Careful questioning as to the onset of vocal problems is needed to separate acute from chronic dysfunction. Often, an upper respiratory tract infection will send a patient to the physician's office, but penetrating inquiry, especially in singers and actors, may reveal a chronic vocal problem that is the patient's real concern. Identifying acute and chronic problems before beginning therapy is important so that both patient and physician may have realistic expectations and make optimal therapeutic selections.

The specific nature of the vocal complaint can provide a great deal of information. Just as dizzy patients rarely walk into the physician's office complaining of "rotary vertigo," voice patients may be unable to articulate their symptoms without guidance. They may use the term *hoarseness* to describe a variety of conditions that the physician must separate. Hoarseness is a coarse or scratchy sound that is most often associated with abnormalities of the leading edge of the vocal folds such as laryngitis or mass lesions. Breathiness is a vocal quality characterized by excessive loss of air during vocalization. In some cases, it is due to improper technique. However, any condition that prevents full approximation of the vocal folds can be responsible. Possible causes include vocal fold paralysis, a mass lesion separating the leading edges of the vocal folds, arthritis of the cricoarytenoid joint, arytenoid dislocation, scarring of the vibratory margin, senile vocal fold atrophy (presbyphonia), psychogenic dysphonia, malingering, and other conditions.

Fatigue of the voice is inability to continue to speak or sing for extended periods without change in vocal quality and/or control. The voice may show fatigue by becoming hoarse, losing range, changing timbre, breaking into different registers, or exhibiting other uncontrolled aberrations. A well-trained singer should be able to sing for several hours without vocal fatigue.

Voice fatigue may occur through more than one mechanism. Most of the time, it is assumed to be due to muscle fatigue. This is often the case in patients who have voice fatigue associated with muscle tension dysphonia. The mechanism is most likely to be peripheral muscle fatigue and due to chemical changes (or depletion) in the muscle fibers. "Muscle fatigue" may also occur on a central (neurologic) basis. This mechanism is common in certain neuropathic disorders, such as some patients with multiple sclerosis; may occur with myasthenia gravis (actually neuromuscular junction pathology); or may be associated with paresis from various causes. However, the voice may also fatigue due to changes in the vibratory margin of the vocal fold. This phenomenon may be described as "lamina propria" fatigue (our description, not universally used). It, too, may be related to chemical or fluid changes in the lamina propria or cellular damage associated with conditions such as phonotrauma and dehydration. Excessive voice use, suboptimal tissue environment (e.g., dehydration, effects of pollution), lack of sufficient time of recovery between phonatory stresses, and genetic or structural tissue weaknesses that predispose to injury or delayed recovery from trauma all may be associated with lamina propria fatigue.

Although it has not been proven, the author (RTS) suspects that fatigue may also be related to the linearity of vocal fold vibrations. However, briefly, voices have linear and nonlinear (chaotic) characteristics. As the voice becomes more trained, vibrations become more symmetrical, and the system becomes more linear. In many pathologic voices, the nonlinear components appear to become more prominent. If a voice is highly linear, slight changes in the vibratory margin may have little effect on the output of the system. However, if the system has substantial nonlinearity due to vocal fold pathology, poor tissue environment, or other causes, slight changes in the tissue (slight swelling, drying, surface cell damage) may cause substantial changes in the acoustic output of the system (the butterfly effect), causing vocal quality changes and fatigue much more quickly with much smaller changes in initial condition in more linear vocal systems.

Fatigue is often caused by misuse of abdominal and neck musculature or oversinging and singing too loudly or too long. However, we must remember that vocal fatigue also may be a sign not only of general tiredness or vocal abuse (sometimes secondary to structural lesions or glottic closure problems) but also of serious illnesses such as myasthenia gravis. So, the importance of this complaint should not be understated.

Volume disturbance may manifest as inability to sing loudly or inability to sing softly. Each voice has its own dynamic range. Within the course of training, singers learn to sing more loudly by singing more efficiently. They also learn to sing softly, a more difficult task, through years of laborious practice. Actors and other trained speakers go through similar training. Most volume problems are secondary to intrinsic limitations of the voice or technical errors in voice use, although hormonal changes, aging, and neurologic disease are other causes. Superior laryngeal nerve paralysis impairs the ability to speak or sing loudly. This is a frequently unrecognized consequence of herpes infection (cold sores) and Lyme disease and may be precipitated by any viral upper respiratory tract infection.

Most highly trained singers require only about 10 minutes to half an hour to "warm up the voice." Prolonged warm-up time, especially in the morning, is most often caused by reflux laryngitis. Tickling or choking during singing is most often a symptom of an abnormality of the vocal fold's leading edge. The symptom of tickling or choking should contraindicate singing until the vocal folds have been examined. Pain while singing can indicate vocal fold lesions, laryngeal joint arthritis, infection, or gastric acid reflux irritation of the arytenoid region. However, pain is much more commonly caused by voice abuse with excessive muscular activity in the neck rather than an acute abnormality on the leading edge of a vocal fold. In the absence of other symptoms, these patients do not generally require immediate cessation of singing pending medical examination. However, sudden onset of pain (usually sharp pain) while singing may be associated with a mucosal tear or a vocal fold hemorrhage and warrants voice conservation pending laryngeal examination.

2.1.3   Do You Have Any Pressing Voice Commitments?

If a singer or professional speaker (e.g., actor, politician) seeks treatment at the end of a busy performance season and has no pressing engagements, management of the voice problem should be relatively conservative and designed to ensure long-term protection of the larynx, the most delicate part of the vocal mechanism. However, the physician and patient rarely have this luxury. Most often, the voice professional needs treatment within a week of an important engagement and sometimes within less than a day. Younger singers fall ill shortly before performances, not because of hypochondria or coincidence, but rather because of the immense physical and emotional stress of the preperformance period. The singer is frequently working harder and singing longer hours than usual. Moreover, he or she may be under particular pressure to learn new material and to perform well for a new audience. The singer may also be sleeping less than usual because of additional time spent rehearsing or because of the discomforts of a strange city. Seasoned professionals make their living by performing regularly, sometimes several times a week. Consequently, any time they get sick is likely to precede a performance. Caring for voice complaints in these situations requires highly skilled judgment and bold management.

2.1.4 Tell Me About Your Vocal Career, Long-Term Goals, and the Importance of Your Voice Quality and Upcoming Commitments

To choose a treatment program, the physician must understand the importance of the patient's voice and his or her long-term career plans, the importance of the upcoming vocal commitment, and the consequences of canceling the engagement. Injudicious prescription of voice rest can be almost as damaging to a vocal career as injudicious performance. For example, although a singer's voice is usually his or her most important commodity, other factors distinguish the few successful artists from the multitude of less successful singers with equally good voices. These include musicianship, reliability, and "professionalism." Canceling a concert at the last minute may seriously damage a performer's reputation. Reliability is especially critical early in a singer's career. Moreover, an expert singer often can modify a performance to decrease the strain on his or her voice. No singer should be allowed to perform in a manner that will permit serious injury to the vocal folds, but in the frequent borderline cases, the condition of the larynx must be weighed against other factors affecting the singer as an artist.

2.1.5 How Much Voice Training Have You Had?

Establishing how long a singer or actor has been performing seriously is important, especially if his or her active performance career predates the beginning of vocal training. Active untrained singers and actors frequently develop undesirable techniques that are difficult to modify. Extensive voice use without training or premature training with inappropriate repertoire may underlie persistent vocal difficulties later in life. The number of years a performer has been training his or her voice may be a fair index of vocal proficiency. A person who has studied voice for 1 or 2 years is somewhat more likely to have gross technical difficulties than is someone who has been studying for 20 years. However, if training has been intermittent or discontinued, technical problems are common, especially among singers. In addition, methods of technical voice use vary among voice teachers. Hence, a student who has had many teachers in a relatively brief period of time commonly has numerous technical insecurities or deficiencies that may be responsible for vocal dysfunction. This is especially true if the singer has changed to a new teacher within the preceding year. The physician must be careful not to criticize the patient's current voice teacher in such circumstances. It often takes years of expert instruction to correct bad habits.

All people speak more often than they sing, yet most singers report little speech training. Even if a singer uses the voice flawlessly while practicing and performing, voice abuse at other times can cause damage that affects singing.

2.1.6   Under What Kinds of Conditions Do You Use Your Voice?

The Lombard effect is the tendency to increase vocal intensity in response to increased background noise. A well-trained singer learns to compensate for this tendency and to avoid singing at unsafe volumes. Singers of classical music usually have such training and frequently perform with only a piano, a situation in which the balance can be controlled well. However, singers performing in large halls, with orchestras, or in operas early in their careers tend to oversing and strain their voices. Similar problems occur during outdoor concerts because of the lack of auditory feedback. This phenomenon is seen even more among "pop" singers. Pop singers are in a uniquely difficult position; often, despite little vocal training, they enjoy great artistic and financial success and endure extremely stressful demands on their time and voices. They are required to sing in large halls or outdoor arenas not designed for musical performance, amid smoke and other environmental irritants, accompanied by extremely loud background music. One frequently neglected key to survival for these singers is the proper use of monitor speakers. These direct the sound of the singer's voice toward the singer on the stage and provide auditory feedback. Determining whether the pop singer uses monitor speakers and whether they are loud enough for the singer to hear is important.

Amateur singers are often no less serious about their music than are professionals, but generally, they have less ability to compensate technically for illness or other physical impairment. Rarely does an amateur suffer a great loss from postponing a performance or permitting someone to sing in his or her place. In most cases, the amateur singer's best interest is served through conservative management directed at long-term maintenance of good vocal health.

A great many of the singers who seek physicians' advice are primarily choral singers. They often are enthusiastic amateurs, untrained but dedicated to their musical recreation. They should be handled as amateur solo singers, educated specifically about the Lombard effect, and cautioned to avoid the excessive volume so common in a choral environment. One good way for a singer to monitor loudness is to cup a hand to his or her ear. This adds about 6 dB [7] to the singer's perception of his or her own voice and can be a very helpful guide in noisy surroundings. Young professional singers are often hired to augment amateur choruses. Feeling that the professional quartet has been hired to "lead" the rest of the choir, they often make the mistake of trying to accomplish that goal by singing louder than others in their sections. These singers should be advised to lead their section by singing each line as if they were soloists giving a voice lesson to the people standing next to them and as if there was a microphone in front of them recording their choral performance for their voice teacher. This approach usually not only preserves the voice but also produces a better choral sound.

2.1.7   How Much Do You Practice and Exercise Your Voice? How, When, and Where Do You Use Your Voice?

Vocal exercise is as essential to the vocalist as exercise and conditioning of other muscle systems is to the athlete. Proper vocal practice incorporates scales and specific exercises designed to maintain and develop the vocal apparatus. Simply acting or singing songs or giving performances without routine studious concentration on vocal technique is not adequate for the vocal performer. The physician should know whether the vocalist practices daily, whether he or she practices at the same time daily, and how long the practice lasts. Actors generally practice and warm up their voices for 10–30 minutes daily, although more time is recommended. Most serious singers practice for at least 1–2 hours per day. If a singer routinely practices in the late afternoon or evening but frequently performs in the morning (religious services, school classes, teaching voice, choir rehearsals, etc.), one should inquire into the warm-up procedures preceding such performances as well as cooldown procedures after voice use. Singing "cold," especially early in the morning, may result in the use of minor muscular alterations to compensate for vocal insecurity produced by inadequate preparation. Such crutches can result in voice dysfunction. Similar problems may result from instances of voice use other than formal singing. School teachers, telephone receptionists, salespeople, and others who speak extensively also often derive great benefit from 5 to 10 minutes of vocalization of scales first thing in the morning. Although singers rarely practice their scales too long, they frequently perform or rehearse excessively. This is especially true immediately before a major concert or audition, when physicians are most likely to see acute problems. When a singer has hoarseness and vocal fatigue and has been practicing a new role for 14 hours a day for the last 3 weeks, no simple prescription will solve the problem. However, a treatment regimen can usually be designed to carry the performer safely through his or her musical obligations.

The physician should be aware of common habits and environments that are often associated with abusive voice behavior and should ask about them routinely. Screaming at sports events and at children is among the most common. Extensive voice use in noisy environments also tends to be abusive. These include noisy rooms, cars, airplanes, sports facilities, and other locations where background noise or acoustic design impairs auditory feedback. Dry, dusty surroundings may alter vocal fold secretions through dehydration or contact irritation, altering voice function. Activities such as cheerleading, teaching, choral conducting, amateur singing, and frequent communication with hearing-impaired persons are likely to be associated with voice abuse, as is extensive professional voice use without formal training. The physician should inquire into the patient's routine voice use and should specifically ask about any activities that frequently lead to voice change such as hoarseness or discomfort in the neck or throat. Laryngologists should ask specifically about other activities that may be abusive to the vocal folds such as weight lifting, aerobics, and the playing of some wind instruments.

2.1.8 *Are You Aware of Misusing or Abusing Your Voice During Singing?*

A detailed discussion of vocal technique in singing is beyond the scope of this chapter. The most common technical errors involve excessive muscle tension in the tongue, neck, and larynx; inadequate abdominal support; and excessive volume. Inadequate preparation can be a devastating source of voice abuse and may result from limited practice, limited rehearsal of a difficult piece, or limited vocal training for a given role. The latter error is common. In some situations, voice teachers are at fault; both the singer and teacher must resist the impulse to "show off" the voice in works that are either too difficult for the singer's level of training or simply not suited to the singer's voice. Singers are habitually unhappy with the limitations of their voices. At some time or another, most baritones wish they were tenors and walk around proving they can sing high Cs in "Vesti la giubba." Singers with other vocal ranges have similar fantasies. Attempts to make the voice something that it is not, or at least that it is not yet, frequently are harmful.

2.1.9 *Are You Aware of Misusing or Abusing Your Voice During Speaking?*

Common patterns of voice abuse and misuse will not be discussed in detail in this chapter. Voice abuse and/or misuse should be suspected particularly in patients who complain of voice fatigue associated with voice use, whose voices are worse at the end of a working day or week, and in any patient who is chronically hoarse. Technical errors in voice use may be the primary etiology of a voice complaint, or it may develop secondarily due to a patient's effort to compensate for voice disturbance from another cause.

Dissociation of one's speaking and singing voices is probably the most common cause of voice abuse problems in excellent singers. Too frequently, all the expert training in support, muscle control, and projection is not applied to a singers' speaking voice. Unfortunately, the resultant voice strain affects the singing voice as well as the speaking voice. Such damage is especially likely to occur in noisy rooms and in cars, where the background noise is louder than it seems. Backstage greetings after a lengthy performance can be particularly devastating. The singer usually is exhausted and distracted; the environment is often dusty and dry; and generally, a noisy crowd is present. Similar conditions prevail at postperformance parties, where smoking and alcohol worsen matters. These situations should be avoided by any singer with vocal problems and should be controlled through awareness at other times.

Three particularly abusive and potentially damaging vocal activities are worthy of note. *Cheerleading* requires extensive screaming under the worst possible physical and environmental circumstances. It is a highly undesirable activity for anyone considering serious vocal endeavor. This is a common conflict in younger singers because the teenager who is the high school choir soloist often is also student council president, yearbook editor, captain of the cheerleaders, and so on.

Conducting, particularly choral conducting, can also be deleterious. An enthusiastic conductor, especially of an amateur group, frequently sings all four parts intermittently, at volumes louder than the entire choir, during lengthy rehearsals. Conducting is a common avocation among singers but must be done with expert technique and special precautions to prevent voice injury. Hoarseness or loss of soft voice control after conducting a rehearsal or concert suggests voice abuse during conducting. The patient should be instructed to record his or her voice throughout the vocal range singing long notes at dynamics from soft to loud to soft. Recordings should be made prior to rehearsal and following rehearsal. If the voice has lost range, control, or quality during the rehearsal, voice abuse has occurred. A similar test can be used for patients who sing in choirs, teach voice, or perform other potentially abusive vocal activities. Such problems in conductors can generally be managed by additional training in conducting techniques and by voice training, including warm-up and cooldown exercises.

Teaching singing may also be hazardous to vocal health. It can be done safely but requires skill and thought. Most teachers teach while seated at the piano. Late in a long, hard day, this posture is not conducive to maintenance of optimal abdominal and back support. Usually, teachers work with students continually positioned to the right or left of the keyboard. This may require the teacher to turn his or her neck at a particularly sharp angle, especially when teaching at an upright piano. Teachers also often demonstrate vocal works in their students' vocal ranges rather than their own, illustrating bad as well as good technique. If a singing teacher is hoarse or has neck discomfort or his or her soft singing control deteriorates at the end of a teaching day (assuming that the teacher warms up before beginning to teach voice lessons), voice abuse should be suspected. Helpful modifications include teaching with a grand piano, sitting slightly sideways on the piano bench, or alternating student position to the right and left of the piano to facilitate better neck alignment. Retaining an accompanist so that the teacher can stand rather than teach from sitting behind a piano and many other helpful modifications are possible.

2.2   Do You Have Pain When You Talk or Sing?

Odynophonia, or pain caused by phonation, can be a disturbing symptom. It is not uncommon, but relatively, little has been written or discussed on this subject. A detailed review of odynophonia is beyond the scope of this publication. However, laryngologists should be familiar with the diagnosis and treatment of at least a few of the most common causes, at least, as discussed elsewhere in this book.

2.2.1   What Kind of Physical Condition Are You In?

Phonation is an athletic activity that requires good conditioning and coordinated interaction of numerous physical functions. Maladies of any part of the body may be reflected in the voice. Failure to maintain good abdominal muscle tone and respiratory endurance through exercise is particularly harmful because deficiencies in these areas undermine the power source of the voice. Patients generally attempt to compensate for such weaknesses by using inappropriate muscle groups, particularly in the neck, causing vocal dysfunction. Similar problems may occur in the well-conditioned vocalist in states of fatigue. These are compounded by mucosal changes that accompany excessively long hours of hard work. Such problems may be seen even in the best singers shortly before important performances in the height of the concert season.

A popular but untrue myth holds that great opera singers must be obese. However, the vivacious, gregarious personality that often distinguishes the great performer seems to be accompanied frequently by a propensity for excess, especially culinary excess. This excess is as undesirable in the vocalist as it is in most other athletic artists, and it should be prevented from the start of one's vocal career. Appropriate and attractive body weight has always been valued in the pop music world and is becoming particularly important in the opera world as this formerly theater-based art form moves to television and film media. However, attempts at weight reduction in an established speaker or singer are a different matter. The vocal mechanism is a finely tuned, complex instrument and is exquisitely sensitive to minor changes. Substantial fluctuations in weight frequently cause deleterious alterations of the voice, although these are usually temporary. Weight reduction programs for people concerned about their voices must be monitored carefully and designed to reduce weight in small increments over long periods. A history of sudden recent weight change may be responsible for almost any vocal complaint.

2.2.2   How Is Your Hearing?

Hearing loss can cause substantial problems for singers and other professional voice users. This may be true especially when the voice patient is unaware that he or she has hearing loss. Consequently, not only should voice patients be asked about hearing loss, tinnitus, vertigo, and family history of hearing loss, but it is also helpful to inquire of spouses, partners, friends, or others who may have accompanied the patient to the office whether they have suspected a hearing impairment in the patient.

2.2.3   Have You Noted Voice or Bodily Weakness, Tremor, Fatigue, or Loss of Control?

Even minor neurologic disorders may be extremely disruptive to vocal function. Specific questions should be asked to rule out neuromuscular and neurologic diseases such as myasthenia gravis, Parkinson disease, tremors, other movement disorders, spasmodic dysphonia, multiple sclerosis, central nervous system neoplasm, and other serious maladies that may be present with voice complaints.

2.2.4   Do You Have Allergy or Cold Symptoms?

Acute upper respiratory tract infection causes inflammation of the mucosa, alters mucosal secretions, and makes the mucosa more vulnerable to injury. Coughing and throat clearing are particularly traumatic vocal activities and may worsen or provoke hoarseness associated with a cold. Postnasal drip and allergy may produce the same response. Infectious sinusitis is associated with discharge and diffuse mucosal inflammation, resulting in similar problems, and may actually alter the sound of a voice, especially the patient's own perception of his or her voice. Futile attempts to compensate for disease of the supraglottic vocal tract in an effort to return the sound to normal frequently result in laryngeal strain. The expert singer or speaker should compensate by monitoring technique by tactile rather than by auditory feedback or singing "by feel" rather than "by ear."

2.2.5   Do You Have Breathing Problems, Especially After Exercise?

Voice patients usually volunteer information about upper respiratory tract infections and postnasal drip, but the relevance of other maladies may not be obvious to them. Consequently, the physician must seek out pertinent history.

Respiratory problems are especially important in voice patients. Even mild respiratory dysfunction may adversely affect the power source of the voice [8]. Occult asthma may be particularly troublesome [9]. A complete respiratory history should be obtained in most patients with voice complaints, and pulmonary function testing is often advisable.

2.2.6   Have You Been Exposed to Environmental Irritants?

Any mucosal irritant can disrupt the delicate vocal mechanism. Allergies to dust and mold are aggravated commonly during rehearsals and performances in concert halls, especially older theaters and concert halls, because of numerous curtains, backstage trappings, and dressing room facilities that are rarely cleaned thoroughly. Nasal obstruction and erythematous conjunctivae suggest generalized mucosal irritation. The drying effects of cold air and dry heat may also affect mucosal secretions, leading to decreased lubrication, a "scratchy" voice, and tickling cough. These symptoms may be minimized by nasal breathing, which allows inspired air to be filtered, warmed, and humidified. Nasal breathing, whenever possible, rather than mouth breathing, is a proper vocal technique. While the performer is backstage between appearances or during rehearsals, inhalation of dust and other irritants may be controlled by wearing a protective mask, such as those used by carpenters, or a surgical mask that does not contain fiberglass. This is especially helpful when sets are being constructed in the rehearsal area.

A history of recent travel suggests other sources of mucosal irritation. The air in airplanes is extremely dry, and airplanes are noisy [10]. One must be careful to avoid talking loudly and to maintain good hydration and nasal breathing during air travel. Environmental changes can also be disruptive. Las Vegas is infamous for the mucosal irritation caused by its dry atmosphere and smoke-filled rooms. In fact, the resultant complex of hoarseness, vocal "tickle," and fatigue is referred to as "Las Vegas voice." A history of recent travel should also suggest jet lag and generalized fatigue, which may be potent detriments to good vocal function.

Environmental pollution is responsible for the presence of toxic substances and conditions encountered daily. Inhalation of toxic pollutants may affect the voice adversely by direct laryngeal injury, by causing pulmonary dysfunction that results in voice maladies, or through impairments elsewhere in the vocal tract. Ingested substances, especially those that have neurolaryngologic effects, may also adversely affect the voice. Nonchemical environmental pollutants such as noise can cause voice abnormalities, as well. Laryngologists should be familiar with the laryngologic effects of the numerous potentially irritating substances and conditions found in the environment. We must also be familiar with special pollution problems encountered by performers. Numerous materials used by artists to create sculptures, drawings, and theatrical sets are toxic and have adverse voice effects. In addition, performers are exposed routinely to chemicals encountered through stage smoke and pyrotechnic effects. Although it is clear that some of the "special effects" may result in serious laryngologic consequences, much additional study is needed to clarify the nature and scope of these occupational problems.

2.2.7   Do You Smoke, Live with a Smoker, or Work Around Smoke?

The effects of smoking on voice performance were reviewed recently in the *Journal of Singing* [11], and that review is recapitulated here. Smoking tobacco is the number one cause of preventable death in the United States as well as the leading cause of heart disease, stroke, emphysema, and cancer. The Centers for Disease Control and Prevention (CDC) attributes approximately 442,000 premature (shortened life expectancy) deaths annually in the United States to smoking, which is more than the combined incidence of deaths caused by highway accidents, fires, murders, illegal drugs, suicides, and AIDS [12]. Approximately four million deaths per year worldwide result from smoking, and if this trend continues, by 2030, this figure will increase to about ten million deaths globally [13]. In addition to causing life-threatening diseases, smoking impairs a great many body systems, including the vocal tract. Harmful consequences of smoking or being exposed to smoke influence voice performance adversely.

Singers need good vocal health to perform well. Smoking tobacco can irritate the mucosal covering of the vocal folds, causing redness and chronic inflammation, and can have the same effect on the mucosal lining of the lungs, trachea, nasopharynx (behind the nose and throat), and mouth. In other words, the components of voice production—the generator, the oscillator, the resonator, and the articulator—all can be compromised by the harmful effects of tobacco use. The onset of effects from smoking may be immediate or delayed.

Individuals who have allergies and/or asthma are usually more sensitive to cigarette smoke with potential for an immediate adverse reaction involving the lungs, larynx, nasal cavities, and/or eyes. Chronic use of tobacco, or exposure to it, causes the toxic chemicals in tobacco to accumulate in the body, damaging the delicate linings of the vocal tract, as well as the lungs, heart, and circulatory system.

The lungs are critical components of the power source of the vocal tract. They help generate an airstream that is directed superiorly through the trachea toward the undersurface of the vocal folds. The vocal folds respond to the increase in subglottic pressure by producing sounds of variable intensities and frequencies. The number of times per second the vocal fold vibrate influences the pitch, and the amplitude of the mucosal wave influences the loudness of the sound. The sound produced by the vibration (oscillation) of the vocal folds passes upward through the oral cavity and nasopharynx where it resonates, giving the voice its richness and timbre, and eventually, it is articulated by the mouth, teeth, lips, and tongue into speech or song.

Any condition that adversely affects lung function such as chronic exposure to smoke or uncontrolled asthma can contribute to dysphonia by impairing the strength, endurance, and consistency of the airstream responsible for establishing vocal fold oscillation. Any lesion that compromises vocal fold vibration and glottic closure can cause hoarseness and breathiness. Inflammation of the cover layer of the vocal folds and/or the mucosal lining of the nose, sinuses, and oral nasopharyngeal cavities can affect the quality and clarity of the voice.

Tobacco smoke can damage the lungs' parenchyma and the exchange of air through respiration. Cigarette manufacturers add hundreds of ingredients to their tobacco products to improve taste, to make smoking seem milder and easier to inhale, and to prolong burning and shelf life [14]. More than 3000 chemical compounds have been identified in tobacco smoke, and more than 60 of these compounds are carcinogens [15]. The tobacco plant, *Nicotiana tabacum*, is grown for its leaves, which can be smoked, chewed, or sniffed with various effects. The nicotine in tobacco is the addictive component and rivals crack cocaine in its ability to enslave its users. Most smokers want to stop, yet only a small percentage is successful in quitting cigarettes; the majority who quit relapses into smoking once again [16]. Tar and carbon monoxide are among the disease-causing components in tobacco products. The tar in cigarettes exposes the individual to a greater risk of bronchitis, emphysema, and lung cancer. These chemicals affect the entire vocal tract as well as the cardiovascular system (Table 2.1).

Table 2.1   Chemical additives found in tobaccos and commercial products

Tobacco chemical additives	Also found in
Acetic acid	Vinegar, hair dye
Acetone	Nail polish remover
Ammonia	Floor cleaner, toilet cleaner
Arsenic	Poison
Benzene	A leukemia-producing agent in rubber cement
Butane	Cigarette lighter fluid
Cadmium	Batteries, some oil paints
Carbon monoxide	Car exhaust
DDT	Insecticides
Ethanol	Alcohol
Formaldehyde	Embalming fluid, fabric, laboratory animals
Hexamine	Barbecue lighter
Hydrazine	Jet fuel, rocket fuel
Hydrogen cyanide	Gas chamber poison
Methane	Swamp gas
Methanol	Rocket fuel
Naphthalene	Explosives, mothballs, paints
Nickel	Electroplating
Nicotine	Insecticides
Nitrobenzene	Gasoline additive
Nitrous oxide phenols	Disinfectant
Phenol	Disinfectants, plastics
Polonium-210	A radioactive substance
Stearic acid	Candle wax
Styrene	Insulation materials
Toluene	Industrial solvent, embalmer's glue
Vinyl chloride	Plastic manufacturing, garbage bags

Cigarette smoke in the lungs can lead also to increased vascularity, edema, and excess mucous production, as well as epithelial tissue and cellular changes. The toxic agents in cigarette smoke have been associated with an increase in the number and severity of asthma attacks, chronic bronchitis, emphysema, and lung cancer, all of which can interfere with the lungs' ability to generate the stream of air needed for voice production.

Chronic bronchitis due to smoking has been associated with an increase in the number of goblet (mucous) cells, an increase in the size (hyperplasia) of the mucosal secreting glands, and a decrease in the number of ciliated cells, the cells used to clean the lungs. Chronic cough and sputum production are also seen more commonly in smokers compared with nonsmokers. Also, the heat and chemicals of unfiltered cigarette and marijuana smoke are especially irritating to the lungs and larynx.

An important component of voice quality is the symmetrical, unencumbered vibration of the true vocal folds. Anything that prevents the epithelium covering the vocal folds from vibrating or affects the loose connective tissue under the epithelium (in the superficial layer of the lamina propria known as Reinke's space) can cause dysphonia. Cigarette smoking can cause the epithelium of the true vocal folds to become red and swollen, develop whitish discolorations (leukoplakia), undergo chronic inflammatory changes, or develop squamous metaplasia or dysplasia (tissue changes from normal to a potentially malignant state). In chronic smokers, the voice may become husky due to the accumulation of fluid in Reinke's space (Reinke's edema). These alterations in structure can interfere with voice production by changing the biomechanics of the vocal folds and their vibratory characteristics. In severe cases, cancer can deform and paralyze the vocal folds.

Vocal misuse often follows in an attempt to compensate for dysphonia and an alerted self-perception of one's voice. The voice may feel weak, breathy, raspy, or strained. There may be a loss of range, vocal breaks, long warm-up time, and fatigue. The throat may feel raw, achy, or tight. As the voice becomes unreliable, bad habits increase as the individual struggles harder and harder to compensate vocally. As selected sound waves move upward, from the larynx toward and through the pharynx, nasopharynx, mouth, and nose (the resonators), sounds gain a unique richness and timbre. Exposing the pharynx to cigarette smoke aggravates the linings of the oropharynx, mouth, nasopharynx, sinuses, and nasal cavities. The resulting erythema, swelling, and inflammation predispose one to nasal congestion and impaired mucosal function; there may be predisposition to sinusitis and pharyngitis, in which the voice may become hyponasal, the sinus achy, and the throat painful.

Although relatively rare in the United States, cancer of the nasopharynx has been associated with cigarette smoking [17], and one of the presenting symptoms is unilateral hearing loss due to fluid in the middle ear caused by eustachian tube obstruction from the cancer. Smoking-induced cancers of the oral cavity, pharynx, larynx, and lung are common throughout the world, including in the United States.

The palate, tongue, cheeks, lips, and teeth articulate the sound modified by the resonators into speech. Cigarettes, cigar, or pipe smoking may cause a "black hairy tongue," precancerous oral lesions (leukoplakia), and/or cancer of the tongue and lips [18]. Any irritation that causes burning or inflammation of the oral mucosa can affect phonation, and all tobacco products are capable of causing these effects.

Smokeless "spit" tobacco is highly addictive, and users who dip eight to ten times a day may get the same nicotine exposure as those who smoke 1½ to two packs of cigarettes per day [19]. Smokeless tobacco has been associated with gingivitis, cheek carcinoma, and cancer of the larynx and hypopharynx.

Exposure to environmental tobacco smoke (ETS), also called secondhand smoke, sidestream smoke, or passive smoke, accounts for an estimated 3000 lung cancer deaths and approximately 35,000 deaths in the United States from heart disease in nonsmoking adults [20].

Secondhand smoke is the "passive" inhalation of tobacco smoke from environmental sources such as smoke given off by pipes, cigars, cigarettes (sidestream), or the smoke exhaled from the lungs of smokers and inhaled by other people (mainstream). This passive smoke contains a mixture of thousands of chemicals, some of which are known to cause cancer. The National Institutes of Health (NIH) lists ETS as a "known" carcinogen, and the more you are exposed to secondhand smoke, the greater your risk [21].

Infants and young children are affected particularly by secondhand smoke with increased incidences of otitis media (ear infections), bronchitis, and pneumonia. If small children are exposed to secondhand smoke, the child's resulting illness can have a stressful effect on the parent who frequently catches the child's illness. Both the illness and the stress of caring for the sick child may interfere with voice performance. People who are exposed routinely to secondhand smoke are at risk for lung cancer, heart disease, respiratory infection, and an increased number of asthma attacks [22].

There is an intricate relationship between the lungs, larynx, pharynx, nose, and mouth in the production of speech and song. Smoking can have deleterious effects on any part of the vocal tract, causing the respiratory system to lose power, damaging the vibratory margins of the vocal folds, and detracting from the richness and beauty of a voice.

The deleterious effects of tobacco smoke on mucosa are indisputable. Anyone concerned about the health of his or her voice should not smoke. Smoking causes erythema, mild edema, and generalized inflammation throughout the vocal tract. Both smoke itself and the heat of the cigarette appear to be important. Marijuana produces a particularly irritating, unfiltered smoke that is inhaled directly, causing considerable mucosal response. Voice patients who refuse to stop smoking marijuana should at least be advised to use a water pipe to cool and partially filter the smoke. Some vocalists are required to perform in smoke-filled environments and may suffer the same effects as the smokers themselves. In some theaters, it is possible to place fans upstage or direct the ventilation system so as to create a gentle draft toward the audience, clearing the smoke away from the stage. "Smoke eaters" installed in some theaters are also helpful.

2.2.8   Do Any Foods Seem to Affect Your Voice?

Various foods are said to affect the voice. Traditionally, singers avoid milk and ice cream before performances. In many people, these foods seem to increase the amount and viscosity of mucosal secretions. Allergy and casein have been implicated, but no satisfactory explanation has been established. In some cases, restriction of these foods from the diet before a voice performance may be helpful. Chocolate may have the same effect and should be viewed similarly. Chocolate also contains caffeine, which may aggravate reflux or cause tremor. Voice patients should be asked about eating nuts. This is important not only because some people experience effects similar to those produced by milk products and chocolate but also because they are extremely irritating if aspirated. The irritation produced by aspiration of even a small organic foreign body may be severe and impossible to correct rapidly enough to permit performance. Highly spiced foods may also cause mucosal irritation. In addition, they seem to aggravate reflux laryngitis. Coffee and other beverages containing caffeine also aggravate gastric reflux and may promote dehydration and/or alter secretions and necessitate frequent throat clearing in some people. Fad diets, especially rapid weight-reducing diets, are notorious for causing voice problems. Eating a full meal before a speaking or singing engagement may interfere with abdominal support or may aggravate upright reflux of gastric juice during abdominal muscle contraction. Lemon juice and herbal teas are considered beneficial to the voice. Both may act as demulcents, thinning secretions, and may very well be helpful.

2.2.9   Do You Have Morning Hoarseness, Bad Breath, Excessive Phlegm, a Lump in Your Throat, or Heartburn?

Reflux laryngitis is especially common among singers and trained speakers because of the high intra-abdominal pressure associated with proper support and because of lifestyle. Singers frequently perform at night. Many vocalists refrain from eating before performances because a full stomach can compromise effective abdominal support. They typically compensate by eating heartily at postperformance gatherings late at night and then go to bed with a full stomach.

Chronic irritation of arytenoid and vocal fold mucosa by reflux of gastric secretions may occasionally be associated with dyspepsia or pyrosis. However, the key features of this malady are bitter taste and halitosis on awakening in the morning, a dry or "coated" mouth, often a scratchy sore throat or a feeling of a "lump in the throat," hoarseness, and the need for prolonged vocal warm-up. The physician must be alert to these symptoms and ask about them routinely; otherwise, the diagnosis will often be overlooked, because people who have had this problem for many years or a lifetime do not even realize it is abnormal.

2.2.10 Do You Have Trouble with Your Bowels or Belly?

Any condition that alters abdominal function, such as muscle spasm, constipation, or diarrhea, interferes with support and may result in a voice complaint. These symptoms may accompany infection, anxiety, various gastroenterological diseases, and other maladies.

2.2.11 Are You Under Particular Stress or in Therapy?

The human voice is an exquisitely sensitive messenger of emotion. Highly trained voice professionals learn to control the effects of anxiety and other emotional stress on their voices under ordinary circumstances. However, in some instances, this training may break down or a performer may be inadequately prepared to control the voice under specific stressful conditions. Preperformance anxiety is the most common example, but insecurity, depression, and other emotional disturbances are also generally reflected in the voice. Anxiety reactions are mediated in part through the autonomic nervous system and result in a dry mouth, cold clammy skin, and thick secretions. These reactions are normal, and good vocal training coupled with assurance that no abnormality or disease is present generally overcomes them. However, long-term, poorly compensated emotional stress and exogenous stress (from agents, producers, teachers, parents, etc.) may cause substantial vocal dysfunction and may result in permanent limitations of the vocal apparatus. These conditions must be diagnosed and treated expertly. Hypochondriasis is uncommon among professional singers, despite popular opinion to the contrary.

Recent publications have highlighted the complexity and importance of psychological factors associated with voice disorders [23]. A comprehensive discussion of this subject is also presented elsewhere in this book. It is important for the physician to recognize that psychological problems may not only cause voice disorders but also delay recovery from voice disorders that were entirely organic in etiology. Professional voice users, especially singers, have enormous psychological investment and personality identifications associated with their voices. A condition that causes voice loss or permanent injury often evokes the same powerful psychological responses seen following death of a loved one. This process may be initiated even when physical recovery is complete if an incident (injury or surgery) has made the vocalist realize that voice loss is possible. Such a "brush with death" can have profound emotional consequences in some patients. It is essential for laryngologists to be aware of these powerful factors and manage them properly if optimal therapeutic results are to be achieved expeditiously.

2.2.12   Do You Have Problems Controlling Your Weight? Are You Excessively Tired? Are You Cold When Other People Are Warm?

Endocrine problems warrant special attention. The human voice is extremely sensitive to endocrinologic changes. Many of these are reflected in alterations of fluid content of the lamina propria just beneath the laryngeal mucosa. This causes alterations in the bulk and shape of the vocal folds and results in voice change. Hypothyroidism [24–28] is a well-recognized cause of such voice disorders, although the mechanism is not fully understood. Hoarseness, vocal fatigue, muffling of the voice, loss of range, and a sensation of a lump in the throat may be present even with mild hypothyroidism. Even when thyroid function tests results are within the low normal range, this diagnosis should be entertained, especially if thyroid-stimulating hormone levels are in the high normal range or are elevated. Thyrotoxicosis may result in similar voice disturbances [25].

2.2.13   Do You Have Menstrual Irregularity, Cyclical Voice Changes Associated with Menses, Recent Menopause, or Other Hormonal Changes or Problems?

Voice changes associated with sex hormones are encountered commonly in clinical practice and have been investigated more thoroughly than have other hormonal changes [29, 30]. Although a correlation appears to exist between sex hormone levels and depth of male voices (higher testosterone and lower estradiol levels in basses than in tenors) [29], the most important hormonal considerations in males occur during or related to puberty [31, 32]. Voice problems related to sex hormones are more common in female singers (C. Carroll, 1992, Arizona State University at Tempe, "Personal communication with Dr. Hans von Leden") [32–48].

2.2.14   Do You Have Jaw Joint or Other Dental Problems?

Dental disease, especially temporomandibular joint (TMJ) dysfunction, introduces muscle tension in the head and neck, which is transmitted to the larynx directly through the muscular attachments between the mandible and the hyoid bone and indirectly as generalized increased muscle tension. These problems often result in decreased range, vocal fatigue, and change in the quality or placement of a voice. Such tension often is accompanied by excess tongue muscle activity, especially pulling of the tongue posteriorly. This hyperfunctional behavior acts through hyoid attachments to disrupt the balance between the intrinsic and extrinsic laryngeal musculature. TMJ problems are also problematic for wind instrumentalists and some string players, including violinists. In some cases, the problems may actually be caused by instrumental technique. The history should always include information about musical activities, including instruments other than the voice.

2.2.15   Do You or Your Blood Relatives Have Hearing Loss?

Hearing loss is often overlooked as a source of vocal problems. Auditory feedback is fundamental to speaking and singing. Interference with this control mechanism may result in altered vocal production, particularly if the person is unaware of the hearing loss. Distortion, particularly pitch distortion (diplacusis), may also pose serious problems for the singer. This appears to be due not only to aesthetic difficulties in matching pitch but also to vocal strain that accompanies pitch shifts [49].

In addition to determining whether the patient has hearing loss, inquiry should also be made about hearing impairment occurring in family members, roommates, and other close associates. Speaking loudly to people who are hard of hearing can cause substantial, chronic vocal strain. This possibility should be investigated routinely when evaluating voice patients.

2.2.16   Have You Suffered Whiplash or Other Bodily Injury?

Various bodily injuries outside the confines of the vocal tract may have profound effects on the voice. Whiplash, for example, commonly causes changes in technique, with consequent voice fatigue, loss of range, difficulty singing softly, and other problems. These problems derive from the neck muscle spasm, abnormal neck posturing secondary to pain, and consequent hyperfunctional voice use. Lumbar, abdominal, head, chest, supraglottic, and extremity injuries may also affect vocal technique and be responsible for the dysphonia that prompted the voice patient to seek medical attention.

2.2.17   Did You Undergo Any Surgery Prior to the Onset of Your Voice Problems?

A history of laryngeal surgery in a voice patient is a matter of great concern. It is important to establish exactly why the surgery was done, by whom it was done, whether intubation was necessary, and whether voice therapy was instituted pre- or postoperatively if the lesion was associated with voice abuse (vocal nodules). If the vocal dysfunction that sent the patient to the physician's office dates from the immediate postoperative period, surgical trauma must be suspected.

Otolaryngologists frequently are asked about the effects of tonsillectomy on the voice. Singers especially may consult the physician after tonsillectomy and complain of vocal dysfunction. Certainly, removal of tonsils can alter the voice [50, 51]. Tonsillectomy changes the configuration of the supraglottic vocal tract. In addition, scarring alters pharyngeal muscle function, which is trained meticulously in the professional singer. Singers must be warned that they may have permanent voice changes after tonsillectomy; however, these can be minimized by dissecting in the proper plane to lessen scarring. The singer's voice generally requires 3–6 months to stabilize or return to normal after surgery, although it is generally safe to begin limited singing within 2–4 weeks following surgery. As with any procedure for which general anesthesia may be needed, the anesthesiologist should be advised preoperatively that the patient is a professional singer. Intubation and extubation should be performed with great care, and the use of nonirritating plastic rather than rubber or ribbed metal endotracheal tubes is preferred. Use of a laryngeal mask may be advisable for selected procedures for mechanical reasons, but this device is often not ideal for tonsillectomy, and it can cause laryngeal injury such as arytenoid dislocation.

Surgery of the neck, such as thyroidectomy, may result in permanent alterations in the vocal mechanism through scarring of the extrinsic laryngeal musculature. The cervical (strap) muscles are important in maintaining laryngeal position and stability of the laryngeal skeleton, and they should be retracted rather than divided whenever possible. A history of recurrent or superior laryngeal nerve injury may explain a hoarse, breathy, or weak voice. However, in rare cases, even a singer can compensate for recurrent laryngeal nerve paralysis and have a nearly normal voice.

Thoracic and abdominal surgery interferes with respiratory and abdominal support. After these procedures, singing and projected speaking should be prohibited until pain has subsided and healing has occurred sufficiently to allow normal support. Abdominal exercises should be instituted before resumption of vocalizing. Singing and speaking without proper support are often worse for the voice than not using the voice for performance at all.

Other surgical procedures may be important factors if they necessitate intubation or if they affect the musculoskeletal system so that the person has to change stance or balance. For example, balancing on one foot after leg surgery may decrease the effectiveness of the support mechanism.

2.2.18   What Medications and Other Substances Do You Use?

A history of alcohol abuse suggests the probability of poor vocal technique. Intoxication results in incoordination and decreased awareness, which undermine vocal discipline designed to optimize and protect the voice. The effect of small amounts of alcohol is controversial. Although many experts oppose its use because of its vasodilatory effect and consequent mucosal alteration, many people do not seem to be adversely affected by small amounts of alcohol such as a glass of wine with a meal. However, some people have mild sensitivities to certain wines or beers. Patients who develop nasal congestion and rhinorrhea after drinking beer, for example, should be made aware that they probably have a mild allergy to that particular beverage and should avoid it before voice commitments.

Patients frequently acquire antihistamines to help control "postnasal drip" or other symptoms. The drying effect of antihistamines may result in decreased vocal fold lubrication, increased throat clearing, and irritability leading to frequent coughing. Antihistamines may be helpful to some voice patients, but they must be used with caution.

When a voice patient seeking the attention of a physician is already taking antibiotics, it is important to find out the dose and the prescribing physician, if any, as well as whether the patient frequently treats himself or herself with inadequate courses of antibiotics often supplied by colleagues. Singers, actors, and other speakers sometimes have a "sore throat" shortly before important vocal presentations and start themselves on inappropriate antibiotic therapy, which they generally discontinue after their performance.

Diuretics are also popular among some performers. They are often prescribed by gynecologists at the vocalist's request to help deplete excess water in the premenstrual period. They are not effective in this scenario, because they cannot diurese the protein-bound water in the laryngeal ground substance. Unsupervised use of these drugs may cause dehydration and consequent mucosal dryness.

Hormone use, especially use of oral contraceptives, must be mentioned specifically during the physician's inquiry. Women frequently do not mention them routinely when asked whether they are taking any medication. Vitamins are also frequently not mentioned. Most vitamin therapy seems to have little effect on the voice. However, high-dose vitamin C (5–6 g/day), which some people use to prevent upper respiratory tract infections, seems to act as a mild diuretic and may lead to dehydration and xerophonia [52].

Cocaine use is common, especially among pop musicians. This drug can be extremely irritating to the nasal mucosa, causes marked vasoconstriction, and may alter the sensorium, resulting in decreased voice control and a tendency toward vocal abuse.

Many pain medications (including aspirin and ibuprofen), psychotropic medications, and others may be responsible for a voice complaint. So far, no adverse vocal effects have been reported with selective COX-2 inhibiting anti-inflammatory medications (which do not promote bleeding, as do other nonsteroidal anti-inflammatory medicines and aspirin) such as celecoxib (Celebrex; Pfizer Inc., New York, New York) and valecoxib (Bextra; Pharmacia Corp., New York, New York). However this group of drugs has been demonstrated to have other side effects and should in our view only be taken under the care of a physician [53]. The effects of other new medications such as sildenafil citrate (Viagra; Pfizer Inc.) and medications used to induce abortion remain unstudied and unknown, but it seems plausible that such medication may affect voice function, at least temporarily. Laryngologists should be familiar with the laryngologic effects of the many substances ingested medically and recreationally.

Acknowledgments Modified in part from Sataloff RT. *Professional Voice: The Science and Art of Clinical Care, 4th Edition*. San Diego, CA: Plural Publishing; 2017, with permission.

References

1. Sataloff RT. Professional singers: the science and art of clinical care. Am J Otolaryngol. 1981;2:251–66.
2. Sataloff RT. The human voice. Sci Am. 1992;267:108–15.
3. Sundberg J. The science of the singing voice. DeKalb: Northern Illinois University Press; 1987.
4. Sataloff RT. Efficient history taking in professional singers. Laryngoscope. 1984;94:1111–4.
5. Ackerman R, Pfan W. Gerontology studies on the susceptibility to voice disorders in professional speakers. Folia Phoniatr (Basel). 1974;26:95–9.
6. von Leden H. Speech and hearing problems in the geriatric patient. J Am Geriatr Soc. 1977;25:422–6.
7. Schiff M. Comment. Presented at: seventh symposium on care of the professional voice; June 15–16, 1978. New York: The Juilliard School.
8. Spiegel JR, Cohn JR, Sataloff RT, et al. Respiratory function in singers: medical assessment, diagnoses, treatments. J Voice. 1988;2:40–50.
9. Cohn JR, Sataloff RT, Spiegel JR, et al. Airway reactivity-induced asthma in singers (ARIAS). J Voice. 1991;5:332–7.
10. Feder RJ. The professional voice and airline flight. Otolaryngol Head Neck Surg. 1984;92:251–4.
11. Anticaglia A, Hawkshaw M, Sataloff RT. The effects of smoking on voice performance. J Singing. 2004;60:161–7.
12. Centers for Disease Control and Prevention (CDC). Annual smoking-attributable, mortality, years of potential life lost, and economic costs, United States—1995–1999. MMWR Morb Mortal Wkly Rep. 2002;51(14):300–3.
13. World Health Organization. World health report 1999. Geneva: World Health Organization; 1999.
14. United States Department of Health Services (USDHHS). Tobacco products fact sheet. Washington: Government Printing Office; 2000.
15. National Cancer Institute. Environmental tobacco smoke. Fact sheet 3.9; 1999. http://cis.nci.nih.gov/fact/3_9.htm.
16. Centers for Disease Control and Prevention. Cigarette smoking among adults—United States, 1993. MMWR Morb Mortal Wkly Rep. 1994;3:925–9.
17. Chow WH, McLaughlin JK, Hrubec Z, et al. Tobacco use and nasopharyngeal carcinoma in a cohort of US veterans. Int J Cancer. 1993;55(4):538–40.
18. Casiglia J, Woo SB. A comprehensive view of oral cancer. Gen Dent. 2001;49(1):72–82.
19. Centers for Disease Control and Prevention. Determination of nicotine pH and moisture content of six U.S. commercial moist snuff products. MMWR Morb Mortal Wkly Rep. 1999;48(19):398.
20. American Cancer Society. Cancer facts and figures 2002. Atlanta: American Cancer Society; 2002.
21. National Toxicology Program (NTP). Report on carcinogens. 10th ed. Research Triangle Park, NC: U.S. Department Health and Human Services, Public Health Service, National Toxicology Program; 2002. http://ehp.niehs.nih.gov/roc/toc10.html.

22. Academy of Pediatrics, Committee on Environmental Health. Environmental tobacco smoke; a hazard to children. Pediatrics. 1997;99(4):639–42.
23. Rosen DC, Sataloff RT. Psychology of voice disorders. 2nd ed. San Diego: Plural Publishing, Inc.; 2020.
24. Gupta OP, Bhatia PL, Agarwal MK, et al. Nasal pharyngeal and laryngeal manifestations of hypothyroidism. Ear Nose Throat J. 1997;56:10–21.
25. Malinsky M, Chevrie-Muller C, Cerceau N. Etude clinique et electrophysiologique des altera- tions de la voix au cours des thyrotoxioses. Ann Endocrinol (Paris). 1997;38:171–2.
26. Michelsson K, Sirvio P. Cry analysis in congenital hypothyroidism. Folia Phoniatr (Basel). 1976;28:40–7.
27. Ritter FN. The effect of hypothyroidism on the larynx of the rat. Ann Otol Rhinol Laryngol. 1964;67:404–16.
28. Ritter FN. Endocrinology. In: Paparella M, Shumrick D, editors. Otolaryngology, vol. I. Philadelphia: Saunders; 1973. p. 727–34.
29. Meuser W, Nieschlag E. Sex hormones and depth of voice in the male [in German]. Dtsch Med Wochenschr. 1977;102:261–4.
30. Schiff M. The influence of estrogens on connective tissue. In: Asboe-Hansen G, editor. Hormones and connective tissue. Copenhagen: Munksgaard Press; 1967. p. 282–341.
31. Brodnitz F. The age of the castrato voice. J Speech Hear Disord. 1975;40:291–5.
32. Brodnitz F. Hormones and the human voice. Bull N Y Acad Med. 1971;47:183–91.
33. von Gelder L. Psychosomatic aspects of endocrine disorders of the voice. J Commun Disord. 1974;7:257–62.
34. Lacina O. Der Einfluss der Menstruation auf die Stimme der Sangerinnen. Folia Phoniatr (Basel). 1968;20:13–24.
35. Wendler J. The influence of menstruation on the voice of the female singer. Folia Phoniatr (Basel). 1972;24:259–77.
36. Brodnitz F. Medical care preventive therapy (Panel). In: Lawrence VL, editor. Transcripts of the seventh annual symposium, care of the professional voice, vol. 3. New York: The Voice Foundation; 1978. p. 86.
37. Dordain M. Etude Statistique de l'influence des contraceptifs hormonaux sur la voix. Folia Phoniatr (Basel). 1972;24:86–96.
38. Pahn J, Goretzlehner G. Voice changes following the use of oral contraceptives [in German]. Zentralbl Gynakol. 1978;100:341–6.
39. Schiff M. "The pill" in otolaryngology. Trans Am Acad Ophthalmol Otolaryngol. 1968;72:76–84.
40. von Deuster CV. Irreversible vocal changes in pregnancy [in German]. HNO. 1977;25:430–2.
41. Flach M, Schwickardi H, Simen R. Welchen Einfluss haben Menstruation und Schwangerschaft auf die augsgebildete Gesangsstimme? Folia Phoniatr (Basel). 1968;21:199–210.
42. Arndt HJ. Stimmstorungen nach Behandlung mit Androgenen und anabolen Hormonen. Munch Med Wochenschr. 1974;116:1715–20.
43. Bourdial J. Les troubles de la voix provoques par la therapeutique hormonale androgene. Ann Otolaryngol Chir Cervicofac. 1970;87:725–34.
44. Damste PH. Virilization of the voice due to anabolic steroids [in Dutch]. Ned Tijdschr Geneeskd. 1963;107:891–2.
45. Damste PH. Voice changes in adult women caused by virilizing agents. J Speech Hear Disord. 1967;32:126–32.
46. Saez S, Francoise S. Recepteurs d'androgenes: mise en evidence dans la fraction cytosolique de muqueuse normale et d'epitheliomas phryngolarynges humains. C R Acad Hebd Seances Acad Sci D. 1975;280:935–8.
47. Vuorenkoski V, Lenko HL, Tjernlund P, et al. Fundamental voice frequency during normal and abnormal growth, and after androgen treatment. Arch Dis Child. 1978;53:201–9.
48. Imre V. Hormonell bedingte Stimmstorungen. Folia Phoniatr (Basel). 1968;20:394–404.

49. Sundberg J, Prame E, Iwarsson J. Replicability and accuracy of pitch patterns in professional singers. In: Davis PJ, Fletcher NH, editors. Vocal fold physiology: controlling chaos and complexity. San Diego: Singular Publishing Group; 1996. p. 291–306.
50. Gould WJ, Alberti PW, Brodnitz F, Hirano M. Medical care preventive therapy [Panel]. In: Lawrence VL, editor. Transcripts of the seventh annual symposium; care of the professional voice, vol. 3. New York: The Voice Foundation; 1978. p. 74–6.
51. Wallner LJ, Hill BJ, Waldrop W, Monroe C. Voice changes following adenotonsillectomy. Laryngoscope. 1968;78:1410–8.
52. Lawrence VL. Medical care for professional voice (Panel). In: Lawrence VL, editor. Transcripts from the annual symposium, care of the professional voice, vol. 3. New York: The Voice Foundation; 1978. p. 17–8.
53. Cannon CP. COX-2 inhibitors and cardiovascular risk. Science. 2012;336(6087):1386–7.

Chapter 3
Physical Examination

A detailed history frequently reveals the cause of a voice problem even before a physical examination is performed. However, a comprehensive physical examination, often including objective assessment of voice function, also is essential [1–3].

Physical examination must include a thorough ear, nose, and throat evaluation and assessment of general physical condition. A patient who is extremely obese or appears fatigued, agitated, emotionally stressed, or otherwise generally ill has increased potential for voice dysfunction. This could be due to any number of factors: altered abdominal support, loss of fine motor control of laryngeal muscles, decreased bulk of the submucosal vocal fold ground substance, change in the character of mucosal secretions, or other similar mechanisms. Any physical condition that impairs the normal function of the abdominal musculature is suspect as cause for dysphonia. Some conditions, such as pregnancy, are obvious; however, a sprained ankle or broken leg that requires the singer to balance in an unaccustomed posture may distract him or her from maintaining good abdominal support and thereby result in voice dysfunction. A tremorous neurologic disorder, endocrine disturbances such as thyroid dysfunction or menopause, the aging process, and other systemic conditions also may alter the voice. The physician must remember that maladies of almost any body system may result in voice dysfunction, and the doctor must remain alert for conditions outside the head and neck. If the patient uses his or her voice professionally for singing, acting, or other vocally demanding professions, physical examination should also include assessment of the patient during typical professional vocal tasks. For example, a singer should be asked to sing. Evaluation techniques for assessing performance are described in greater detail elsewhere in this book.

A.-L. Hamdan et al., *Voice Disorders in Athletes, Coaches and other Sports Professionals*, https://doi.org/10.1007/978-3-030-69831-7_3

3.1 Complete Ear, Nose, and Throat Examination

Examination of the ears must include assessment of hearing acuity. Even a relatively slight hearing loss may result in voice strain as a singer tries to balance his or her vocal intensity with that of associate performers. Similar effects are encountered among speakers, but they are less prominent in the early stages of hearing loss. This is especially true of hearing losses acquired after vocal training has been completed. The effect is most pronounced with sensorineural hearing loss. Diplacusis, distortion of pitch perception, makes vocal strain even worse. With conductive hearing loss, singers tend to sing more softly than appropriate rather than too loudly, and this is less harmful.

During an ear, nose, and throat examination, the conjunctivae and sclerae should be observed routinely for erythema that suggests allergy or irritation, pallor that suggests anemia, and other abnormalities such as jaundice. These observations may reveal the problem reflected in the vocal tract even before the larynx is visualized. Hearing loss in a spouse may be problematic as well if the voice professional strains vocally to communicate.

The nose should be assessed for patency of the nasal airway, character of the nasal mucosa, and nature of secretions, if any. A patient who is unable to breathe through the nose because of anatomic obstruction is forced to breathe unfiltered, unhumidified air through the mouth. Pale gray allergic mucosa or swollen infected mucosa in the nose suggests abnormal mucosa elsewhere in the respiratory tract.

Examination of the oral cavity should include careful attention to the tonsils and lymphoid tissue in the posterior pharyngeal wall, as well as to the mucosa. Diffuse lymphoid hypertrophy associated with a complaint of "scratchy" voice and irritative cough may indicate infection. The amount and viscosity of mucosal and salivary secretions also should be noted. Xerostomia is particularly important. The presence of scalloping of the lateral aspects of the tongue should be noted. This finding is caused commonly by tongue thrust and may be associated with inappropriate tongue tension and muscle tension dysphonia. Dental examination should focus not only on oral hygiene but also on the presence of wear facets suggestive of bruxism. Bruxism is a clue to excessive tension and may be associated with dysfunction of the temporomandibular joints, which should also be assessed routinely. Thinning of the enamel of the central incisors in a normal or underweight patient may be a clue to bulimia. However, it may also result from excessive ingestion of lemons, which some singers eat to help thin their secretions.

The neck should be examined for masses, restriction of movement, excess muscle tension and/or spasm, and scars from prior neck surgery or trauma. Laryngeal vertical mobility is also important. For example, tilting of the larynx produced by partial fixation of cervical muscles cut during previous surgery may produce voice dysfunction, as may fixation of the trachea to overlying neck skin. Particular attention should be paid to the thyroid gland. Examination of posterior neck muscles and range of motion should not be neglected. The cranial nerves should also be examined. Diminished fifth nerve sensation, diminished gag reflex, palatal deviation, or other mild cranial nerve deficits may indicate cranial polyneuropathy. Postviral, infectious neuropathies may involve the superior laryngeal nerve(s) and cause weakness of the vocal fold muscle secondary to decreased neural input, fatigability, and loss of range and projection in the voice. The recurrent laryngeal nerve also is affected in some cases. More serious neurologic disease may also be associated with such symptoms and signs.

3.2 Laryngeal Examination

Examination of the larynx begins when the singer or other voice patient enters the physician's office. The range, ease, volume, and quality of the speaking voice should be noted. If the examination is not being conducted in the patient's native language, the physician should be sure to listen to a sample of the patient's mother tongue, as well. Voice use is often different under the strain or habits of foreign language use. Rating scales of the speaking voice may be helpful [4, 5]. The classification proposed by the Japan Society of Logopedics and Phoniatrics is one of the most widely used. It is known commonly as the GRBAS voice rating scale and is discussed below in the section on psychoacoustic evaluation [6].

Physicians are not usually experts in voice classification. However, the physicians should at least be able to discriminate substantial differences in range and timbre, such as between bass and tenor or alto and soprano. Although the correlation between speaking and singing voices is not perfect, a speaker with a low, comfortable bass voice who reports that he is a tenor may be misclassified and singing inappropriate roles with consequent voice strain. This judgment should be deferred to an expert, but the observation should lead the physician to make the appropriate referral. Excessive volume or obvious strain during speaking clearly indicates that voice abuse is present and may be contributing to the patient's singing complaint. The speaking voice can be evaluated more consistently and accurately using standardized reading passages, and such assessments are performed routinely by speech-language pathologists, phoniatricians, and sometimes laryngologists.

The definition of "register" or "registration" is controversial, and many different terms are used by musicians and scientists. Often, the definitions are unclear. Terms to describe register include chest, creek, falsetto, head, heavy, light, little, low, middle, modal, normal, pulse, upper, vocal fry, voce di petto, voce di mista, voce di testa, and whistle (also called flageolet and flute register). A register is a range of frequencies that has a consistent quality or timbre. The break between registers is an area of instability called the passaggio. During vocal training, singers are taught to integrate qualities of their various registers and to smooth and obscure the transition between registers. Registers occur not only in voices but also in some instruments, notably the organ. Vocal register changes are associated with changes in laryngeal musculature and in vocal fold shape. For example, in chest register, contraction of the thyroarytenoid muscles causes thickening of the vocal folds, with a square-shaped glottis and large vibratory margin contact area. In falsetto in men and head voice in women, cricothyroid muscle contraction is dominant, vocal folds are elongated, and the contact area is much thinner and more triangular than in chest voice. Vertical phase differences are diminished in head voice in comparison with chest voice. Controversy remains on the use of traditional terms in males such as chest, middle, head, and falsetto register or chest and head register in females. Voice scientists commonly prefer terms such as modal register. In any case, healthcare professionals should understand that there is a difference between the terms *register* and *range*. For example, if a singer complains of inability to sing high notes, this should be described as a loss of upper range, not a loss of upper register. Register and range difficulties should be noted.

Vibrato is a fluctuation of the fundamental frequency of a note. It is produced by the vocal mechanism under neural control and is present naturally in adult voices. The primary components of vibrato include rate (the number of frequency fluctuations per second), extent (number of hertz of fluctuation above and below the center frequency), regularity (consistency of frequency variations from one cycle to the next), and waveform. Rate and extent have been studied most extensively and are arguably the most important components in determining how the vibrato is perceived. Natural vibrato generally is about 6 Hz. Vibrato rate is slower in males than in females, and vocal pitch and effort do not have a substantial influence on vibrato. However, singers are able to alter vibrato rate and pitch oscillation voluntarily for stylistic purposes. The athletic choice of vibrato rate varies over time. For example, vibrato rates of 6–7 Hz were popular in classical Western (operatic) singing in the early twentieth century, but a vibrato rate of 5.5–6 Hz was considered more attractive by the end of the twentieth century. In general, pitch fluctuation covers about one semitone (half a semitone above and half a semitone below the center frequency) at present. A prominent wobble, as may be heard in some elderly singers who are not in ideal physical and vocal condition generally, is referred to as a tremolo. The excessive pitch (and sometimes intensity) fluctuations are caused by muscle activity, sometimes with a respiratory component, and are superimposed on the individual's vibrato in most cases, rather than actually being a widened, distorted vibrato. The true source of natural vibrato is uncertain, although the larynx, pharynx, tongue, and other components of the vocal tract may move in concert with vibrato, as well as with tremolo. Vibrato is thought not to be due primarily to phonatory structural activity rather than to respiratory source. The pressure of vibrato abnormalities or tremolo should be documented.

Any patient with a voice complaint should be examined by indirect laryngoscopy at least. It is not possible to judge voice range, quality, or other vocal attributes by inspection of the vocal folds. However, the presence or absence of nodules, mass lesions, contact ulcers, hemorrhage, erythema, paralysis, arytenoid erythema (reflux), and other anatomic abnormalities must be established. Erythema and edema of the laryngeal surface of the epiglottis are seen often in association with muscle tension dysphonia and with frequent coughing or clearing of the throat. It is caused by direct trauma from the arytenoids during these maneuvers. The mirror or a laryngeal telescope often provides a better view of the posterior portion of the endolarynx than is obtained with flexible endoscopy. Stroboscopic examination

Fig. 3.1 Normal larynx showing the true vocal folds (V), false vocal folds (F), arytenoids (A), and epiglottis (E)

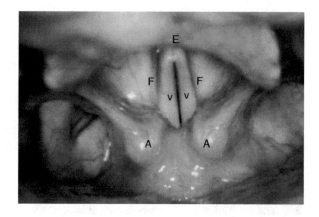

adds substantially to diagnostic abilities (Fig. 3.1), as discussed below. Another occasionally helpful adjunct is the operating microscope. Magnification allows visualization of small mucosal disruptions and hemorrhages that may be significant but overlooked otherwise. This technique also allows photography of the larynx with a microscope camera. Magnification may also be achieved through magnifying laryngeal mirrors or by wearing loupes. Loupes usually provide a clearer image than do most of the magnifying mirrors available.

A laryngeal telescope may be combined with a stroboscope to provide excellent visualization of the vocal folds and related structures. The author usually uses a 70-degree laryngeal telescope, although 90-degree telescopes are required for some patients. The combination of a telescope and stroboscope provides optimal magnification and optical quality for assessment of vocal fold vibration. However, it is generally performed with the tongue in a fixed position, and the nature of the examination does not permit assessment of the larynx during normal phonatory gestures.

Flexible fiber-optic laryngoscopy can be performed as an office procedure and allows inspection of the vocal folds in patients whose vocal folds are difficult to visualize indirectly. In addition, it permits observation of the vocal mechanism in a more natural posture than does indirect laryngoscopy, permitting sophisticated dynamic voice assessment. In the hands of an experienced endoscopist, this method may provide a great deal of information about both speaking and singing techniques. The combination of a fiber-optic laryngoscope with a laryngeal stroboscope may be especially useful. This system permits magnification, photography, and detailed inspection of vocal fold motion. Sophisticated systems that permit flexible or rigid fiber-optic strobovideolaryngoscopy are currently available commercially. They are invaluable assets for routine clinical use. The video system also provides a permanent record, permitting reassessment, comparison over time, and easy consultation. A refinement not currently available commercially is stereoscopic fiber-optic laryngoscopy, accomplished by placing a laryngoscope through each nostril, fastening the two together in the pharynx, and observing the larynx through the eyepieces [7]. This method allows visualization of laryngeal motion in three dimensions. However, it is used primarily in a research setting.

Rigid endoscopy under general anesthesia may be reserved for the rare patient whose vocal folds cannot be assessed adequately by other means or for patients who need surgical procedures to remove or biopsy laryngeal lesions. In some cases, this may be done with local anesthesia, avoiding the need for intubation and the traumatic coughing and vomiting that may occur even after general anesthesia administered by mask. Coughing after general anesthesia may be minimized by using topical anesthesia in the larynx and trachea. However, topical anesthetics may act as severe mucosal irritants in a small number of patients. They may also predispose the patient to aspiration in the postoperative period. If a patient has had difficulty with a topical anesthetic administered in the office, it should not be used in the operating room. When used in general anesthesia cases, topical anesthetics should usually be applied at the end of the procedure. Thus, if inflammation occurs, it will not interfere with performance of microsurgery. Postoperative duration of anesthesia is also optimized. The author has had the least difficulty with 4% Xylocaine.

3.3   Objective Tests

Reliable, valid, objective analysis of the voice is extremely important and is an essential part of a comprehensive physical examination [2]. It is as valuable to the laryngologist as audiometry is to the otologist [8, 9]. Familiarity with some of the measures and technological advances currently available is helpful. This information is covered in greater detail elsewhere in this book but is included here as a brief overview for the convenience of the reader.

3.3.1   Strobovideolaryngoscopy

Integrity of the vibratory margin of the vocal fold is essential for the complex motion required to produce good vocal quality. Under continuous light, the vocal folds vibrate approximately 250 times per second while phonating at middle C. Naturally, the human eye cannot discern the necessary details during such rapid motion. The vibratory margin may be assessed through high-speed photography, strobovideolaryngoscopy, high-speed video, videokymography, electroglottography (EGG), or photoglottography. Strobovideolaryngoscopy provides the necessary clinical information in a practical fashion. Stroboscopic light allows routine slow-motion evaluation of the mucosal cover layer of the leading edge of the vocal fold. This state-of-the-art physical examination permits detection of vibratory asymmetries, structural abnormalities, small masses, submucosal scars, and other conditions that are invisible under ordinary light [10, 11]. Documentation of the procedure by

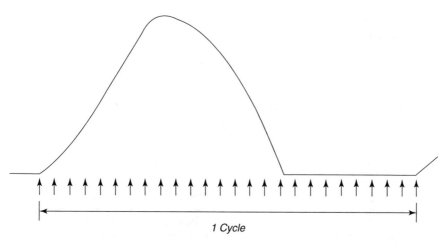

Fig. 3.2 The principle of ultrahigh-speed photography. Numerous images are taken during each vibratory cycle. This technique is a true slow-motion representation of each vocal fold vibration

coupling stroboscopic light with the video camera allows later reevaluation by the laryngologist or other healthcare providers.

Stroboscopy does not provide a true slow-motion image, as obtained through high-speed photography (Fig. 3.2). The stroboscope actually illuminates different points on consecutive vocal fold waves, each of which is retained on the retina for 0.2 seconds. The stroboscopically lighted portions of the successive waves are fused visually, and thus, the examiner is actually evaluating simulated cycles of phonation. The slow-motion effect is created by having the stroboscopic light desynchronized with the frequency of vocal fold vibration by approximately 2 Hz. When vocal fold vibration and the stroboscope are synchronized exactly, the vocal folds appear to stand still, rather than move in slow motion (Fig. 3.3). In most instances, this approximation of slow motion provides all the clinical information necessary. Our routine stroboscopy protocol is described elsewhere [11]. We use a modification of the standardized method of subjective assessment of strobovideolaryngoscopic images, as proposed by Bless et al. [12] and Hirano [13]. Characteristics evaluated include the fundamental frequency, symmetry of movements, periodicity, glottic closure, amplitude of vibration, mucosal wave, presence of nonvibrating portions of the vocal fold, and other unusual findings. With practice, perceptual judgments of stroboscopic images provide a great deal of information. However, it is easy for the inexperienced observer to draw unwarranted conclusions because of normal variations in vibration. Vibrations depend on fundamental frequency, intensity, and vocal register. For example, failure of glottic closure occurs normally in falsetto phonation. Consequently, it is important to note these characteristics and to examine each voice under a variety of conditions.

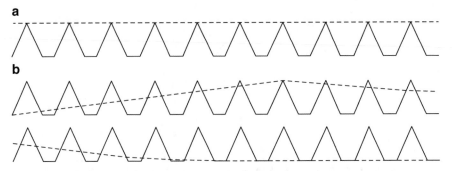

Fig. 3.3 The principle of stroboscopy. The stroboscopic light illuminates portions of successive cycles. The eye fuses the illuminated points into an illusion of slow motion. (**a**) If the stroboscope is synchronized with vocal fold vibration, a similar point is illuminated on each successive cycle, and the vocal fold appears to stand still. (**b**) If the stroboscope is slightly desynchronized, each cycle is illuminated at a slightly different point, and the slow-motion effect is created

3.3.2   Other Techniques to Examine Vocal Fold Vibration

Other techniques to examine vocal fold vibration include ultrahigh-speed photography, EGG, photoelectroglottography, and ultrasound glottography and most recently videokymography [14] and high-speed video (digital or analog). Ultrahigh-speed photography provides images that are in true slow motion, rather than simulated. High-speed video offers similar advantages without most of the disadvantages of high-speed motion pictures. Videokymography offers high-speed imaging of a single line along the vocal fold. EGG uses two electrodes placed on the skin of the neck above the thyroid laminae. It traces the opening and closing of the glottis and can be compared with stroboscopic images [15]. EGG allows objective determination of the presence or absence of glottic vibrations and easy determination of the fundamental period of vibration and is reproducible. It reflects the glottic condition more accurately during its closed phase. Photo electroglottography and ultrasound glottography are less useful clinically [16].

3.3.3   Measures of Phonatory Ability

Objective measures of phonatory ability are easy to use, readily available to the laryngologist, helpful in the treatment of professional vocalists with specific voice disorders, and quite useful in assessing the results of surgical therapies. Maximum phonation time is measured with a stopwatch. The patient is instructed to sustain the vowel /a/ for as long as possible after deep inspiration and vocalizing at a comfortable frequency and intensity. The frequency and intensity may be determined and controlled by an inexpensive frequency analyzer and sound level meter. The test is repeated three times, and the greatest value is recorded. Normal values have been determined [16]. Frequency range of phonation is recorded in semitones and documents the vocal range from the lowest note in the modal register (excluding vocal fry) to the highest falsetto note. This is the physiologic frequency range of phonation and disregards quality. The musical frequency range of phonation measures lowest to highest notes of musically acceptable quality. Tests for maximum phonation time, frequency ranges, and many of the other parameters discussed later (including spectrographic analysis) may be preserved on a tape recorder or digitized and stored for analysis at a convenient future time and used for pre- and posttreatment comparisons. Recordings should be made in a standardized, consistent fashion.

Frequency limits of vocal register also may be measured. The registers are (from low to high) vocal fry, chest, mid, head, and falsetto. However, classification of registers is controversial, and many other classifications are used. Although the classification listed above is common among musicians, at present, most voice scientists prefer to classify registers as pulse, modal, and loft. Overlap of frequency among registers occurs routinely.

Testing the speaking fundamental frequency often reveals excessively low pitch, an abnormality associated with chronic voice abuse and development of vocal nodules. This parameter may be followed objectively throughout a course of voice therapy. Intensity range of phonation (IRP) has proven to be a less useful measure than frequency range. It varies with fundamental frequency (which should be recorded) and is greatest in the middle frequency range. It is recorded in sound pressure level (SPL) (re 0.0002 microbar). For healthy adults who are not professional vocalists, measuring at a single fundamental frequency, IRP averages 54.8 dB for males and 51 dB for females [17]. Alterations of intensity are common in voice disorders, although IRP is not the most sensitive test to detect them. Information from these tests may be combined in a fundamental frequency-intensity profile [16], also called a *phonetogram*.

Glottic efficiency (ratio of the acoustic power at the level of the glottis to subglottic power) provides useful information but is not clinically practical because measuring acoustic power at the level of the glottis is difficult. Subglottal power is the product of subglottal pressure and airflow rate. These can be determined clinically. Various alternative measures of glottic efficiency have been proposed, including the ratio of radiated acoustic power to subglottal power [18], airflow intensity profile [19], and ratio of the root mean square value of the AC component to the mean volume velocity (DC component) [20]. Although glottic efficiency is of great interest, none of these tests are particularly helpful under routine clinical circumstances.

3.3.4 Aerodynamic Measures

Traditional pulmonary function testing provides the most readily accessible measure of respiratory function. The most common parameters measured include (1) tidal volume, the volume of air that enters the lungs during inspiration and leaves during expiration in normal breathing; (2) functional residual capacity, the volume of air remaining in the lungs at the end of inspiration during normal breathing, which can be divided into expiratory reserve volume (maximal additional volume that can be exhaled) and residual volume (the volume of air remaining in the lungs at the end of maximal exhalation); (3) inspiratory capacity, the maximal volume of air that can be inhaled starting at the functional residual capacity; (4) total lung capacity, the volume of air in the lungs following maximal inspiration; (5) vital capacity, the maximal volume of air that can be exhaled from the lungs following maximal inspiration; (6) forced vital capacity, the rate of airflow with rapid, forceful expiration from total lung capacity to residual volume; (7) FEV_1, the forced expiratory volume in 1 second; (8) FEV_3, the forced expiratory volume in 3 seconds; and (9) maximal mid-expiratory flow, the mean rate of airflow over the middle half of the forced vital capacity (between 25% and 75% of the forced vital capacity). For singers and professional speakers with an abnormality caused by voice abuse, abnormal pulmonary function tests may confirm deficiencies in aerobic conditioning or reveal previously unrecognized asthma [21]. Flow glottography with computer inverse filtering is also a practical and valuable diagnostic for assessing flow at the vocal fold level, evaluating the voice source, and imaging the results of the balance between adductory forces and subglottal pressure [22]. It also has therapeutic value as a biofeedback tool.

The spirometer, readily available for pulmonary function testing, can also be used for measuring airflow during phonation. However, the spirometer does not allow simultaneous display of acoustic signals, and its frequency response is poor. A pneumotachograph consists of a laminar air resistor, a differential pressure transducer, and an amplifying and recording system. It allows measurement of airflow and simultaneous recording of other signals when coupled with a polygraph. A hot-wire anemometer allows determination of airflow velocity by measuring the electrical drop across the hot wire. Modern hot-wire anemometers containing electrical feedback circuitry that maintains the temperature of the hot wire provide a flat response up to 1 kHz and are useful clinically.

The four parameters traditionally measured in the aerodynamic performance of a voice are subglottal pressure (P_{sub}), supraglottic pressure (P_{sup}), glottic impedance, and the volume velocity of airflow at the glottis. These parameters and their rapid variations can be measured under laboratory circumstances. However, clinically, their mean value is usually determined as follows:

$$P_{sub} - P_{sup} = MFR \times GR$$

where *MFR* is the mean (root mean square) flow rate and *GR* is the mean (root mean square) glottic resistance. When vocalizing the open vowel /a/, the supraglottic pressure equals the atmospheric pressure, reducing the equation to the following:

$$P_{sub} = MFR \times GR$$

The mean flow rate is a useful clinical measure. While the patient vocalizes the vowel /a/, the mean flow rate is calculated by dividing the total volume of air used during phonation by the duration of phonation. The subject phonates at a comfortable pitch and loudness either over a determined period of time or for a maximum sustained period of phonation.

Air volume is measured by the use of a mask fitted tightly over the face or by phonating into a mouthpiece while wearing a nose clamp. Measurements may be made using a spirometer, pneumotachograph, or hot-wire anemometer. The normal values for mean flow rate under habitual phonation, with changes in intensity or register, and under various pathologic circumstances were determined in the 1970s [16]. Normal values are available for both adults and children. Mean flow rate also can be measured and is a clinically useful parameter to follow during treatment for vocal nodules, recurrent laryngeal nerve paralysis, spasmodic dysphonia, and other conditions.

Glottic resistance cannot be measured directly, but it may be calculated from the mean flow rate and mean subglottal pressure. Normal glottic resistance is 20–100 dyne-seconds/cm^5 at low and medium pitches and 150 dyne-seconds/cm^5 at high pitches [18]. The normal values for subglottal pressure under various healthy and pathologic voice conditions have also been determined by numerous investigators [16]. The phonation quotient is the vital capacity divided by the maximum phonation time. It has been shown to correlate closely with maximum flow rate [23] and is a more convenient measure. Normative data determined by various authors have been published [16]. The phonation quotient provides an objective measure of the effects of treatment and is particularly useful in cases of recurrent laryngeal nerve paralysis and mass lesions of the vocal folds, including nodules.

3.3.5   Acoustic Analysis

Acoustic analysis equipment can determine frequency, intensity, harmonic spectrum, cycle-to-cycle perturbations in frequency (jitter), cycle-to-cycle perturbations in amplitude (shimmer), harmonics/noise ratios, breathiness index, and many other parameters. The DSP Sona-Graph Sound Analyzer Model 5500 (Kay Elemetrics, Lincoln Park, New Jersey) is an integrated voice analysis system. It is equipped for sound spectrography capabilities. Spectrography provides a visual record of the voice. The acoustic signal is depicted using time (x-axis), frequency (y-axis), and intensity (z-axis), shading of light vs dark. Using the band-pass filters, generalizations about quality, pitch, and loudness can be made. These observations are used in formulating the voice therapy treatment plan. Formant structure and strength can be determined using the narrow-band filters, of which a variety of configurations are possible. In clinical settings in which singers and other professional voice users are evaluated and treated routinely, this feature is extremely valuable. A sophisticated voice analysis program (an optional program) may be combined with the Sona-Graph and is an especially valuable addition to the clinical laboratory. The voice analysis program (Computer Speech Lab, Kay Elemetrics) measures speaking fundamental frequency, frequency perturbation (jitter), amplitude perturbation (shimmer), and harmonics/noise ratio and provides many other useful values. An electroglottograph may be used in conjunction with the Sona-Graph to provide some of these voicing parameters. Examining the EGG waveform alone is possible with this setup, but its clinical usefulness has not yet been established. An important feature of the Sona-Graph is the long-term average (LTA) spectral capability, which permits analysis of longer voice samples (30–90 seconds). The LTA analyzes only voiced speech segments and may be useful in screening for hoarse or breathy voices. In addition, computer interface capabilities (also an optional program) have solved many data storage and file maintenance problems.

In analyzing acoustic signals, the microphone may be placed at the level of the mouth or positioned in or over the trachea, although intratracheal recordings are used for research purposes only. The position should be standardized in each office or laboratory [24]. Various techniques are being developed to improve the usefulness of acoustic analysis. Because of the enormous amount of information carried in the acoustic signal, further refinements in objective acoustic analysis should prove particularly valuable to the clinician.

3.3.6   Laryngeal Electromyography

Electromyography (EMG) requires an electrode system, an amplifier, an oscilloscope, a loudspeaker, and a recording system [25]. Electrodes are placed transcutaneously into laryngeal muscles. EMG can be extremely valuable in confirming cases of vocal fold paresis, differentiating paralysis from arytenoid dislocation, distinguishing recurrent laryngeal nerve paralysis from combined recurrent and superior nerve paralysis, diagnosing other more subtle neurolaryngologic pathology, and documenting functional voice disorders and malingering. It is also recommended for needle localization when using botulinum toxin for treatment of spasmodic dysphonia and other conditions.

3.3.7   Psychoacoustic Evaluation

Because the human ear and brain are the most sensitive and complex analyzers of sound currently available, many researchers have tried to standardize and quantify psychoacoustic evaluation. Unfortunately, even definitions of basic terms such as hoarseness and breathiness are still controversial. Psychoacoustic evaluation protocols and interpretations are not standardized. Consequently, although subjective psychoacoustic analysis of voice is of great value to the individual skilled clinician, it remains generally unsatisfactory for comparing research among laboratories or for reporting clinical results.

The GRBAS scale [6] helps standardize perceptual analysis for clinical purposes. It rates the voice from a scale of 0 to 3, with regard to grade, roughness, breathiness, asthenia, and strain. Grade 0 is normal, 1 is slightly abnormal, 2 is moderately abnormal, and 3 is extremely abnormal. Grade refers to the degree of hoarseness or voice abnormality. Roughness refers to the acoustic/auditory impression of irregularity of vibration and corresponds with gear and shimmer. Breathiness refers to the acoustic/auditory impression of air leakage and corresponds to turbulence. Asthenic evaluation assesses weakness or lack of power and corresponds to vocal intensity and energy in higher harmonics. Strain refers to the acoustic/auditory impression of hyperfunction and may be related to fundamental frequency, noise in the high-frequency range, and energy in higher harmonics. For example, a patient's voice might be graded as G2, R2, B1, A1, and S2.

3.4 Outcomes Assessment

Measuring the impact of a voice disorder has always been challenging. However, recent advances have begun to address this problem. Validated instruments such as the Voice Handicap Index (VHI) [26] are currently in clinical use and are likely to be used widely in future years.

3.5 Voice Impairment and Disability

Quantifying voice impairment and assigning a disability rating (percentage of whole person) remain controversial. This subject is still not addressed comprehensively even in the most recent editions (2008, 6th edition) of the American Medical Association's *Guidelines for the Evaluation of Impairment and Disability* (The Guides). The Guides still do not take into account the person's profession when calculating disability. Alternative approaches have been proposed [27], and advances in this complex arena are anticipated over the next few years.

3.6 Evaluation of the Singing Voice

The physician must be careful not to exceed the limits of his or her expertise, especially in caring for singers. However, if voice abuse or technical error is suspected or if a difficult judgment must be reached on whether to allow a sick singer to perform, a brief observation of the patient's singing may provide invaluable information. This is accomplished best by asking the singer to stand and sing scales either in the examining room or in the soundproof audiology booth. Similar maneuvers may be used for professional speakers, including actors (who can vocalize and recite lines), clergy and politicians (who can deliver sermons and speeches), and virtually all other voice patients. The singer's stance should be balanced, with the weight slightly forward. The knees should be bent slightly, and the shoulders, torso, and neck should be relaxed. The singer should inhale through the nose whenever possible allowing filtration, warming, and humidification of inspired air. In general, the chest should be expanded, but most of the active breathing is abdominal. The chest should not rise substantially with each inspiration, and the supraclavicular musculature should not be involved obviously in inspiration. Shoulder and neck muscles should not be tensed even with deep inspiration. Abdominal musculature should be contracted shortly before the initiation of the tone. This may be evaluated visually or by palpation (Fig. 3.4). Muscles of the neck and face should be relaxed. Economy is a basic principle of all art forms. Wasted energy and motion and muscle tension are incorrect and usually deleterious.

The singer should be instructed to sing a scale (a five-note scale is usually sufficient) on the vowel /a/, beginning on any comfortable note. Technical errors are usually most obvious as contraction of muscles in the neck and chin, retraction of the lower lip, retraction of the tongue, or tightening of the muscles of mastication.

Fig. 3.4 Bimanual palpation of the support mechanism. The singer should expand posteriorly and anteriorly with inspiration. Muscles should tighten prior to onset of sung tone

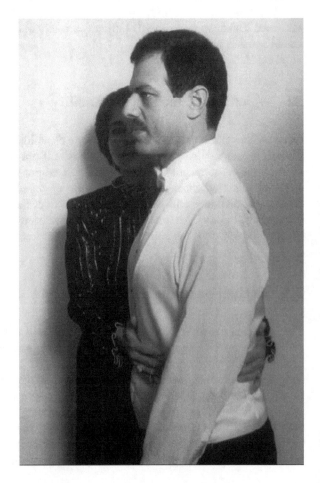

The singer's mouth should be open widely but comfortably. When singing /a/, the singer's tongue should rest in a neutral position with the tip of the tongue lying against the back of the singer's mandibular incisors. If the tongue pulls back or demonstrates obvious muscular activity as the singer performs the scales, improper voice use can be confirmed on the basis of positive evidence (Fig. 3.5). The position of the larynx should not vary substantially with pitch changes. Rising of the larynx with ascending pitch is evidence of technical dysfunction. This examination also gives the physician an opportunity to observe any dramatic differences between the qualities and ranges of the patient's speaking voice and singing voice. A physical examination summary form has proven helpful in organization and documentation [3].

Remembering the admonition not to exceed his or her expertise, the physician who examines many singers can often glean valuable information from a brief attempt to modify an obvious technical error. For example, deciding whether to allow a singer with mild or moderate laryngitis to perform is often difficult. On one hand, an expert singer has technical skills that allow him or her to compensate safely. On the other hand, if a singer does not sing with correct technique and does not have the discipline to modify volume, technique, and repertoire as necessary, the risk of vocal injury may be increased substantially even by mild inflammation of the vocal folds. In borderline circumstances, observation of the singer's technique may greatly help the physician in making a judgment.

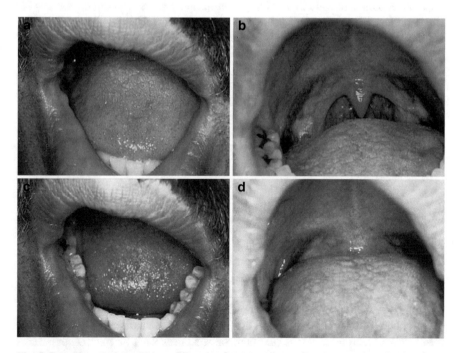

Fig. 3.5 Proper relaxed position of the anterior (**a**) and posterior (**b**) portions of the tongue. Common improper use of the tongue pulled back from the teeth (**c**) and raised posteriorly (**d**)

If the singer's technique appears flawless, the physician may feel somewhat more secure in allowing the singer to proceed with performance commitments. More commonly, even good singers demonstrate technical errors when experiencing voice difficulties. In a vain effort to compensate for dysfunction at the vocal fold level, singers often modify their technique in the neck and supraglottic vocal tract. In the good singer, this usually means going from good technique to bad technique. The most common error involves pulling back the tongue and tightening the cervical muscles. Although this increased muscular activity gives the singer the illusion of making the voice more secure, this technical maladjustment undermines vocal efficiency and increases vocal strain. The physician may ask the singer to hold the top note of a five-note scale; while the note is being held, the singer may simply be told, "Relax your tongue." At the same time, the physician points to the singer's abdominal musculature. Most good singers immediately correct to good technique. If they do and if upcoming performances are particularly important, the singer may be able to perform with a reminder that meticulous technique is essential. The singer should be advised to "sing by feel rather than by ear," consult his or her voice teacher, and conserve the voice except when it is absolutely necessary to use it. If a singer is unable to correct from bad technique to good technique promptly, especially if he or she uses excessive muscle tension in the neck and ineffective abdominal support, it is generally safer not to perform with even a mild vocal fold abnormality. With increased experience and training, the laryngologist may make other observations that aid in providing appropriate treatment recommendations for singer patients. Once these skills have been mastered for the care of singers, applying them to other patients is relatively easy, so long as the laryngologist takes the time to understand the demands of the individual's professional, avocational, and recreational vocal activities.

If treatment is to be instituted, making at least a tape recording of the voice is advisable in most cases and essential before any surgical intervention. The author routinely uses strobovideolaryngoscopy for diagnosis and documentation in virtually all cases as well as many of the objective measures discussed. Pretreatment testing is extremely helpful clinically and medicolegally.

3.7   Additional Examinations

A general physical examination should be performed whenever the patient's systemic health is questionable. Debilitating conditions such as mononucleosis may be noticed first by the singer as vocal fatigue. A neurologic assessment may be particularly revealing. The physician must be careful not to overlook dysarthrias and dysphonias, which are characteristic of movement disorders and of serious neurologic disease. Dysarthria is a defect in rhythm, enunciation, and articulation that usually results from neuromuscular impairment or weakness such as may occur after a stroke. It may be seen with oral deformities or illness, as well. Dysphonia is an abnormality of vocalization usually caused by problems at the laryngeal level.

Physicians should be familiar with the six types of dysarthria, their symptoms, and their importance [28, 29]. Flaccid dysarthria occurs in lower motor neuron or primary muscle disorders such as myasthenia gravis and tumors or strokes involving the brainstem nuclei. Spastic dysarthria occurs in upper motor neuron disorders (pseudobulbar palsy) such as multiple strokes and cerebral palsy. Ataxic dysarthria is seen with cerebellar disease, alcohol intoxication, and multiple sclerosis. Hypokinetic dysarthria accompanies Parkinson disease. Hyperkinetic dysarthria may be spasmodic, as in the Gilles de la Tourette syndrome, or dystonic, as in chorea and cerebral palsy. Mixed dysarthria occurs in amyotrophic lateral sclerosis (ALS) or Lou Gehrig's disease. The preceding classification actually combines dysphonic and dysarthric characteristics but is very useful clinically. The value of a comprehensive neurolaryngologic evaluation [30] cannot be overstated. More specific details of voice changes associated with neurologic dysfunction and their localizing value are available elsewhere [2, 31].

It is extremely valuable for the laryngologist to assemble an arts-medicine team that includes not only a speech-language pathologist, singing voice specialist, acting voice specialist, and voice scientist but also medical colleagues in other disciplines. Collaboration with an expert neurologist, pulmonologist, endocrinologist, psychologist, psychiatrist, internist, physiatrist, and others with special knowledge of, and interest in, voice disorders is invaluable in caring for patients with voice disorders. Such interdisciplinary teams not only have changed the standard of care in voice evaluation and treatment but also are largely responsible for the rapid and productive growth of voice as a subspecialty.

Acknowledgments Modified in part from Sataloff RT. *Professional Voice: The Science and Art of Clinical Care, 4th Edition.* San Diego, CA: Plural Publishing; 2017, with permission.

References

1. Sataloff RT. Professional singers: the science and art of clinical care. Am J Otolaryngol. 1981;2:251–66.
2. Rubin J, Sataloff R, Korovin G. Diagnosis and treatment of voice disorders. 4th ed. San Diego: Plural Publishing; 2014.
3. Sataloff RT. The professional voice: part II, physical examination. J Voice. 1987;1:91–201.
4. Fuazawa T, Blaugrund SM, El-Assuooty A, Gould WJ. Acoustic analysis of hoarse voice: a preliminary report. J Voice. 1988;2(2):127–31.
5. Gelfer M. Perceptual attributes of voice: development and use of rating scales. J Voice. 1988;2(4):320–6.
6. Hirano M. Clinical examination of the voice. New York: Springer-Verlag; 1981. p. 83–4.
7. Fujimura O. Stereo-fiberoptic laryngeal observation. J Acoust Soc Am. 1979;65:70–2.
8. Sataloff RT, Spiegel JR, Carroll LM, Darby KS, Hawkshaw MJ, Rulnick RK. The clinical voice laboratory: practical design and clinical application. J Voice. 1990;4:264–79.
9. Sataloff RT, Heuer RH, Hoover C, Baroody MM. Laboratory assessment of voice. In: Gould WJ, Sataloff RT, Spiegel JR. Voice surgery. St. Louis: Mosby; 1993. p. 203–16.

10. Sataloff RT, Spiegel JR, Carroll LM, Schiebel BR, Darby KS, Rulnick RK. Strobovideolaryngoscopy in professional voice users: results and clinical value. J Voice. 1986;1:359–64.
11. Sataloff RT, Spiegel JR, Hawkshaw MJ. Strobovideolaryngoscopy: results and clinical value. Ann Otol Rhinol Laryngol. 1991;100:725–7.
12. Bless D, Hirano M, Feder RJ. Video stroboscopic evaluation of the larynx. Ear Nose Throat J. 1987;66:289–96.
13. Hirano M. Phonosurgery: basic and clinical investigations. Otologia (Fukuoka). 1975;21:239–442.
14. Svec J, Shutte H. Videokymography: high-speed line scanning of vocal fold vibration. J Voice. 1996;10:201–5.
15. Leclure FLE, Brocaar ME, Verscheeure J. Electroglottography and its relation to glottal activity. Folia Phoniatr (Basel). 1975;27:215–24.
16. Hirano M. Clinical examination of the voice. New York: Springer-Verlag; 1981:25–7, 85–98.
17. Coleman RJ, Mabis JH, Hinson JK. Fundamental frequency sound pressure level profiles of adult male and female voices. J Speech Hear Res. 1977;20:197–204.
18. Isshiki N. Regulatory mechanism of voice intensity variation. J Speech Hear Res. 1964;7:17–29.
19. Saito S. Phonosurgery: basic study on the mechanisms of phonation and endolaryngeal microsurgery. Otologia (Fukuoka). 1977;23:171–384.
20. Isshiki N. Functional surgery of the larynx. Report of the 78th annual convention of the Oto-Rhino-Laryngological Society of Japan. Fukuoka: Kyoto University; 1977.
21. Cohn JR, Sataloff RT, Spiegel JR, Fish JE, Kennedy K. Airway reactivity-induced asthma in singers (ARIAS). J Voice. 1991;5:332–7.
22. Sundberg J. The science of the singing voice. Dekalb: Northern Illinois University Press; 1987:11, 66, 77–89.
23. Hirano M, Koike Y, von Leden H. Maximum phonation time and air usage during phonation. Folia Phoniatr (Basel). 1968;20:185–201.
24. Price DB, Sataloff RT. A simple technique for consistent microphone placement in voice recording. J Voice. 1988;2:206–7.
25. Sataloff RT, Mandel S, Heman-Ackah YD, Abaza M. Laryngeal electromyography. 3rd ed. San Diego: Plural Publishing, Inc; 2017.
26. Benninger MS, Syamal MN, Gardner GM, Jacobson BH. New dimensions in measuring voice treatment outcomes and quality of life. In: Sataloff RT, editor. Professional voice: the science and art of clinical care. 4th ed. San Diego: Plural Publishing, Inc; 2017. p. 547–58.
27. Sataloff RT. Voice impairment, disability, handicap, and medical-legal evaluation. In: Sataloff RT. Professional voice: the science and art of clinical care. 4th ed. San Diego: Plural Publishing, Inc; 2017. p. 1741–54.
28. Darley FL, Aronson AE, Brown JR. Differential diagnostic of patterns of dysarthria. J Speech Hear Res. 1969;12(2):246–9.
29. Darley FL, Aronson AE, Brown JR. Clusters of deviant speech dimensions in the dysarthrias. J Speech Hear Res. 1969;12(3):462–96.
30. Rosenfield DB. Neurolaryngology. Ear Nose Throat J. 1987;66:323–6.
31. Raphael BN, Sataloff RT. Increasing vocal effectiveness. In: Sataloff RT. Professional voice: the science and art of clinical care. 4th ed. San Diego: Plural Publishing, Inc; 2017. p. 1201–12.

Chapter 4
Professional Voice Users: An Overview of Medical Disorders and Treatments

Laryngologists specializing in voice devote the majority of their practices to the medical management of benign voice disorders. Although most of us are active surgeons, a good voice specialist takes pride in avoiding the need for laryngeal surgery through expert medical management. Success depends not only on a good laryngologist but also on the availability of a voice team, including a speech-language pathologist, voice scientist, singing voice specialist, and medical consultants who have acquired special knowledge about voice disorders (neurologists, pulmonologists, endocrinologists, internists, allergists, and others). This chapter provides an overview of many of the benign voice problems encountered by healthcare providers and current nonsurgical management concepts.

Numerous medical conditions affect the voice adversely. Many have their origins primarily outside the head and neck. This chapter is not intended to be all-inclusive but rather to highlight some of the more common and important conditions found in professional voice users and wind instrumentalists seeking medical care.

In the 2286 cases of all forms of voice disorders reported by Brodnitz in 1971 [1], 80% were attributed to voice abuse or to psychogenic factors resulting in vocal dysfunction. Of these patients, 20% had organic voice disorders. Of women with organic problems, about 15% had identifiable endocrine causes. A much higher incidence of organic disorders, particularly reflux laryngitis, acute infectious laryngitis, and benign vocal fold masses, is found in the author's (RTS) practice.

4.1 Voice Abuse

When voice abuse is suspected or observed in a patient with vocal complaints, he or she should be referred to a laryngologist who specializes in voice, preferably a physician affiliated with a voice care team.

A.-L. Hamdan et al., *Voice Disorders in Athletes, Coaches and other Sports Professionals*, https://doi.org/10.1007/978-3-030-69831-7_4

Common patterns of voice abuse and misuse will not be discussed in detail in this chapter. They are covered elsewhere in the literature [2]. Voice abuse and/or misuse should be suspected particularly in patients who complain of voice fatigue associated with voice use, whose voices are worse at the end of a working day or week, and in any patient who is chronically hoarse. Technical errors in voice use may be the primary etiology of a voice complaint or may develop secondarily as a result of a patient's efforts to compensate for voice disturbance from another cause.

Speaking in noisy environments such as cars and airplanes is particularly abusive to the voice, as are backstage greetings, post-performance parties, choral conducting, voice teaching, cheerleading, and many other activities. With proper training, all these vocal activities can be done safely. However, most patients, surprisingly even singers, have little or no training for their speaking voice.

If voice abuse is caused by speaking, treatment should be provided by a licensed, certified speech-language pathologist in the United States or by a phoniatrist in many other countries. In many cases, training the speaking voice will benefit singers greatly not only by improving speech but also by indirectly helping singing technique. Physicians should not hesitate to recommend such training, but it should be performed by an expert speech-language pathologist who specializes in voice. Many speech-language pathologists who are well trained in swallowing rehabilitation, articulation therapy, and other techniques are not trained in voice therapy for the speaking voice, and virtually, none are trained through their speech and language programs to work with singing unless they are also singing teachers or singing voice specialists.

Specialized singing training also may be helpful to many voice patients who are not singers, and it is invaluable for patients who are singers. Initial singing training teaches relaxation techniques, develops muscle strength, and is symbiotic with standard voice therapy. Abuse of the voice during singing is an even more complex problem, as discussed elsewhere in this book.

4.2 Infection and Inflammation

4.2.1 Upper Respiratory Tract Infection Without Laryngitis

Although mucosal irritation usually is diffuse, patients sometimes have marked nasal obstruction with little or no sore throat and a "normal" voice. If the laryngeal examination showed no abnormality, a singer or professional speaker with a "head cold" should be permitted to use his or her voice and be advised not to try to duplicate his or her usual sound but rather accept the insurmountable alterations in self-perception caused by the change in the supraglottic vocal tract and auditory system. The decision as to whether performing under the circumstances is advisable professionally rests with the voice professional and his or her musical associates. The patient should be cautioned against throat clearing, as this is traumatic and may produce laryngitis. If a cough is present, nonnarcotic medications should be used to suppress it. In addition, the patient should be taught how to "silent cough," which is less traumatic. "Cold sores" or dry, split lips or tongue also may interfere with singing, although they are far more troublesome for wind instrumentalists, as are dental braces which can traumatize mucosal surfaces and affect instrument or voice performance.

4.2.2 Laryngitis with Serious Vocal Fold Injury

Hemorrhage in the vocal folds and mucosal disruption associated with acute laryngitis are contraindications to speaking and singing. When these are observed, treatment includes strict voice rest in addition to correction of any underlying disease. If the patient also plays a wind instrument, laryngoscopy while playing will determine whether there is vocal fold contact during wind performance (there is in many players, but not all). If so, instrument playing should be stopped during the period of voice rest. Vocal fold hemorrhage in voice professionals is most common in premenstrual women who are using aspirin products or nonsteroidal anti-inflammatory drugs (NSAIDS) for dysmenorrhea. Severe hemorrhage or mucosal scarring may result in permanent alternations in vocal fold vibratory function. In rare instances, surgical intervention may be necessary. The potential gravity of these conditions must be stressed, for singers are generally reluctant to cancel an appearance. As von Leden observed, it is a pleasure to work with "people who are determined that the show must go on when everyone else is determined to goof off" [3]. However, patient compliance is essential when serious damage has occurred. At present, acute treatment of vocal fold hemorrhage is controversial. Most laryngologists allow the hematoma to resolve spontaneously. Because this sometimes results in an organized hematoma and scar formation requiring surgery, some physicians advocate incision along the superior edge of the vocal fold and drainage of the hematoma in selected cases. Further study is needed to determine optimal therapy guidelines (Figs. 4.1 and 4.2).

4.2.3 Laryngitis Without Serious Damage

Mild to moderate edema and erythema of the vocal folds may result from infection or from noninfectious causes. In the absence of mucosal disruption or hemorrhage, they are not absolute contraindications to voice use (including wind instrument performance in selected cases). Noninfectious laryngitis commonly is associated with excessive voice use in pre-performance rehearsals. It also may be caused by other forms of voice abuse and by mucosal irritation produced by allergy, smoke inhalation, and other causes. Mucous stranding between the anterior and middle thirds of the vocal folds is seen commonly in inflammatory laryngitis. Laryngitis sicca (dry

Fig. 4.1 Video print obtained from a strobovideolaryngoscopic examination shows diffuse erythema from acute laryngitis. Additionally, there is a left sulcus vocalis. Also visible is an ecstatic vessel on the superior surface of the left vocal fold (straight arrow). (Republished from Sataloff et al. [118]; with permission)

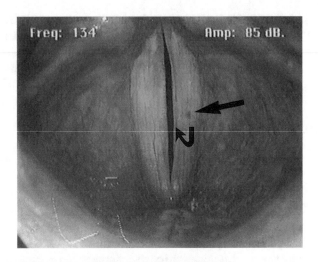

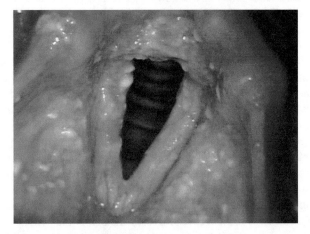

Fig. 4.2 Strobovideolaryngoscopy in this 65-year-old female shows the white, lacy, diffuse plaques embedded in inflamed mucosal surfaces. This appearance is typical of fungal laryngitis, caused most commonly by *Candida albicans*. (Republished from Sataloff et al. [118]; with permission)

voice) is associated with dehydration, dry atmosphere, mouth breathing, and anti-histamine therapy (although antihistamines actually cause more mucous thickening than dehydration). Deficiency of mucosal lubrication causes irritation and coughing and results in mild inflammation. If no pressing professional need for performance exists, inflammatory conditions of the larynx are treated best with relative voice rest in addition to other modalities. However, in some instances, speaking and singing may be permitted. The patient should be instructed to avoid all forms of irritation and to rest the voice at all times except during warm-up and performance. Corticosteroids and other medications discussed later may be helpful. If mucosal secretions are copious, low-dose antihistamine therapy may be beneficial, but it must be prescribed with caution and generally should be avoided. Copious, thin secretions are better than scant, thick secretions or excessive dryness. The patient with laryngitis must be kept well hydrated to maintain the desired character of mucosal lubrication. The patient should be instructed to "pee pale," consuming enough water to keep urine diluted. Psychologic support is crucial. For example, it is often helpful for the physician to intercede on a singer's behalf and to convey "doctor's orders" directly to agents or theater management. Such mitigation of exogenous stress can be highly therapeutic.

Infectious laryngitis may be caused by bacteria or viruses. Subglottic involvement frequently indicates a more severe infection, which may be difficult to control in a short period of time. Indiscriminate use of antibiotics must be avoided; however, when the physician is in doubt as to the cause and when a major voice commitment is imminent, vigorous antibiotic treatment is warranted. In this circumstance, the damage caused by allowing progression of a curable condition is greater than the damage that might result from a course of therapy for an unproven microorganism while culture results are pending. When a major concert or speech is not imminent, indications for therapy are the same as for the nonsinger or nonprofessional speaker.

Voice rest (absolute or relative) is an important therapeutic consideration in any case of laryngitis. When no professional commitments are pending, a short course of absolute voice rest may be considered, as it is the safest and most conservative therapeutic intervention. This means absolute silence and communication with a writing pad or electronic device. The patient must be instructed not to whisper, as this may be an even more traumatic vocal activity than speaking softly. However, exceptions can be made for patients who do not make vocal fold contact when they whisper, as determined during flexible laryngoscopy. Whistling through the lips also involves vocal fold contact in many people and should not be permitted unless laryngoscopy has confirmed that the instrumentalist does not make vocal fold contact while playing. The playing of many musical wind instruments also should not be permitted. Absolute voice rest is necessary only for serious vocal fold injury such as hemorrhage or mucosal disruption (Fig. 4.3). Even then, it is virtually never indicated for more than 7–10 days. Three days are often sufficient. Some excellent laryngologists do not believe voice rest should be used at all. However, absolute voice rest for a few days may be helpful in patients with laryngitis, especially those gregarious, verbal singers who find it difficult to moderate their voice use to comply with relative voice rest instructions. In many instances, considerations of finances and reputation mitigate against a recommendation of voice rest. In advising performers to minimize vocal use, Punt counseled, "Don't say a single word for which you are not being paid" [4].

This admonition frequently guides the ailing singer or speaker away from pre-performance conversations and backstage greetings and allows a successful series of performances. Patients also should be instructed to speak softly and as infrequently as possible, often at a slightly higher pitch than usual; to avoid excessive

Fig. 4.3 Mucosal tear (arrow) of the vibratory margin of the left vocal fold in a 27-year-old tenor with sudden voice change. This lesion resolved completely with voice rest. (Republished from Sataloff et al. [118]; with permission)

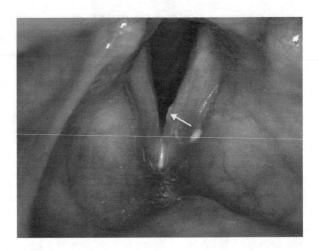

telephone use; and to speak with abdominal support as they would in singing. This is relative voice rest, and it is helpful in most cases. An urgent session with a speech-language pathologist is extremely helpful for discussing vocal hygiene and providing guidelines to prevent voice abuse. Nevertheless, the patient must be aware that some risk is associated with performing with laryngitis even when performance is possible. Inflammation of the vocal folds is associated with increased capillary fragility and increased risk of vocal fold injury or hemorrhage. Many factors must be considered in determining whether a given speech or concert is important enough to justify the potential consequences.

Steam inhalations deliver moisture and heat to the vocal folds and tracheobronchial tree and may be useful. Some people use nasal irrigations, although these have little proven value for voice disorders. Gargling has no proven efficacy, but it is probably harmful only if it involves loud, abusive vocalization as part of the gargling process. Some physicians and patients believe it to be helpful in "moistening the throat," and it may have some relaxing or placebo effect. Ultrasonic treatments, local massage, psychotherapy, and biofeedback directed at relieving anxiety and decreasing muscle tension may be helpful adjuncts to a broader therapeutic program. However, psychotherapy and biofeedback, in particular, must be expertly supervised if used at all.

Voice lessons given by an expert teacher are invaluable. When technical dysfunction is suggested, the singer or actor should be referred to his or her teacher or to a singing voice specialist in a medical setting. Even when an obvious organic abnormality is present, referral to a voice teacher is appropriate, especially for younger actors and singers. Numerous "tricks of the trade" permit a voice professional to overcome some of the impairments of mild illness safely. If a singer plans to proceed with a performance during an illness, he or she should not cancel voice lessons as part of the relative voice rest regimen; rather, a short lesson to ensure optimal technique is extremely useful.

4.2.4 Sinusitis

Chronic inflammation of the mucosa lining the sinus cavities commonly produces thick secretions known as postnasal drip. Postnasal drip can be particularly problematic because it causes excessive phlegm, which interferes with phonation, and because it leads to frequent throat clearing, which may inflame the vocal folds. Sometimes, chronic sinusitis is caused by allergies and can be treated with medications. However, many medications used for this condition cause side effects that are unacceptable in professional voice users, particularly mucosal drying. When medication management is not satisfactory, functional endoscopic sinus surgery may be appropriate [5]. Acute purulent sinusitis is a different matter. It requires aggressive treatment with antibiotics, sometimes surgical drainage, treatment of underlying conditions (such as dental abscess), and occasionally surgery [5].

4.2.5 Lower Respiratory Tract Infection

Lower respiratory tract infection may be almost as disruptive to a voice as upper respiratory tract infection. Bronchitis, pneumonitis, pneumonia, and especially reactive airway disease impair the power source of the voice and lead to vocal strain and sometimes injury. Lower respiratory tract infections should be treated aggressively, pulmonary function tests should be considered, and bronchodilators (preferably oral rather than inhaled) should be used as necessary. Coughing is also a very traumatic vocal activity, and careful attention should be paid to cough suppression. If extensive voice use is anticipated, nonnarcotic antitussive agents are preferable because narcotics may dull the sensorium and lead to potentially damaging voice or instrument performance technique.

4.2.6 COVID-19

COVID-19 or SARS-CoV-2 infection, also known as the novel coronavirus, may be asymptomatic, may cause mild URI symptoms, or may cause devastating symptoms including death. Cough, fever and chills, shortness of breath, sore throat, fatigue, nausea and vomiting, diarrhea, and other symptoms are common. Loss of taste and smell was recognized early as symptoms of COVID-19. However, COVID-19 also may cause many other neurologic effects including vocal fold paresis and paralysis. When the disease affects the lower respiratory tract severely, it can impair respiratory function permanently. This undermines the support needed to provide power for phonation (speaking, as well as singing) and wind instrument performance. Such problems lead commonly to compensatory hyperfunction. If the respiratory compromise is severe enough, it may disable a performer permanently, and since excellent respiratory function is required for singing, projected speech, and wind performance (as well as for high-level athletic activity), relatively "mild" pulmonary compromise can be severe enough to impair or end a performance career.

4.2.7   Tonsillitis

Tonsillitis also impairs the voice through alterations of the resonator system and through technical changes secondary to pain. Although there is a tendency to avoid tonsillectomy, especially in professional voice users, the operation should not be withheld when clear indications for tonsillectomy are present. These include documented severe bacterial tonsillitis six times per year. However, patients must be warned that tonsillectomy may alter the sound of the voice, even though there is no change at the vocal fold (oscillator) level.

4.2.8   Lyme Disease

Lyme disease, as it is known today, has been reported for over a 100 years, but the bacteria responsible for the disease was not identified until 1982. It was discovered in Lyme, Connecticut, when a group of children contracted arthritis inexplicably, and research was initiated to identify the cause [6]. Due to its ability to appear similar to many other diseases and its wide range of nonspecific symptoms, Lyme disease often goes undiagnosed. If not recognized and treated, this condition can have profound consequences including damage to the inner ear, the 8th cranial nerve, and the facial nerve as reviewed by Sataloff and Sataloff (from which a portion of this section has been modified, with permission) [7]. It also can affect laryngeal nerves. Lyme disease is one of many common illnesses that can cause special problems for singers and other voice professionals. Lyme disease is an increasingly prevalent infection in many parts of the United States and elsewhere. It can affect the larynx directly by causing unilateral or bilateral vocal fold paresis/paralysis or interfere with other parts of the vocal tract by causing joint pains that impair posture and support, temporomandibular joint pain that leads to technical changes, and in other ways [8]. It is important for healthcare providers and music professionals to be familiar with this common problem in order to improve the chances of prompt diagnosis and treatment.

4.2.8.1   Epidemiology

In the United States, Lyme disease is known to be endemic particularly in northeastern, mid-Atlantic, and North Central states, with expansion into some parts of the Southwest [9]. Approximately 60% of initial infections occur during the summer when it's warm and people are outside [10]. Lyme disease has no sex or age predilection.

4.2.8.2 Etiology

Lyme disease is an illness caused by a spirochete infection. Like syphilis, another spirochete infection, the clinical presentations may vary. Sir William Osler once termed syphilis "the great imitator," and likewise, Lyme disease has a broad clinical spectrum.

Lyme disease had many different names given to it until Steere, in 1977, recognized it as a multistage systemic disease [11]. In 1982, Burgdorfer et al. isolated the infectious organism from the belly of a tick while studying a group of children with unexplained arthritis in Lyme, Connecticut [12]. He named this spirochete *Borrelia burgdorferi*. *Borrelia burgdorferi* is the primary cause of Lyme disease. However, *Borrelia garinii* and *Borrelia afzelii* also have been implicated and reported as common causes of Lyme neuroborreliosis in Europe [13]. Many different vectors have been listed as contributors to this disease. However, the tick seems to be the main culprit transmitting the spirochete. In the Northeast, the tick *Ixodes dammini* is the most common, and in the West, *Ixodes pacificus* has been implicated [9]. The ticks carry the disease in their stomachs and transmit it while feeding on the blood of their victims which can take up to 2 days. In many cases, the ticks are noticed and removed or washed away before the disease can be spread, but sometimes, a tick is small enough to avoid notice. Even when definitive symptoms occur, the tick often is not found, and the classic target rash may have been absent or gone unnoticed. Therefore, the opportunity for early diagnosis often is missed, and many people carry Lyme disease into later stages of the disorder, during which nerve and vascular problems can occur, before the condition is diagnosed [7].

The tick life cycle has three stages: larva, nymph, and adult [11]. In each stage, the tick acquires a blood meal and may obtain the spirochete from an infected host such as the white-tailed deer or white-footed mouse.

The exact nature of injury to humans is not known, but evidence exists for three possible mechanisms. These theories include direct invasion, immunological attack, and vasculitis [14].

4.2.8.3 Otolaryngologic Findings

The clinical spectrum of Lyme disease is broken down into three stages. In stage 1, a rash named erythema chronicum migrans follows the tick bite in 6–80% of cases [15]. The rash has an outer red circular or oval border with a clear central area. These lesions are called "target rash." The outer red zone is felt to represent the best area for biopsy when trying to isolate the organism for culture. This rash may follow or precede cold or flu-like symptoms. The rash usually occurs within a few days of the tick bite but may show up as long as a month later [16].

Other symptoms during this stage include fatigue, fever, chills, sore throat, headache, cough, chest pain, abdominal pain, muscle aches, loss of appetite, dizziness, lymphadenopathy, backache, conjunctivitis, enlarged liver and spleen, arthritis, and low-grade fever.

The patient usually calls on an otolaryngologist during stage 2 of Lyme disease. Although facial paralysis is the most common complaint in these patients, other symptoms may occur [10, 17]. They include hoarseness from involvement of the recurrent laryngeal nerve or inability to sustain a high note or project the voice due to injury to the superior laryngeal nerve. In 1988, Schroeter reported a case of a 45-year-old singer who developed left vocal fold paralysis and had positive antibodies to *Borrelia burgdorferi* [18]. The patient was treated with antibiotics for 6 weeks, during which time there was resolution of the vocal fold paralysis and dramatic reduction of the Lyme titers.

Stage 2 also may include a skin lesion called lymphadenosis benigna cutis. This lesion has another name, *Borrelia* lymphocytoma, and is characterized by lymphocytic infiltration of the dermis or subcutaneous tissue [19]. The lesion has a blue-red color with gross swelling.

Patients may have involvement of the temporomandibular joint and complain of ear pain or pain when chewing. Other joints may be involved such as the neck, knees, hips, shoulders, ankles, and elbows. Finger, wrist, elbow, shoulder, and neck involvement can be troubling particularly for wind and other instrumentalists.

Patients also may have involvement of the cardiovascular system and may develop arrhythmias and/or lightheadedness. Failure to recognize these lesions may lead to increased morbidity and possible death.

Another skin lesion is seen in stage 3 of Lyme disease. It is termed acrodermatitis chronic atrophicans [19]. This lesion usually is seen in elderly patients and is often misdiagnosed as scleroderma or vascular insufficiency.

4.2.8.4   Diagnosis and Treatment

The ELISA test is the most sensitive and is used widely for Lyme disease [14]. Western blot technique is used to confirm the diagnosis. Other assays such as immunofluorescence antibody and cultures have been utilized with varying success. Results of all of these studies vary from lab to lab, and blood samples should be sent to labs that do large volumes of testing and have experience. The IgM antibody is seen early and is less specific. However, it is useful when reinfection or reactivation is suspected. The IgG antibody may take 6 weeks to appear and is good for assessing stages 2 and 3. False-positive tests occur in patients with mononucleosis, syphilis, or rheumatic fever [9, 14]. False negatives may be seen in patients on antibiotics or patients who are immunocompromised by diseases such as cancer or AIDS.

Antibiotics are the recommended treatment. For adults, doxycycline or tetracycline is effective. When intolerance to these medications is encountered, amoxicillin is used. Amoxicillin is preferred in children. Chloramphenicol may be used when there is allergy to cephalosporin or penicillin. When resistance to these medications is found, intravenous medication such as ceftriaxone is used. Lyme disease is complex; with proper recognition, it is treatable and has an excellent prognosis.

4.3 Systemic Conditions

4.3.1 Aging

This subject is so important that is has been covered extensively in other literature [20]. Many characteristics associated with vocal aging are actually deficits in conditioning, rather than irreversible aging changes. For example, in singers, such problems as a "wobble," pitch inaccuracies (singing flat), and inability to sing softly are rarely caused by irreversible aging changes, and these problems usually can be managed easily through voice therapy and training.

4.3.2 Hearing Loss

Hearing loss is often overlooked as a source of vocal problems. Auditory feedback is fundamental to speaking and singing. Interference with this control mechanism may result in altered vocal production, particularly if the person is unaware of the hearing loss. Distortion, particularly pitch distortion (diplacusis), also may pose serious problems for the singer. This appears to cause not only aesthetic difficulties in matching pitch but also vocal strain, which accompanies pitch shifts [21]. Hearing impairment can cause vocal strain, particularly if a person has sensorineural hearing loss (involving the nerve or inner ear) and is unaware of it. This condition may lead people to speak or sing more loudly than they realize.

4.3.3 Respiratory Dysfunction

The importance of "the breath" has been well recognized in the field of voice pedagogy. Respiratory disorders are discussed at length in other literature [22].

Even a mild degree of obstructive pulmonary disease can result in substantial voice problems. Unrecognized exercise-induced asthma is especially problematic in singers and actors, because bronchospasm may be precipitated by the exercise and airway drying that occurs during voice performance. In such cases, the bronchospastic obstruction on exhalation impairs support. This commonly results in compensatory hyperfunction.

Treatment requires skilled management and collaboration with a pulmonologist and a voice team [23]. Whenever possible, patients should be managed primarily with oral medications; the use of inhalers should be minimized. Steroid inhalers should be avoided altogether whenever possible for professional voice users. It is particularly important to recognize that asthma can be induced by the exercise of phonation itself [24], and in many cases, a high index of suspicion and methacholine challenge test are needed to avoid missing this important diagnosis.

4.3.4 Allergy

Even mild allergies are more incapacitating to professional voice users than to others. This subject can be reviewed elsewhere [25]. Briefly, patients with mild intermittent allergies can usually be managed with antihistamines, although they should never be tried for the first time immediately prior to a voice performance. Because antihistamines commonly produce unacceptable side effects, trial and error may be needed in order to find a medication with an acceptable balance between effect and side effect for any individual patient, especially a voice professional. Patients with allergy-related voice disturbances may find hyposensitization a more effective approach than antihistamine use if they are candidates for such treatment. For voice patients with unexpected allergic symptoms immediately prior to an important voice commitment, corticosteroids should be used rather than antihistamines, in order to minimize the risks of side effects (such as drying and thickening of secretions) that might make voice performance difficult or impossible. Allergies commonly cause voice problems by altering the mucosa and secretions and causing nasal obstruction.

4.3.5 Laryngopharyngeal Reflux

Laryngopharyngeal reflux (LPR) is extremely common among voice patients, especially singers [26]. This is a condition in which the sphincter between the stomach and esophagus is inefficient and acidic stomach secretions reflux (reach the laryngeal tissues), causing inflammation. The most typical symptoms are hoarseness in the morning, prolonged vocal warm-up time, postnasal drip, halitosis and a bitter taste in the morning, a feeling of a "lump in the throat," frequent throat clearing, chronic irritative cough, and frequent tracheitis or tracheobronchitis. Any or all of these symptoms may be present. Heartburn is not common in these patients, so the diagnosis is often missed. Prolonged reflux also is associated with the development of Barrett esophagus, esophageal carcinoma, and laryngeal carcinoma [26].

Physical examination usually reveals erythema (redness) of the arytenoid mucosa. A barium swallow radiographic study with water siphonage may provide additional information but is not needed routinely. However, if a patient complies strictly with treatment recommendations and does not show marked improvement within a month or if there is a reason to suspect more serious pathology, a more comprehensive evaluation should be carried out. Twenty-four hour pH impedance monitoring of the esophagus or pharyngeal pH monitoring is often effective in establishing a diagnosis. The results are correlated with a diary of the patient's activities and symptoms. Endoscopic examination of the esophagus should be considered for many patients. Bulimia should also be considered in the differential diagnosis when symptoms are refractory to treatment and other physical and psychologic signs are suggestive.

The mainstays of treatment for reflux laryngitis are elevation of the head of the bed (not just sleeping on pillows), antacids, proton-pump inhibitors and H2 blockers, low-acid diet, alkaline water, alginate, and avoidance of eating for 3–4 hours before going to sleep. This is often difficult for singers and actors because of their performance schedules, but if they are counseled about minor changes in eating habits (such as eating larger meals at breakfast and lunch), usually, they can comply. Avoidance of alcohol, caffeine, and specific foods is beneficial. Medications that decrease or block acid production may be necessary. It must be recognized that control of acidity is not the same as control of reflux. In many cases, reflux is provoked during singing because of the increased abdominal pressure associated with support. In these instances, it often causes excessive phlegm and throat clearing during the first 10 or 15 minutes of a performance or lesson, as well as other common laryngopharyngeal symptoms, even when acidity has been neutralized effectively. Laparoscopic Nissen fundoplication has proven extremely effective and should be considered a reasonable alternative to lifelong medication in this relatively young patient population [26].

4.3.6 Endocrine Dysfunction

Endocrine (hormonal) problems warrant special attention. The human voice is extremely sensitive to endocrinologic changes. Many of these are reflected in alterations of fluid content of the lamina propria just beneath the laryngeal mucosa. This causes alterations in the bulk and shape of the vocal folds and results in voice change. Hypothyroidism is a well-recognized cause of such voice disorders, although the mechanism is not understood fully [27–30]. Hoarseness, voice fatigue, muffling of the voice, loss of range, and a sensation of a lump in the throat may be present even with mild hypothyroidism. Even when thyroid function tests results are within the low normal range, this diagnosis should be considered, especially if thyroid-stimulating hormone levels are in the high-normal range or are elevated. Thyrotoxicosis may result in similar voice disturbances [30, 31].

Voice changes associated with sex hormones are encountered commonly in clinical practice and have been investigated more thoroughly than have other hormonal changes. Although a correlation appears to exist between sex hormone levels and depth of male voices (higher testosterone and lower estradiol levels in basses than in tenors) [32], the most important hormonal considerations in males occur during the maturation process.

When castrato singers were in vogue, castration at about age 7 or 8 years resulted in failure of laryngeal growth during puberty and voices that stayed in the soprano or alto range and boasted a unique quality of sound [33]. Failure of a male voice to change at puberty is uncommon today and is often psychogenic in etiology [1]. However, hormonal deficiencies such as those seen in cryptorchidism, delayed sexual development, Klinefelter syndrome, or Fröhlich syndrome may be responsible.

In these cases, the persistently high voice may be the complaint that causes the patient to seek medical attention.

Voice problems related to sex hormones are most common in female singers [34]. Although voice changes associated with the normal menstrual cycle may be difficult to quantify with current experimental techniques, unquestionably, they occur [2, 34–38]. Most of the ill effects seen in the immediate premenstrual period are known as laryngopathia premenstrualis. This common condition is caused by physiologic, anatomic, and psychologic alterations secondary to endocrine changes. The vocal dysfunction is characterized by decreased vocal efficiency, loss of the highest notes in the voice, voice fatigue, slight hoarseness, and some muffling of the voice. It is often more apparent to the singer than to the listener. It was recognized long ago that submucosal hemorrhages in the larynx are more common in the premenstrual period [36], and premenstrual vascular changes have been confirmed over the ensuing decades. In many European opera houses, singers used to be excused from singing during the premenstrual and early menstrual days ("grace days"). This practice was not followed in the United States and is no longer in vogue anywhere. Premenstrual changes cause significant vocal symptoms in approximately one-third of singers. Although ovulation inhibitors were shown long ago to mitigate some of these symptoms [37], in some women (about 5%), first-generation birth control pills used to deleteriously alter voice range and character even after only a few months of therapy [39–43]. However, modern oral contraceptives usually do not produce such problems and may even improve voice [42]. Under crucial performance circumstances, oral contraceptives may be used to alter the time of menstruation, but this practice is justified only in unusual situations. Symptoms similar to laryngopathia premenstrualis also occur in some women at the time of ovulation.

Pregnancy results frequently in voice alterations known as laryngopathia gravidarum. The changes may be similar to premenstrual symptoms or may be perceived as desirable changes. In some cases, alterations produced by pregnancy are permanent [44, 45]. Although hormonally induced changes in the larynx and respiratory mucosa secondary to menstruation and pregnancy are discussed widely in the literature, references to the important alterations in abdominal support are scarce. Abdominal distention during pregnancy also interferes with abdominal muscle function. Any singer whose abdominal support is compromised substantially should be discouraged from strenuous practice or performance until the abdominal impairment has resolved.

Estrogens are helpful in postmenopausal singers and should be administered under the supervision of a gynecologist or endocrinologist as potential systemic side effects have been described. Under no circumstances should androgens be given to female singers even in small amounts if any reasonable therapeutic alternative exists. Clinically, these drugs are used most commonly to treat endometriosis or postmenopausal loss of libido. Androgens cause unsteadiness of the voice, rapid changes of timbre, and lowering of the fundamental frequency (masculinization) [46–50]. These changes have been known for decades but still occur not only from illicit drug use for bodybuilding but also iatrogenically. These changes are usually permanent.

Recently, we have seen increasing abuse of anabolic steroids among bodybuilders and other athletes. In addition to their many other hazards, these medications may alter the voice. They are (or are closely related to) male hormones; consequently, they are capable of producing masculinization of the voice. Lowering of the fundamental frequency and coarsening of the voice produced in this fashion are similar to a boy's voice change at puberty and generally are irreversible.

Other hormonal disturbances may also produce voice dysfunction. In addition to the thyroid gland and the gonads, the parathyroid, adrenal, pineal, and pituitary glands are included in this system. Other endocrine disturbances may alter voice, as well. For example, pancreatic dysfunction may cause xerophonia (dry voice), as in diabetes mellitus. Thymic abnormalities can lead to feminization of the voice [51], and thymomas may cause laryngeal myasthenia gravis that produces voice instability and fatigue.

4.3.7 Neurologic Disorders

Numerous neurologic conditions may adversely affect the voice. They are discussed in other literature [2]. Some of them, such as myasthenia gravis, are amenable to medical therapy with drugs such as pyridostigmine (Mestinon). Such therapy frequently restores the voice to normal. An exhaustive neurolaryngologic discussion is beyond the scope of this chapter. Nevertheless, when evaluating voice dysfunction, healthcare providers must consider numerous neurologic problems, including Parkinson disease, essential tremor, various other disorders that produce tremor, drug-induced tremor, multiple sclerosis, dystonias, and many other conditions. Spasmodic dysphonia (SD), a laryngeal dystonia, presents particularly challenging problems. This subject is covered in detail elsewhere [2]. Focal dystonias that effect the mouth and lips can be troublesome for singers and other voice professionals, but they can be devastating for wind instrumentalists. The same is true for velopharyngeal insufficiency, a condition that is common among instrumentalists who play clarinet, oboe, saxophone, bassoon, French horn, trumpet, coronet, and other wind instruments. People who play these instruments often develop velopharyngeal insufficiency (VPI) which also is more likely to disable a wind player than a singer. In addition, wind instrumentalists (some of whom are also singers) develop a variety of other problems such as pneumoparotitis. Stuttering also provides unique challenges. Although still poorly understood, this condition is noted for its tendency to affect speech while sparing singing.

4.3.8 Vocal Fold Hypomobility

Vocal fold hypomobility may be caused by paralysis (no movement), paresis (partial movement), arytenoid dislocation, cricoarytenoid joint dysfunction, tumor, laryngeal fracture, and other causes. Differentiating among these conditions is often more complicated than it appears to be at first glance. A comprehensive discussion is beyond the scope of this chapter, and the reader is referred to other literature [2]. In addition to a comprehensive history and physical examination, evaluation commonly includes strobovideolaryngoscopy, objective voice assessment, laryngeal electromyography, and high-resolution computed tomography (CT) or magnetic resonance imaging (MRI) of the larynx and related neurologic structures. Most vocal fold motion disorders are amenable to treatment. Voice therapy should be used first in virtually all cases. Even in many patients with recurrent laryngeal nerve paralysis, voice therapy alone is often sufficient. When therapy fails to produce adequate voice improvement in the patient's opinion, surgical intervention is appropriate and usually is effective.

4.3.9 Autoimmune Deficiency Syndrome (AIDS)

AIDS is a potentially lethal disease that has become common. Its incidence in the artistic community is probably somewhat higher than in the general public. Physicians should consider this diagnosis along with other causes of chronic debilitation and recurrent infections in the proper clinical setting in professional voice users. Dry mouth and hoarseness are common complaints in patients with HIV infection. *Candida* infection of the oral cavity or tracheobronchial tree should make the clinician particularly suspicious. When fungal infections are encountered, particularly fungal laryngitis, it is important not only to treat the infection but also to rule out serious predisposing causes such as HIV infection and other conditions that suppress the immune system. Recurrent respiratory tract infection and infection with unusual organisms also raise one's suspicions, but it should be remembered that infections with *Haemophilus influenzae, Streptococcus pneumoniae*, and common viruses are the most frequent pathogens in HIV-infected patients, just as they are in patients without HIV. Acute infectious laryngitis and epiglottis may occur in AIDS patients, but they are less common than mild chronic laryngitis, dry mouth, and frequent or persistent symptoms of a "cold."

4.4 General Health

As with any other athletic activity, optimal voice use requires reasonably good general health and physical conditioning. Abdominal and respiratory strength and endurance are particularly important. If a person becomes short of breath from climbing two flights of stairs, he or she certainly does not have the physical stamina necessary for proper respiratory support for a speech, let alone a strenuous musical production. This deficiency usually results in abusive vocal habits used in vain attempts to compensate for the deficiencies.

Systemic illnesses, such as anemia, Lyme disease, mononucleosis, AIDS, chronic fatigue syndrome, or other diseases associated with malaise and weakness, may impair the ability of vocal musculature to recover rapidly from heavy use and may also be associated with alterations of mucosal secretions. Other systemic illnesses may be responsible for voice complaints, particularly if they impair the abdominal muscles necessary for breath support. For example, diarrhea and constipation that prohibit sustained abdominal contraction may be reasons for the physician to prohibit a strenuous singing or acting engagement. Healthcare providers should be familiar with laryngeal manifestations of systemic disease [52].

Any extremity injury, such as a sprained ankle, may alter posture and therefore interfere with customary abdominothoracic support. Voice patients are often unaware of this problem and develop abusive, hyperfunctional compensatory maneuvers in the neck and tongue musculature as a result. These technical flaws may produce voice complaints such as voice fatigue and neck pain that bring the performer to the physician's office for assessment and care. They even can produce structural lesions such as hemorrhage and nodules.

4.4.1   Obesity

Singers, actors, and many other professional voice users are verbal, oral people. Most enjoy singing, talking, and a good bowl of pasta after the show. However, before indulging our passions for culinary excess, it is important to understand the impact of obesity not only on singing performance but also on general health and longevity [53].

For medical reasons, when obesity becomes extreme, serious measures may be necessary to accomplish weight loss. The most severely overweight patients have an entity called "morbid obesity." This condition is diagnosed when a person is more than 100 pounds or 100% over ideal body weight. Morbid obesity is extremely common in our society. It is estimated that 34 million adult Americans (one in every five people over the age of 19) have significant obesity. As little as 20% excess over desirable body weight may be enough to constitute a health hazard. Doctors have long been aware of the difficulty in controlling weight problems with medical treatment alone. Of all patients who lose weight, 90% regain it at some point in their lives, and many even exceed their original weight. This led doctors to consider surgery as an option in treating this problem in selected cases.

In February 1985, a panel of experts from the National Institutes of Health looked at health problems associated with obesity [54]. Opinions have not changed substantially since that time. They concluded that obesity has adverse effects on health and longevity:

1. Obesity creates enormous psychologic stress, which is a problem not well understood by the general population. Large people are unpopular, discriminated against in the workplace, and considered lazy.
2. Obesity is associated with high blood pressure. Obese people have high blood pressure three times more often than nonobese people.
3. Obesity is associated with higher levels of cholesterol.

4. Obesity is associated with diabetes. As with high blood pressure, this is seen three times more commonly in obese individuals.
5. Obesity is a factor in the development of heart disease.
6. Obesity increases the risk of developing certain cancers, specifically those of the uterus, breast, cervix, and gallbladder in women and the colon, rectum, and prostate in men.
7. Obese individuals have a shorter life span.
8. Obesity is related to respiratory problems and arthritis.

With weight loss, all of these problems can be improved substantially, and prolongation of life is possible.

The best treatment for obesity is avoidance of the problem. Early in training, singers and other voice professionals, as well as all other performers, should learn the importance of good physical and aerobic conditioning. This is important to the voice professional's general health, vocal health, and art. Even a moderate degree of obesity may affect the respiratory system adversely, undermining support. Weight reduction is recommended for people who are 20% or more above ideal weight. In the singer, weight should be lost slowly through modification of eating and lifestyle habits. Loss of 2 or 3 pounds per week is plenty. More rapid loss of weight causes fluid shifts and hormonal alterations that may result in changes in vocal quality and endurance. Although these changes appear to be temporary, the effects of weight loss on vocal function have not been studied adequately; therefore, we do not have answers to all the pertinent questions. It is certainly possible for a singer to lose weight too quickly, but we are not yet sure how much weight loss is too much. Studies should be encouraged to learn more about this problem. However, it appears that maintenance of ideal body weight is probably as healthy for the voice as it is for the rest of the body. For people 20–100% above ideal body weight, weight loss can be accomplished with a medically supervised diet and exercise. However, people who are morbidly obese frequently are unable to lose weight by dietary or medical means alone. Morbidly obese patients may be candidates for surgery to help control their weight problems.

Although several kinds of obesity operations exist, the older procedures have troublesome side effects. At present, the best methods are a form of gastric restrictive surgery, known as the gastric bypass and gastric banding. Postoperatively, weight loss occurs over 12–18 months and stops as ideal body weight is approached. In most cases, singing may be resumed at about 6 weeks following abdominal surgery. Although the effects on the voice are not yet documented fully, there does not appear to be any significant problem associated with slow weight loss in patients with morbid obesity. Although further study is necessary to confirm these impressions, in singers or actors with this degree of weight problem, considerations of longevity, heart condition, blood pressure, and other critical health matters may outweigh immediate voice concerns.

For most singers, an extra 10, 20, or 30 pounds is not perceived as much of a problem. However, as 20 becomes 30 and 30 becomes 40, substantial adverse effects occur in the body in general and the vocal tract specifically. In training, singers and actors should be encouraged to treat their entire bodies with the same reverence with which they regard their vocal folds. Self-respect as a professional athlete is a sound basis for a long vocal career—and a long life.

4.4.2   Anxiety

Voice professionals, especially singers and actors, are frequently sensitive and communicative people. When the principal cause of vocal dysfunction is anxiety, the physician often can accomplish much by assuring the patient that no organic problem is present and by stating the diagnosis of anxiety reaction. The patient should be counseled that anxiety is normal and that recognition of it as the principle problem frequently allows the performer to overcome it. Tranquilizers and sedatives are rarely necessary and often are undesirable because they may interfere with fine motor control. For example, beta-adrenergic blocking agents such as propranolol hydrochloride have become popular among performers for the treatment of pre-performance anxiety. Beta-blockers are not recommended for regular use; they have significant effects on the cardiovascular system and many potential complications, including hypotension, thrombocytopenic purpura, mental depression, agranulocytosis, laryngospasm with respiratory distress, and bronchospasm. In addition, their efficacy is controversial. Although they may have a favorable effect in relieving performance anxiety, beta-blockers may produce a noticeable adverse effect on singing performance [55].

Although these drugs have a place under occasional, extraordinary circumstances, their routine use for this purpose not only is potentially hazardous but also violates an important therapeutic principle. Performers have chosen a career that exposes them to the public. If such persons are so incapacitated by anxiety that they are unable to perform the routine functions of their chosen profession without chemical help, this should be considered symptomatic of an important underlying psychologic problem. For a performer to depend on drugs to perform is neither routine nor healthy, whether the drug is a benzodiazepine, a barbiturate, a beta-blocker, or an alcohol. If such dependence exists, psychologic evaluation by an experienced arts-medicine psychologist or psychiatrist should be considered [56, 57]. Obscuring the symptoms by fostering the dependence is insufficient. However, if the patient is on tour and will only be under a particular otolaryngologist's care for a week or so, the physician should not try to make major changes in his or her customary regimen. Rather, the physician should communicate with the performer's primary otolaryngologist or family physician to coordinate appropriate long-term care.

As professional voice users constitute a subset of society as a whole, all the psychiatric disorders encountered among the general public are seen from time to time in voice professionals. In some cases, professional voice users require modification of the usual psychologic treatment, particularly with regard to psychotropic medications. Detailed discussion of this and related subjects can be found elsewhere [56, 57].

When voice professionals, especially singers and actors, have a significant vocal impairment that results in voice loss (or the prospect of voice loss), they often go through a psychologic process similar to grieving [56]. In some cases, fear of discovering that the voice is lost forever may unconsciously prevent patients from trying to use their voices optimally following injury or treatment. This can dramatically impede or prevent recovery of function following a perfect surgical result, for example. It is essential that otolaryngologists, performers, and their teachers are familiar with this fairly common scenario, and it is ideal to include an arts-medicine psychologist and/or psychiatrist as part of the voice team.

Psychogenic voice disorders, incapacitating psychologic reactions to organic voice disorders, and other psychologic problems are encountered commonly in young voice patients. They are discussed in other literature [56].

4.4.3　Substance Abuse

The list of substances ingested, smoked, or "snorted" by many people is disturbingly long. Whenever possible, patients who care about vocal quality and longevity should be educated about the deleterious effects of such habits upon their voice and upon the longevity of their careers by their physicians and teachers. A few specific substances have already been discussed.

4.4.4　Other Diseases that May Affect the Voice

The larynx is subject to numerous acute and chronic infections. Some of them may be mistaken for malignancy and may be biopsied unnecessarily, exposing the patient (and sometimes the physician) to unnecessary risk. Tuberculosis, for example, is still seen in modern practice. Although laryngeal lesions used to be associated with extensive pulmonary infection, they are now usually associated with much less virulent disease, often only a mild cough. Laryngeal tuberculosis lesions usually are localized [58, 59]. Sarcoidosis, another granulomatous disease, causes laryngeal symptoms in roughly 3–5% of cases [60]. Noncaseating granulomas are found in the larynx, and the false vocal folds are frequently involved, producing airway obstruction rather than dysphonia. Less common diseases including leprosy [61, 62], syphilis [63], scleroderma [64], typhoid [65], typhus, anthrax, and other conditions can produce laryngeal lesions that might lead the laryngologist to obtain a possibly unnecessary biopsy. Confusing lesions also may be caused by a variety of mycotic infections including histoplasmosis [66–68], coccidioidomycosis [69], cryptococcosis [70], blastomycosis [68–72], actinomycosis [73, 74], candidiasis [75], aspergillosis [76–78], mucormycosis [79], rhinosporidiosis [80], and sporotrichosis [81]. Parasitic diseases may also produce laryngeal masses. The most prominent example is leishmaniasis [82]. More detailed information about most of the conditions discussed above is available in a text by Michaels [83] and elsewhere in this book [2].

Collagen vascular diseases and other unusual problems may produce laryngeal masses. Rheumatoid arthritis may produce not only fixation of the cricoarytenoid and cricothyroid joints but also consequent neuropathic muscle atrophy [84] and rheumatoid nodules of the larynx [85]. Rheumatoid arthritis with or without nodules may produce respiratory obstruction. Gout may cause laryngeal arthritis. In addition, gouty tophi may appear as white submucosal masses of the true vocal fold. They consist of sodium urate crystals in fibrous tissue and have been documented well [86–88]. Amyloidosis of the larynx is rare but well recognized [89–91]. Urbach-Wiethe disease (lipoid proteinosis) [92] often involves the mucous membrane of the larynx, usually the vocal folds, aryepiglottic fold, and epiglottis. Other conditions, such as granulomatosis with polyangiitis (Wegener granulomatosis) and relapsing polychondritis, also may involve the larynx. They are less likely to produce discrete nodules, but the diffuse edema associated with chondritis and necrotizing granulomas may produce substantial laryngeal and voice abnormalities. Amyloidosis of the larynx is rare and usually involves the false vocal folds, but it can extend onto the true vocal folds. Unusual laryngeal masses also may be caused by trauma. Trauma is discussed in detail elsewhere [2], but the physician must be careful to inquire about laryngeal trauma, the consequences of which may not be recognized until months or years after the injury.

A few rare skin lesions also may involve the larynx producing symptomatic lesions and sometimes airway obstruction. These include pemphigus vulgaris, seen in adults between 40 and 60 years of age. Pemphigus lesions may involve the mucosa, including the epiglottis [93]. Epidermolysis bullosa describes a group of congenital vesicular disorders usually seen at birth or shortly thereafter. This condition may cause laryngeal stenosis or large, bleb-like vocal fold masses with detachment of the epithelium. Some viral conditions may cause laryngeal structural pathology, most notably papillomas. However, herpes, variola, and other organisms also have been implicated in laryngeal infection.

There are numerous other conditions, many of which are not covered comprehensively in this chapter, that may affect voices adversely. Most of them are not common problems among professional voice users. However, the laryngologist should remember that laryngeal manifestations of many systemic diseases may cause voice changes that bring the patient to medical attention for the first time [52, 53]. We must remain alert for their presence and think of them particularly when more common, obvious etiologies are not identified or when patients do not respond to treatment as expected. The voice may be affected by the following problems not discussed above (among others): acromegaly, Arnold-Chiari malformations, blood dyscrasias, neurologic disease (vocal fold paralysis), collagen vascular disease (including rheumatoid arthritis, systemic lupus erythematosus, scleroderma, and Sjögren's syndrome), deafness, gout, Hodgkin's disease, leprosy, lymphoma, Madelung's disease, malignancies, myopathies, a myriad of infectious diseases (bacterial, viral, granulomatous, and fungal), mononucleosis, numerous syndromes (Basedow's disease, adrenogenital syndrome, Down's syndrome, hereditary angioedema, Kleinfelter's syndrome, Melkersson-Rosenthal syndrome, pachyonychia congenita, short stature syndromes, Shy-Drager syndrome, and many others), syphilis, sarcoidosis, tuberculosis, Crohn's disease, Wilson's disease, and other chronic diseases.

Dentofacial anomalies also may impact voice substantially, as reviewed elsewhere [119].

4.5 Structural Abnormalities of the Larynx

4.5.1 Nodules

Nodules are callous-like masses of the vocal folds that are caused by vocally abusive behaviors and are a dreaded malady of singers and actors. Occasionally, laryngoscopy reveals asymptomatic vocal nodules that do not appear to interfere with voice production; in such cases, the nodules need not be treated. Some famous and successful singers have had untreated vocal nodules throughout their careers. However, in most cases, nodules result in hoarseness, breathiness, loss of range, and voice fatigue. They may be caused by abusive speaking rather than improper singing technique. Voice therapy always should be tried as the initial therapeutic modality and will cure the vast majority of patients even if the nodules look firm and have been present for many months or years. Even apparently large, fibrotic nodules often shrink, disappear, or become asymptomatic with 6–12 weeks of expert voice therapy with good patient compliance. Even in those who eventually need surgical excision of the nodules, preoperative voice therapy is essential to prevent recurrence. Care must be taken in diagnosing nodules.

It is almost impossible to make the diagnosis accurately and consistently without strobovideolaryngoscopy and good optical magnification. Vocal fold cysts are commonly misdiagnosed as nodules, and treatment strategies are different for the two lesions. Vocal nodules are confined to the superficial layer of the lamina propria and are composed primarily of edematous tissue or collagenous fibers. Basement membrane reduplication is common. They are usually bilateral and fairly symmetric.

Caution must be exercised in diagnosing small nodules in patients who have been singing or speaking actively. In many singers, for example, bilateral, symmetric soft swellings at the junction of the anterior and middle thirds of the vocal folds develop after heavy voice use. No evidence suggests that patients with such "physiologic swelling" are predisposed to develop vocal nodules. At present, the condition is generally considered to be within normal limits. The physiologic swelling usually disappears with 24–48 hours of rest from heavy voice use. The physician must be careful not to frighten the patient by misdiagnosing physiologic swellings as vocal nodules. Nodules carry a great stigma among voice professionals, and the psychologic impact of the diagnosis should not be underestimated. When nodules are present, these patients should be informed with the same gentle caution used in telling a patient that he or she has a life-threatening mass.

4.5.2   Submucosal Cysts

Submucosal cysts of the vocal folds are probably also traumatic lesions that are the result of a blocked mucous gland duct in many cases. However, they also may be congenital or occur from other causes. They often cause contact swelling on the contralateral side and can be misdiagnosed as nodules. They usually can be differentiated from nodules by strobovideolaryngoscopy when the mass is observed to be fluid filled. They also may be suspected when the nodule (contact swelling) on one vocal fold resolves with voice therapy while the mass on the other vocal fold does not resolve. Cysts may be discovered on one side (occasionally both sides) when surgery is performed for apparent nodules that have not resolved with voice therapy. The surgery should be performed superficially and with minimal trauma, as discussed in a separate chapter. Ordinarily, cysts are lined with thin squamous epithelium. Retention cysts contain mucus. Epidermoid cysts contain caseous material. Generally, cysts are located in the superficial layer of the lamina propria. In some cases, they may be attached to the vocal ligament.

4.5.3   Polyps

Vocal fold polyps, another type of vocal fold mass, usually occur on only one vocal fold. They often have a feeding blood vessel coursing along the superior surface of the vocal fold and joining (or originating from) the base of the polyp. The pathogenesis of polyps cannot be proven in many cases, but the lesion is thought to be traumatic and sometimes starts as a hemorrhage. Polyps may be sessile or pedunculated. Typically, they are located in the superficial layer of the lamina propria and do not involve the vocal ligament. In those arising from an area of hemorrhage, the vocal ligament may be involved with posthemorrhagic fibrosis that is contiguous with the polyp. Histologic evaluation most commonly reveals collagenous fibers, hyaline degeneration, edema, thrombosis, and often bleeding within the polypoid tissue. Cellular infiltration also may be present. In some cases, even sizable polyps resolve with relative voice rest and a few weeks of low-dose steroid therapy (e.g., methylprednisone 4 mg twice a day). However, most require surgical removal. If polyps are not treated, they may produce contact injury on the contralateral vocal fold. Voice therapy should be used to ensure good relative voice rest and prevent abusive voice behavior before and after surgery. When surgery is performed, care must be taken not to damage the leading edge of the vocal fold, especially if a laser is used. In all laryngeal surgery, delicate microscopic dissection is the standard of care. Vocal fold "stripping" is an out-of-date surgical approach formerly used for benign lesions, and it often resulted in scar and/or poor unserviceable voice function. It is no longer an acceptable surgical technique in most situations.

4.5.4 Granulomas

Granulomas usually occur in the cartilaginous portion of the vocal fold near the vocal process or on the medial surface of the arytenoid. They are composed of collagenous fibers, fibroblasts, proliferated capillaries, and leukocytes. They are usually covered with epithelium. Granulomas are associated with gastroesophageal reflux laryngitis and trauma (including trauma from voice abuse and from intubation). The term is a misnomer, since these lesions are inflammatory, not true granulomas as would be seen in tuberculosis or sarcoidosis. Therapy should include reflux control, voice therapy, and surgery if the granuloma continues to enlarge or does not resolve after adequate time and treatment. Granular cell tumors also can occur in the larynx [94].

4.5.5 Reinke's Edema

Severe Reinke's edema is characterized by an "elephant ear," floppy vocal fold appearance. It is often observed during examination in many nonprofessional and professional voice users and is accompanied by a low, coarse, gruff voice. Reinke's edema is a condition in which the superficial layer of lamina propria (Reinke's space) becomes edematous. The lesion does not usually include hypertrophy, inflammation, or degeneration, although other terms for the condition include polypoid degeneration, chronic polypoid corditis, and chronic edematous hypertrophy. Reinke's edema is often associated with smoking, voice abuse, reflux, and hypothyroidism. Underlying conditions should be treated. However, the condition may require surgery if voice improvement is desired. The surgery should be performed only if there is a justified high suspicion of serious pathology such as cancer, if there is airway obstruction, or if the patient is unhappy with his or her vocal quality. For some voice professionals, abnormal Reinke's edema is an important component of the vocal signature. Although the condition is usually bilateral, surgery should generally be performed on one side at a time. Many patients have mild Reinke's edema on one or both vocal folds that does not require treatment.

4.5.6 Sulcus Vocalis

Sulcus vocalis is a groove along the edge of the membranous vocal fold. The majority are congenital, bilateral, and symmetric, although posttraumatic acquired lesions occur. When symptomatic (they often are not), sulcus vocalis can be treated surgically if sufficient voice improvement is not obtained through voice therapy.

4.5.7 Scar

Vocal fold scar is a sequela of trauma and results in fibrosis and obliteration of the layered structure of the vocal fold. It may impede vibration and consequently cause dysphonia. Recent surgical advances have made this condition much more treatable than it used to be [95, 96], but it is still rarely possible to restore voices to normal in the presence of scar.

4.5.8 Hemorrhage

Vocal fold hemorrhage is a potential disaster in singers. Hemorrhages resolve spontaneously in most cases, with restoration of normal voice. However, in some instances, the hematoma organizes and fibroses, resulting in scar [97]. This alters the vibratory pattern of the vocal fold and can result in permanent hoarseness. In selected cases, it may be best to avoid this problem through surgical incision and drainage of the hematoma. In all cases, vocal fold hemorrhage usually is managed with absolute voice rest until the hemorrhage has largely resolved (usually about 1 week) and relative voice rest until normal vascular and mucosal integrity have been restored. This often takes 6 weeks and sometimes longer. Recurrent vocal fold hemorrhages usually are caused by weakness in a specific blood vessel, which may require surgical cauterization of the blood vessel using a laser or microscopic resection of the vessel [98].

4.5.9 Papilloma

Laryngeal papillomas are epithelial lesions caused by human papilloma virus. Histology reveals neoplastic epithelial cell proliferation in a papillary pattern and viral particles. At the present time, symptomatic papillomas are treated surgically, although alternatives have been recommended to the usual laser vaporization approach [99, 100]. Cidofovir injected into the lesion has shown considerable promise [99, 101].

4.5.10 Cancer

A detailed discussion of cancer of the larynx is beyond the scope of this chapter [120]. The prognosis for small vocal fold cancers is good, whether they are treated by radiation or surgery. Although it may seem intuitively obvious that radiation therapy provides a better chance of voice conservation than even limited vocal fold surgery, late radiation changes in the vocal fold may produce substantial hoarseness, xerophonia (dry voice), and voice dysfunction. Consequently, from the standpoint of voice preservation, optimal treatments remain uncertain. Prospective studies using objective voice measures and strobovideolaryngoscopy should answer the relevant questions in the future. Strobovideolaryngoscopy is also valuable for follow-up of patients who have had laryngeal cancers. It permits detection of vibratory changes associated with infiltration by the cancer long before they can be seen with continuous light. Stroboscopy has been used in Europe and Japan for this purpose for many years. In the United States, the popularity of strobovideolaryngoscopy for follow-up of patients with cancer has increased greatly since the mid-to-late 1980s.

The psychologic consequences of vocal fold cancer can be devastating, especially in a professional voice user. They may be overwhelming for nonvoice professionals, as well. These reactions are understandable and expected. In many patients, however, psychologic reactions may be as severe following medically "less significant" vocal fold problems such as hemorrhages, nodules, and other conditions that do not command the public respect and sympathy afforded to a cancer. In many ways, the management of related psychologic problems can be even more difficult in patients with these "lesser" vocal disturbances.

4.5.11   Laryngoceles and Pharyngoceles

The ventricle of Morgagni is located between the true and false vocal folds. The appendix of the ventricle of Morgagni is a blind pouch called the saccule in the anterior superior portion. Laryngoceles are abnormal dilations or herniations of the laryngeal saccule [101–105]. They communicate with the laryngeal lumen and generally are filled with air. They become apparent clinically when they are distended after air is forced into them or when they are filled with fluid. They are connected to the ventricle by a narrow stalk and form a sac lined with pseudostratified, ciliated columnar epithelium. The appendix of the ventricle is considered abnormal if it extends above the upper border of the thyroid cartilage.

Laryngoceles limited to the interior of the larynx are called internal; those that protrude outside the thyroid cartilage into the neck are called external. They also may be mixed (internal and external). Laryngoceles should be distinguished from pharyngoceles, which are not true pouches and which generally diminish in size in the absence of pharyngeal pressure (e.g., when not whistling or playing a wind instrument) [102]. Pharyngoceles are air-filled expansions of the pharynx that can be large enough to require musicians to wear shirts with extra large collar sizes or to play with the collar unbuttoned. Laryngoceles and pharyngoceles are most common in brass instrumentalists. In laryngoceles, outpouchings of the laryngeal ventricle can extend through the openings in the thyrohyoid membrane for the superior laryngeal vessels and nerve and balloon outward and upward toward the submandibular triangle [103]. External and mixed laryngoceles are real variants of the internal laryngocele. Because laryngoceles arise from the region of the saccule within the larynx, if the lesion is a laryngocele, there must be an intralaryngeal component manifested at least as a tract connecting the lateral component with the ventricle, with or without internal dilation. Hence, pure external laryngoceles do not exist. Lesions without an intralaryngeal component should be classified differently (e.g., as pharyngoceles).

There are several proposed mechanisms for laryngocele formation. In neonates, they are presumed to be remnants of the lateral air sacs seen in other primates. In adults, they can represent a congenital enlargement of the saccule or an acquired lesion associated with increased intraluminal pressure. The association of laryngoceles with occupations that involve long periods of forced expiration supports this notion, and they also are associated with laryngeal carcinomas [104].

Brass and woodwind players are at risk for a variety of head and neck abnormalities as a result of increased intraluminal pressure during musical performances. Transient ischemic attacks, temporomandibular joint dysfunction, and dental malocclusion have been reported. Injury to the orbicularis oris in brass players can require surgical repair [106]. Stress velopharyngeal incompetence has been documented in trumpeters, bassoonists, and others as noted above. Young trumpet players are at greatest risk for injury to oral and cervical tissues when they generate peak respiratory pressure averaging 151 torr [107].

Although laryngoceles usually are associated with brass instruments, several authors have examined laryngocele formation in woodwind players. Stephanie and Tarab obtained plain x-rays on 25 wind instrument players and found laryngoceles in all of them [108]. Macfie found laryngoceles in 53 of 94 (56%) woodwind bandsman [109]. Subclinical laryngoceles are common among horn players, and they rarely require surgical intervention.

Surgery for laryngoceles in young musicians poses several problems. The literature offers no definitive guidance regarding the timing of surgery, the healing period before playing can be resumed, and the risk of recurrence with continued performance. Furthermore, the cervical approach used commonly for the treatment of external laryngoceles can disrupt the normal function of the strap muscles, which is important for tone generation for instrumentalists and for singers [110]. The risks of infection and progression of the defect must be balanced against a young performer's desire for musical growth.

Since Ward's early reports on this subject [103], our understanding of laryngoceles and pharyngoceles has changed slightly. Both laryngoceles and pharyngoceles can change size and appearance with variations in internal pressure. Although the classical definitions of laryngocele remain valid, combinations of both can occur. Air-filled masses that arise in the pharynx (commonly in the region of the pyriform sinuses) and lack a laryngeal component or origin should be called pharyngoceles. Those that arise in the laryngeal ventricle should be called laryngoceles. Considering the origins of pharyngeal pouches as reviewed in Ward's 1963 paper [103] as well as the forces involved, it appears likely that most lesions with a laryngeal component originated in the larynx and extended in the neck rather than vice versa, but it is not always possible to prove the origin. It is also important to recognize that the therapeutic implications of the distinctions are not as clear-cut as they once were and that lesions that combine the features of laryngoceles and pharyngoceles occur [111]. The distinctions between laryngoceles and pharyngoceles were quite important when we still believed laryngoceles usually required surgery and pharyngoceles required surgery only rarely. However, as arts-medicine has evolved, experience has shown that, in most cases, neither lesion requires surgery. Contrary to our earlier understandings, the vast majority of laryngoceles are asymptomatic.

4.5.12   Other Conditions

For a more comprehensive discussion of the conditions covered above and numerous others, the reader is referred to other literature [2].

4.6   Medical Management for Voice Dysfunction

Medical management of many problems affecting the voice involves not only care prescribed by an otolaryngologist but also voice therapy, which is provided by an interdisciplinary team. The roles and training of the principal members of the team are covered in detail elsewhere [2]. This chapter provides a brief introduction to their roles in the medical milieu.

4.6.1   Speech-Language Pathologist

An excellent speech-language pathologist is an invaluable asset in caring for professional voice users and other voice patients. However, otolaryngologists and singing teachers should recognize that, like physicians, speech-language pathologists have varied backgrounds and experience in treatment of voice disorders. In fact, most speech-language pathology programs teach relatively little about caring for professional speakers and nothing about professional singers. Moreover, few speech-language pathologists have vast experience in this specialized area, and no fellowships in this specialty exist. Speech-language pathologists often subspecialize. A speech-language pathologist who expertly treats patients who have had strokes, stutter, have undergone laryngectomy, or have swallowing disorders will not necessarily know how to manage professional voice users optimally or even other less demanding voice patients. The otolaryngologist must learn the strengths and weaknesses of the speech-language pathologist with whom he or she works. After identifying a speech-language pathologist who is interested in treating professional voice users, the otolaryngologist should work closely with the speech-language pathologist to develop the necessary expertise. Assistance may be found through otolaryngologists who treat large numbers of singers or through educational programs such as the Voice Foundation's Symposium on Care of the Professional Voice. In general, therapy should be directed toward vocal hygiene, relaxation techniques, voice function exercised breath management, and abdominal support.

Speech (voice) therapy may be helpful even when a singer has no obvious problem in the speaking voice but has significant technical problems singing. Once a person has been singing for several years, a singing teacher may have difficulty convincing him or her to correct certain technical errors. However, singers are much less protective of their speaking voices. A speech-language pathologist may be able to teach proper support, relaxation, and voice placement in speaking. Once mastered, these techniques can be carried over fairly easily into singing through cooperation between the speech-language pathologist and singing teacher or singing voice specialist. This "back door" approach has been extremely useful. For the actor, coordinating speech-language pathology sessions with acting voice lessons, and especially with training of the speaking voice provided by the actor's voice teacher or coach, is often helpful. We have found this combination so helpful that we have added an acting voice trainer to our medical staff. Information from the speech-language pathologist, acting voice trainer, and singing teacher or singing voice specialist should be symbiotic and should not conflict. If major discrepancies exist, bad training from one of the team members should be suspected, and changes should be made.

4.6.2   Singing Voice Specialist

Singing voice specialists are singing teachers who have acquired extra training to prepare them for work with injured voices, in collaboration with a medical voice team. They are indispensable for singers and very valuable for nonsingers with voice disorders.

In selected cases, singing lessons may be extremely helpful to nonsingers with voice problems. The techniques used to develop abdominal and thoracic muscle strength, breath control, laryngeal and neck muscle strength, and relaxation are similar to those used in voice therapy. Singing lessons often expedite therapy and appear to improve the outcome in some patients.

Otolaryngologists who care for singers frequently are often asked to recommend a voice teacher. This may put them in an uncomfortable position, particularly if the singer is already studying with someone in the community. Most physicians do not have sufficient expertise to criticize a voice teacher, and we must be extremely cautious about recommending that a singer changes teachers. However, no certifying agency standardizes or ensures the quality of a singing teacher. Although one may be slightly more confident of a teacher associated with a major conservatory or music school or one who is a member of the National Association of Teachers of Singing (NATS), neither of these credentials ensures excellence, and many expert teachers have neither affiliation. However, with experience, an otolaryngologist can develop valid impressions. The physician should record the name of the voice teacher of every patient and observe whether the same kinds of voice abuse occur with disproportionate frequency in the pupils of any given teacher. Technical problems can cause organic abnormalities such as nodules; therefore, any teacher who has a high incidence of nodules among his or her students should be viewed with cautious concern, but the physician also needs to determine whether the teacher attracts a student cohort that has a high incidence of nodules before the students have started lessons, as may be seen among some populations of rock and popular music singers who have performed extensively without voice training. The physician should be particularly wary of teachers who are reluctant to allow their students to consult a doctor. The best voice teachers usually are quick to refer their students to an otolaryngologist if they hear anything disturbing in a student's voice. Similarly, voice teachers and voice professionals should compare information on the nature and quality of medical care received and its success. No physician cures every voice problem in every patient, just as no singing teacher produces premiere stars from every student who walks into the studio. Nevertheless, voice professionals must be critical, informed consumers and accept nothing less than the best medical care and voice training.

After seeing a voice patient, the otolaryngologist should speak with and/or write a letter to the voice teacher (with the patient's permission) describing the findings and recommendations as he or she would to a physician, speech-language pathologist, or any other referring professional. An otolaryngologist seriously interested in caring for singers should take the trouble to talk with and meet local singing teachers. Taking a lesson or two with each teacher provides enormous insight, as well. Taking voice lessons regularly is even more helpful. In practice, the otolaryngologist will usually identify a few teachers in whom he or she has particular confidence, especially for patients with voice disorders, and should not hesitate to refer singers to these colleagues, especially singers who are not already in training.

Pop singers may be particularly resistant to the suggestion of voice lessons, yet they are in great need of training. The physician should assure patients that a good voice teacher can teach a pop singer how to protect and expand the voice without changing its quality or making it sound "trained" or "operatic." It is helpful to point out that singing, like other athletic activities, requires exercise, warm-up, and coaching for anyone planning to enter the "big league" and stay there. Just as no major league baseball pitcher would play without a pitching coach and warm-up time in the bullpen, no singer should try to build a career without a singing teacher and appropriate strength and agility exercises. This approach has proved palatable and effective. Physicians also should be aware of the difference between a voice teacher and a voice coach.

A voice teacher trains a singer in singing technique and is essential. A voice coach is responsible for teaching songs, interpretation, language, diction, style, operatic roles, and so on, but is not responsible for exercise and basic technical development of the voice.

4.6.3 Acting Voice Trainer

The use of acting voice trainers (drama voice coaches) as members of the medical team is relatively new [2]. This addition to the team has been extremely valuable to patients and other team members. Like singing voice specialists, professionals with education in theater arts use numerous vocal and body movement techniques that not only enhance physical function but also release tension and break down emotional barriers that may impede voice function. Tearful revelations to the acting voice trainer are not uncommon, and like the singing teacher, this individual may identify psychologic and emotional problems that interfere with professional success and have been skillfully hidden from other professionals on the voice team and in the patient's life.

4.6.4 Others

A psychologist, psychiatrist, neurologist, pulmonologist, endocrinologist, gastroenterologist, and others with special interest and expertise in arts-medicine are also invaluable to the voice team. Every comprehensive center should seek out such people and collaborate with them, even if they are not full-time members of the voice team.

4.7 Surgery

A detailed discussion of laryngeal surgery is beyond the scope of this chapter and may be found elsewhere [2, 112]. However, a few points are worthy of special emphasis. Surgery for vocal nodules should be avoided whenever possible and should almost never be performed without an adequate trial of expert voice therapy, including patient compliance with therapeutic suggestions. A minimum of 6–12 weeks of observation should be allowed while the patient is using therapeutically modified voice techniques under the supervision of a speech-language pathologist and ideally a singing voice specialist. Proper voice use rather than voice rest (silence) is correct therapy. The surgeon should not perform surgery prematurely for vocal nodules under pressure from the patient for a "quick cure" and early return to performance. Permanent destruction of voice quality is a very real potential complication.

Even after expert surgery, voice quality may be diminished by submucosal scarring, resulting in an adynamic segment along the vibratory margin of the vocal fold. This situation produces a hoarse voice with vocal folds that appear normal on indirect examination under routine light, although under stroboscopic light the adynamic segment is obvious. No reliable cure exists for this complication. Even large, apparently fibrotic nodules of long standing should be given a chance to resolve without surgery. In some cases, the nodules remain but become asymptomatic, and voice quality is normal. Stroboscopy in such patients usually reveals that the nodules are on the superior surface rather than the leading edge of the vocal folds during proper, relaxed phonation (although they may be on the contact surface and symptomatic when hyperfunctional voice technique is used and the larynx is forced down).

When surgery is indicated for vocal fold lesions, it should be limited as strictly as possible to the area of abnormality. Virtually, no place exists for "vocal fold stripping" in patients with benign disease. Submucosal resection through a laryngeal microflap used to be advocated. The technique was introduced and first published by the author (RTS). Microflap technique involved an incision on the superior surface of the vocal fold, submucosal resection, and preservation of the mucosa along the leading edge of the vocal fold. The concept that led to this innovation was based on the idea that the intermediate layer of the lamina propria should be protected to prevent fibroblast proliferation. Consequently, it seemed reasonable to preserve the mucosa as a biologic dressing. This technique certainly produced better results than vocal fold stripping. However, close scrutiny of outcomes revealed a small number of cases with poor results and stiffness beyond the limits of the original pathology. Consequently, the technique was abandoned in favor of a new technique called minimicroflap or a method of local resection strictly limited to the region of pathology [113]. Lesions such as vocal nodules should be removed to a level even with the vibratory margin rather than deeply into the submucosa. This minimizes scarring and optimizes chances for return to good vocal function. Naturally, if concern about a serious neoplasm exists, proper treatment takes precedence over voice preservation. Surgery should be performed under microscopic control. Preoperative and postoperative objective voice measures are essential to allow outcome assessment and self-critique. Only through such study can we improve surgical technique. Outcome studies are especially important in voice surgery as all our technical pronouncements are anecdotal because there is no experimental model for vocal fold surgery. The human adult is the only species with our complex, layered lamina propria.

Lasers are an invaluable adjunct in the laryngologists' armamentarium, but they must be used knowledgeably and with care. Considerable early evidence suggested that healing time was prolonged and the incidence of adynamic segment formation was higher with the laser on the vibratory margin than with traditional instruments. Two early studies raised serious concerns about dysphonia after laser surgery [114, 115]. Such complications may result from using too low a wattage causing dissipation of heat deeply into the vocal fold; thus, high power density for short duration has been recommended. Small spot size is also helpful. More recent experience has shown that expert laser surgery on the vibratory margin can produce excellent results. Nevertheless, many laryngologists caring for voice professionals avoid laser surgery to eliminate the risk of thermal injury to the vocal ligament. If a laser is used when biopsy specimens are needed, they should be taken before vaporizing the lesion with a laser. If a lesion is to be removed from the leading edge, the laser beam should be centered in the lesion, rather than on the vibratory margin, so that the beam does not create a divot in the vocal fold. The CO_2 laser used to be used for cauterizing isolated blood vessels responsible for recurrent hemorrhage or other problems, and it still is used occasionally. At the suggestion of Jean Abitbol, MD, the author (RTS) has placed a small piece of ice on the vocal fold immediately before CO_2 laser use to help dissipate the heat and help prevent edema (1983, "personal communication"). No studies on the efficacy of this maneuver exist, but the technique appears helpful.

Such vessels are often found at the base of a hemorrhagic polyp. Vascular lasers are better than CO_2 lasers for management of these lesions and other vascular abnormalities. They include the 532 nm KTP (Nd-YAG) laser and the 445 nm blue laser.

Voice rest after vocal fold surgery is controversial. Although some laryngologists do not recognize its necessity at all, many physicians recommend voice rest for approximately 1 week or until the mucosal surface has healed. Even after surgery, silence for more than 7–10 days is nearly never necessary and represents a real hardship for many patients.

Too often, the laryngologist is confronted with a desperate patient whose voice has been "ruined" by vocal fold surgery, recurrent or superior laryngeal nerve paralysis, trauma, or some other tragedy. Occasionally, the cause is as straightforward as a dislocated arytenoid that can be reduced [116, 117]. However, if the problem is an avulsed vocal process, an adynamic segment, decreased bulk of one vocal fold after "stripping," bowing caused by superior laryngeal nerve paralysis, or some other complication in a mobile vocal fold, great conservatism should be exercised. None of the available surgical procedures for these conditions are effective consistently. If surgery is considered, the procedure and prognosis should be explained to the patient realistically and pessimistically. The patient must understand that the chances of returning the voice to professional quality are very slim and that it might be made worse. Nevertheless, procedures for vocal fold scar have improved, and surgery is often possible (including vocal fold injection and other procedures) to at least decrease the severity of dysphonia and to lessen vocal effort.

Occasionally, voice professionals inquire about surgery for pitch alteration. Such procedures have been successful in specially selected patients (such as those undergoing gender modification surgery), but they do not consistently provide good enough voice quality and range to be performed on a professional voice user in most situations.

4.8 Discretion

The excitement and glamour associated with caring for voice patients, particularly a famous performer, naturally tempt the physician to talk about a distinguished patient. However, this tendency must be tempered. Having it known that he or she has consulted a laryngologist, particularly for treatment of a significant vocal problem, is not always in a voice professional's best interest. Famous singers, actors, politicians, and other professional voice users are entitled ethically and legally to the same confidentiality we ensure for our other patients.

4.9 Voice Maintenance

Prevention of voice dysfunction should be the goal of all professionals involved in the care of professional voice users. Good vocal health habits should be encouraged in childhood. Screaming, particularly outdoors at athletic events, should be discouraged. Promising young singers who join choirs should be educated to compensate for the Lombard effect. The youngster interested in singing, acting, debating, or other vocal activities should receive enough training to prevent voice abuse and should receive enthusiastic support for performing works and activities suitable for his or her age and voice. Training should be continued during or after puberty, and the voice should be allowed to develop naturally without pressure to perform operative roles prematurely. Young instrumentalists should be managed with similar care, as discussed in Chap. 4.

Excellent regular training and practice are essential, and avoidance of irritants, particularly smoke, should be stressed early. Educating voice professionals and wind instrumentalists about hormonal and anatomic alterations that may influence the voice allows them to recognize and analyze voice dysfunction, compensating for it intelligently when it occurs. The body is dynamic, changing over a lifetime, and the voice is no exception. Continued voice education, training, and monitoring are necessary throughout a lifetime, even in the most successful and well-established voice professionals and instrumental musicians. Voice problems even in premiere singers commonly are caused by cessation of lessons, excessive schedule demands, and other correctable problems, rather than by irreversible alterations of aging. Anatomic, physiologic, and serious medical problems may affect the voices of patients of any age. Cooperation among the laryngologist, speech-language pathologist, acting teacher, voice specialist, and music teacher and singing teacher provides an optimal environment for cultivation and protection of the vocal artist and for voice presentation in wind instrumentalists.

Acknowledgments Modified in part from Sataloff RT. *Professional Voice: The Science and Art of Clinical Care, 4th ed.* San Diego, CA: Plural Publishing, Inc. 2017; with permission.

References

1. Brodnitz F. Hormones and the human voice. Bull N Y Acad Med. 1971;47:183–91.
2. Sataloff RT. Professional voice: the science and art of clinical care. 4th ed. San Diego: Plural Publishing; 2017. p. 1–2099.
3. von Leden H. Presentation at: seventh symposium on care of the professional voice. New York: The Juilliard School; 1978.

4. Punt NA. Applied laryngology—singers and actors. Proc R Soc Med. 1968;61:1152–6.
5. Anderson TD, Sataloff RT. Rhinosinusitis. In: Sataloff RT. Professional voice: the science and art of clinical care. 4th ed. San Diego: Plural Publishing; 2017. p. 747–50.
6. Nachman SA, Pontrelli L. Central nervous system Lyme disease. Semin Pediatr Infect Dis. 2003;14(2):123–30.
7. Sataloff JB, Sataloff RT. Otologic manifestations of Lyme disease. In: Kountakis SE, editor. Encyclopedia of otolaryngology, head and neck surgery. New Delhi: Springer; 2013. p. 2015–20.
8. Goldfarb D, Sataloff RT. Lyme disease: a review for the otolaryngologist. Ear Nose Throat J. 1994;73(11):824–9.
9. Kugeler KJ, Farley GM, Forrester JD, Mead P. Geographic distribution and expansion of human Lyme disease, United States. Emerg Infect Dis. 2015;21(8):1455–7.
10. Clark JR, Carlson RD, Sasaki CT, Pachner AR, Steere AC. Facial paralysis in Lyme disease. NATS J. 1995;95:1341–5.
11. Steere AC, Grodzick MS, Kornblatt AN, et al. The spirochetal etiology of Lyme disease. N Engl J Med. 1983;308:733–40.
12. Burgdorfer WA, Barbour AG, Hayes SF, Benach JL, Grunwaldt E, David JP. Lyme disease-tick-borne spirochetosis. Science. 1982;216:1317–9.
13. Strle F, Ruzic-Sablijic E, Cimperman J, Lotric-Furlan S, Maraspin V. Comparison of findings for patients with Borrelia garinii and Borrelia afzelii isolated from cerebrospinal fluid. Clin Infect Dis. 2006;43(6):704–10.
14. Magnarelli LA. Serologic diagnostics of Lyme disease. Ann N Y Acad Sci. 1988;539:154–61.
15. Sehgal VN, Khurana A. Lyme disease/borreliosis as a systemic disease. Clin Dermatol. 2015;33:542–50.
16. Barbour AG. Diagnosis of Lyme disease: rewards and perils. Ann Intern Med. 1989;11(7):501–2.
17. Glassock ME, Pensak ML, Gulia AJ, Baker DC. Lyme disease: a cause of bilateral facial paralysis. Arch Otolaryngol. 1985;111:47–9.
18. Schroeter V. Paralysis of recurrent laryngeal nerve in Lyme disease. Lancet. 1988;2(8622):1245.
19. Steere AC, Malaawista SE, Hardin JA, Ruddy S, Askenase PW, Andiman WA. Erythema chronicum migrans and Lyme arthritis: the enlarging clinical spectrum. Ann Intern Med. 1988;86:685–98.
20. Sataloff RT, Johns MM, Kost KM. Geriatric otolaryngology. New York: Thieme; 2015.
21. Sundberg J, Prame E, Iwarsson J. Replicability and accuracy of pitch patterns in professional singers. In: David PJ, Fletcher NH, editors. Vocal fold physiology: controlling chaos and complexity. Sydney: Singular Publishing; 1996. p. 291–306.
22. Sataloff RT, Cohn JR, Hawkshaw M. Respiratory dysfunction. In: Sataloff RT. Professional voice: the science and art of clinical care. 4th ed. San Diego: Plural Publishing; 2017. p. 751–64.
23. Spiegel JR, Sataloff RT, Cohn JR, et al. Respiratory function in singers. Medical assessment, diagnoses and treatments. J Voice. 1988;2(1):40–50.
24. Cohn JR, Sataloff RT, Spiegel JR, et al. Airway reactivity-induced asthma in singers (ARIAS). J Voice. 1991;5(4):332–7.
25. Cohn JR, Padams PA, Hawkshaw MJ, Sataloff RT. Allergy. In: Sataloff RT. Professional voice: the science and art of clinical care. 4th ed. San Diego: Plural Publishing; 2017. p. 737–42.
26. Sataloff RT, Katz PO, Sataloff DM, Hawkshaw MJ. Reflux laryngitis and related disorders. 4th ed. San Diego: Plural Publishing; 2013. p. 1–210.
27. Ritter FN. The effect of hypothyroidism on the larynx of the rat. Ann Otol Rhinol Laryngol. 1964;67:404–16.
28. Ritter RN. Endocrinology. In: Paparella M, Shumrick D, editors. Otolaryngology, vol. 1. Philadelphia: Saunders; 1973. p. 727–34.
29. Michelsson K, Sirvio P. Cry analysis in congenital hypothyroidism. Folia Phoniatr (Basel). 1976;28:40–7.

30. Gupta OP, Bhatia PL, Agarwal MK, Mehrotra ML, Mishr SK. Nasal pharyngeal and laryn-geal manifestations of hypothyroidism. Ear Nose Throat J. 1977;56(9):10–21.
31. Malinsky M, Chevrrie-Muller C, Cerceau N. Etude Clinique et electrophysiologique des alterations de la voix au cours des thyrotoxioses. Ann Endocrinol. 1977;38:171–2.
32. Meuser W, Nieschlag E. Sexual hormone und Stimmlage des Mannes. Dtsch Med Wochenschr. 1977;102:261–4.
33. Brodnitz F. The age of the castrato voice. J Speech Hear Disord. 1975;40:291–5.
34. Anderson TD, Anderson DD, Sataloff RT. Endocrine function. In: Sataloff RT. Professional voice: the science and art of clinical care. 4th ed. San Diego: Plural Publishing; 2017. p. 655–70.
35. Schiff M. The influence of estrogens on connective tissue. In: Asboe-Hansen G, editor. Hormones and connective tissue. Copenhagen: Munksgaard Press; 1967. p. 282–341.
36. Lacina V. Der Einfluss der Menstruation auf die Stimme der Sangerinnen. Folia Phoniatr. 1968;20:13–24.
37. Wendler J. Cyclically dependent variations in efficiency of the voice and its influencing by ovulation inhibitors. Zyklusabhangige Leistungsschwankungen der Stimme und ihre Beeinflussung durch Ovulationshemmer. Folia Phoniatr. 1972;24(4):259–77.
38. Abitbol J, Abitbol P. The larynx: a hormonal target. In: Rubin J, Sataloff RT, Korovin G. Diagnosis and treatment of voice disorders. 4th ed. San Diego: Plural Publishing, Inc.; 2014. p. 431–56.
39. Dordain M. Etude Statistique de l'influence des contraceptifs hormonaux sur la voix. Folia Phoniatr (Basel). 1972;24:86–96.
40. Pahn V, Goretzlehner G. Stimmstorungen durch hormonale Kontrazeptiva. Zentralbl Gynakol. 1978;100:341–6.
41. Schiff M. "The pill" in otolaryngology. Trans Am Acad Opthalmol Otolaryngol. 1968;72:76–84.
42. Rodney JP, Sataloff RT. The effects of hormonal contraception on the voice: history of its evolution in the literature. J Voice. 2016;30(6):726–30.
43. Brodnitz F. Medical care preventative therapy (Panel). In: Lawrence V, editor. Transcripts of the seventh annual symposium, care of the professional voice, vol. 3. New York: Voice Foundation; 1978. p. 86.
44. Flach M, Schwickardi H, Simen R. Welchen Einfluss haben Menstruation and Schwangershaft auf die augsgebildete Gesangsstimme? Folia Phoniatr. 1968;21:199–210.
45. Deuster CV. Irreversible Stimmstorung in der Schwangersheft. HNO. 1977;25:430–2.
46. Damste PH. Virilization of the voice due to anabolic steroids. Folia Phoniatr. 1964;16:10–8.
47. Damste PH. Voice changes in adult women caused by virilizing agents. J Speech Hear Disord. 1967;32:126–32.
48. Saez S, Francoise S. Recepteurs d'androgenes: mise en evidence dans la fraction cytosolique de muqueuse normale et d'epitheliomas pharyngolarynges humains. C R Acad Sci (Paris). 1975;280:935–8.
49. Vuorenkoski V, Lenko HL, Tjernlund P, Vuorenkoski L, Perheentupa J. Fundamental voice frequency during normal and abnormal growth, and after androgen treatment. Arch Dis Child. 1978;53:201–9.
50. Bourdial J. Les troubles de la voix provoques par la therapeutique hormonale androgene. Ann Otolaryngol. 1970;87:725–34.
51. Imre V. Hormonell bedingte Stimmstorungen. Folia Phoniatr. 1968;20:394–404.
52. Hamdan A, Sataloff RT, Hawkshaw MJ. Laryngeal manifestations of systemic diseases. San Diego: Plural Publishing, Inc; 2019.
53. Hamdan A, Sataloff RT, Hawkshaw MJ. Obesity and voice. San Diego: Plural Publishing, Inc; 2020.
54. National Institutes of Health. Health implications of obesity. Bethesda: Consensus Development Conference Statement; 1986.
55. Gates GA, Saegert J, Wilson N, Johnson L, Sheperd A, Hearnd EM. Effects of beta-blockade on singing performance. Ann Otol Rhinol Laryngol. 1985;94:570–4.

56. Rosen DC, Sataloff JB, Sataloff RT. Psychology of Voice Disorders, 2nd ed. San Diego, CA: Plural Publishing; 2020.
57. Sataloff RT, Brandfonbrener A, Lederman R, editors. Performing arts medicine. 3rd ed. Narberth: Science and Medicine; 2010.
58. Bull TR. Tuberculosis of the larynx. Br Med J. 1966;2:991–2.
59. Hunter AM, Millar JW, Wrightman AJ, Horne NW. The changing pattern of laryngeal tuberculosis. J Laryngol Otol. 1981;95:393–8.
60. Divine KD. Sarcoidosis and sarcoidosis of the larynx. Laryngoscope. 1965;75:533–69.
61. Munor MacCormick CE. The larynx in leprosy. Arch Otolaryngol. 1957;66:138–49.
62. Binford CH, Meyers WM. Leprosy. In: Binford CH, Conor DH, editors. Pathology of tropical and extraordinary diseases, vol. 1. Washington, DC: Armed Forces Institute of Pathology; 1976. p. 205–25.
63. MacKenzie M. A manual of diseases of the throat and nose. Diseases of the pharynx, larynx, and trachea, vol. 1. London: J.& A. Churchill; 1884.
64. Astacio JN, Goday GA, Espinosa FJ. Escleroma. Experiences en El Salvador. Seconda Mongrafia de Dermatologia iberolatino-americana. Suplemento AO No. 1, Lisboa, Portugal, 1971.
65. Hajek M. Pathologie unde Therapie der Erkrankungen des Kehlkopfes, der Luftrohre und der Bronchien. Leipzig: Verlag von Curt Kabitzsch; 1932.
66. Withers BT, Pappas JJ, Erickson EE. Histoplasmosis primary in the larynx. Report of a case. Arch Otolaryngol. 1977;77:25–8.
67. Calcaterra TC. Otolaryngeal histoplasmosis. Laryngoscope. 1970;80:111–20.
68. Sataloff RT, Wilborn A, Prestipino A, Hawkshaw MJ, Heuer RJ, Cohn JR. Histoplasmosis of the larynx. Am J Otolaryngol. 1993;14(3):199–205.
69. Friedmann I. Diseases of the larynx. Disorders of laryngeal function. In: Paparella MM, Shumrick DA, editors. Otolaryngology. 2nd ed. Philadelphia: WB Saunders; 1980. p. 2449–69.
70. Reese MC, Conclasure JB. Cryptococcosis of the larynx. Arch Otolaryngol. 1975;101:698–701.
71. Bennett M. Laryngeal blastomycosis. Laryngoscope. 1964;74:498–512.
72. Hoffarth GA, Joseph DL, Shumrick DA. Deep mycoses. Arch Otolaryngol. 1973;97:475–9.
73. Brandenburg JH, Finch WW, Kirkham WR. Actinomycosis of the larynx and pharynx. Otolaryngology. 1978;86:739–42.
74. Shaheen SO, Ellis FG. Actinomycosis of the larynx. J R Soc Med. 1983;76:226–8.
75. Tedeschi LG, Cheren RV. Laryngeal hyperkeratosis due to primary monilial infection. Arch Otolaryngol. 1968;82:82–4.
76. Rao PB. Aspergillosis of the larynx. J Laryngol Otol. 1969;83:377–9.
77. Ferlito A. Clinical records. Primary aspergillosis of the larynx. J Laryngol Otol. 1974;88:1257–63.
78. Keir SM, Flint A, Moss JA. Primary aspergillosis of the larynx simulating carcinoma. Hum Pathol. 1983;14:184–6.
79. Anand CS, Gupta MC, Kothari MG, Anand TS, Singh SK. Laryngeal mucormycosis. Indian J Otolaryngol. 1978;30:90–2.
80. Pillai OS. Rhinosporidiosis of the larynx. J Laryngol Otol. 1974;88:277–80.
81. Khabie N, Boyce TG, Roberts GD, Thompson DM. Laryngeal sporotrichosis causing stridor in young child. Int J Pediatr Otorhinolaryngol. 2003;67(7):819–23.
82. Zinneman HH, Hall WH, Wallace FG. Leishmaniasis of the larynx. Report of a case and its confusion with histoplasmosis. Am J Med. 1961;31:654–8.
83. Michaels L. Pathology of the larynx. New York: Springer-Verlag; 1984.
84. Wolman L, Darke CS, Young A. The larynx in rheumatoid arthritis. J Laryngol. 1965;79:403–34.
85. Bridger MWN, Jahn AF, van Nostrand AWP. Laryngeal rheumatoid arthritis. Laryngoscope. 1980;90:296–303.
86. Virchow R. Seltene gichtablagerungen. Virchows Arch Path Anat. 1868;44:137–8.

87. Marion RB, Alperin JE, Maloney WH. Gouty tophus of the true vocal cord. Arch Otolaryngol. 1972;96:161–2.
88. Epstein SS, Winston P, Friedmann I, Ormerod FC. The vocal cord polyp. J Laryngol Otol Lond. 1957;71:673–88.
89. Stark DB, New GB. Amyloid tumors of larynx, trachea or bronchi: report of 15 cases. Ann Otol Rhinol Laryngol. 1949;58:117–34.
90. Michaels L, Hyams VJ. Amyloid in localized deposits and plasmacytomas of the respiratory tract. J Pathol. 1979;128(1):29–38.
91. Pribtkin E, Friedman O, O'Hara B, et al. Amyloidosis of the upper aerodigestive tract. Laryngoscope. 2003;113:2095–101.
92. Urbach E, Wiethe C. Lipoidosis cutis et mucosae. Virchows Arch Path Anat. 1929;273:285–319.
93. Charow A, Pass F, Ruben R. Pemphigus of the upper respiratory tract. Arch Otolaryngol. 1971;93:209–10.
94. Sataloff RT, Hawkshaw MJ, Ressue J. Granular cell tumor of the larynx. Ear Nose Throat J. 1998;77(8):582–4.
95. Moore JE, Hawkshaw MJ, Sataloff RT. Vocal fold scar. United Kingdom: Compton Publishing, Ltd; 2016.
96. Moore JE, Sataloff RT. Vocal fold scar. In: Sataloff RT. Professional voice: the science and art of clinical care. 4th ed. San Diego: Plural Publishing; 2017. p. 1605–10.
97. Sataloff RT, Hawkshaw M. Vocal fold hemorrhage. In: Sataloff RT. Professional voice: the science and art of clinical care. 4th ed. San Diego: Plural Publishing; 2017. p. 1587–604.
98. Hochman I, Sataloff RT, Hillman R, Zeitels S. Ectasias and varices of the vocal fold: clearing the striking zone. Ann Otol Rhinol Laryngol. 1999;108(1):10–6.
99. Zeitels SM. Phonomicrosurgical techniques. In: Sataloff RT. Professional voice: the science and art of clinical care. 4th ed. San Diego: Plural Publishing; 2017. p. 1479–500.
100. Zeitels SM, Sataloff RT. Phonomicrosurgical resection of glottal papillomatosis. J Voice. 1999;13(1):123–7.
101. Wellens W, Snoeck R, Desloovere C, et al. Treatment of severe laryngeal papillomatosis with intralesional injections of cidofovir [(S)-1-(3-Hydroxy-Phosphonylmethoxypropyl) Cytosine, HPMPC, Vistide]. In: McCafferty G, Coman W, Carroll R, editors. Proceedings of the XVI World Congress of otorhinolaryngology head and neck surgery. Bologna: Monduzzi Editor; 1997. p. 455–549.
102. Holinger LD, Barnes DR, Smid LJ, Holinger PH. Laryngocele and saccular cysts. Ann Otol Rhinol Laryngol. 1978;87:675–85.
103. Ward PH, Frederickson J, Strandjord NM, Valvessori GE. Laryngeal and pharyngeal pouches. Surgical approach and the use of cinefluorographic and other radiologic techniques as diagnostic aids. Laryngoscope. 1963;73:564–82.
104. DeSanto LW. Laryngocele, laryngeal mucocele, large saccules, and laryngeal saccular cysts: a developmental spectrum. Laryngoscope. 1974;84:1291–6.
105. Norris CW. Pharyngoceles of the hypopharynx. Laryngoscope. 1979;89:1788–807.
106. Papsin BC, Maaske LA, McGrail JS. Orbicularis oris muscle injury in brass players. Laryngoscope. 1996;106:757–60.
107. Fiz JA, Aguilar J, Carreras A, et al. Maximum respiratory pressure in trumpet players. Chest. 1993;104:1203–4.
108. Stephani A, Tarab S. Obscure and ventricular laryngocele. Schweiz Rundsch Med Prax. 1972;61:1520–3.
109. Macfie DD. Asymptomatic laryngoceles in wind instrument bandsmen. Arch Otolaryngol. 1966;83:270–5.
110. Backus J. The effect of the player's vocal tract on wood wind instrument tone. J Acoust Soc Am. 1985;78:17–20.
111. Isaacson G, Sataloff RT. Bilateral laryngoceles in a young trumpet player: case report. Ear Nose Throat J. 2000;4:272–4.

112. Sataloff RT, Chowdhury F, Portnoy J, Hawkshaw MJ, Joglekar S. Surgical techniques in otolaryngology – head and neck surgery: laryngeal surgery. New Delhi: Jaypee Brothers Medical Publishers; 2014.
113. Sataloff RT, Spiegel JR, Heuer RJ, et al. Laryngeal mini-microflap: a new technique and reassessment of the microflap saga. J Voice. 1995;9(2):198–204.
114. Abitbol J. Limitations of the laser in microsurgery of the larynx. In: Lawrence VL, editor. Transactions of the twelfth symposium: care of the professional voice. New York: The Voice Foundation; 1984. p. 297–302.
115. Strong MS, Jako GJ. Laser surgery in the larynx. Early clinical experience with continuous CO_2 laser. Ann Otol Rhinol Laryngol. 1972;81:791–8.
116. Sataloff RT, Feldman M, Darby KS, Carroll LM, Spiegel JR. Arytenoid dislocation. J Voice. 1988;1(4):368–77.
117. Sataloff RT, Bough ID, Spiegel JR. Arytenoid dislocation: diagnosis and treatment. Laryngoscope. 1994;104(10):1353–61.
118. Sataloff RT, Hawkshaw MJ, Sataloff JB, DeFatta RA, Eller RL. Atlas of laryngoscopy. 3rd ed. San Diego: Plural Publishing, Inc.; 2012.
119. Hamdan A, Sataloff RT, Trollinger V, Hawkshaw MJ. Dentofacial Anomalies: Implications for Voice and Wind Instrument Performance. Switzerland AG: Springer Nature; in press.
120. Hamdan A, Sataloff RT, Hawkshaw MJ. Non-Laryngeal Cancer and Voice. San Diego, CA: Plural Publishing; 2020.

Chapter 5
Vocal Health Risk Factors in Sports Occupational Voice Users

5.1 Introduction

The fitness industry, like other occupational industry with high vocal demand, increases the risk of voice disorders among its occupational voice users. The risk of dysphonia varies across the different subgroups of sports occupational voice users (SOVU). Athletes often engage in phonotraumatic behavior such as grunting or loud phonation during sports activity leading to change in voice quality [1]. Dysphonia may also be ascribed to vocal fold dysfunction and laryngeal trauma particularly during competitive events [2, 3]. Similarly, coaches and fitness instructors are subject to high voice demand while exercising [4–7]. Fontan et al. reported a positive correlation between "shouting" and Voice Handicap Index (VHI) score in their study of 320 sports and fitness instructors. The results showed that those who shouted had higher VHI score in comparison to those who did not [6]. Note that VHI is a self- report questionnaire on the impact of dysphonia on quality of life. Similarly, in another study of 361 fitness instructors, Rumbach et al. reported loud voice use while instructing as a risk factor for dysphonia. Additional health-related risk factors included sore throat and history of flu and/or a cold [7]. More often than not, the high voice demand in sports occupational voice users is compounded by environmental factors that impose additional burden on the voice apparatus. The need for high voice intensity and prolonged phonation in a noisy environment with suboptimal acoustic conditions has become a significant threat to athletes, coaches, fitness instructors, and announcers.

In this chapter, the authors review the risk factors for voice disorders in SOVU. The risk factors are stratified as individual-related factors such as poor vocal hygiene and dehydration and environment-related factors such as allergens, noise, and poor environmental acoustics. Analyzing these factors is crucial in understanding why athletes, coaches, fitness instructors, and announcers develop voice disorders. This information is important to otolaryngologists, laryngologists,

© The Author(s), under exclusive license to Springer Nature Switzerland AG 2021
A.-L. Hamdan et al., *Voice Disorders in Athletes, Coaches and other Sports Professionals*, https://doi.org/10.1007/978-3-030-69831-7_5

sports medicine professionals, voice teachers, and speech-language pathologists involved in the management of dysphonia in SOVU. It also is useful in defining and implementing preventive measures that help avert sports-related phonatory disturbances.

5.2 Individual-Related Risk Factors for Voice Disorders

Individual-related risk factors are primarily responsible for the variation in the prevalence of phonatory disorders among SOVU. These factors include the level of voice education/health awareness, the extent of dehydration and fluid loss, and the presence of comorbid health conditions such as asthma and/or laryngopharyngeal reflux disease. The prevalence and implications of these risk factors for voice in SOVU should be recognized by healthcare providers, as well as by SOVU.

5.2.1 Voice Educational Health Awareness

The level of voice education/health awareness among athletes, coaches, and fitness instructors has been a subject of thorough discussion in the literature. The consensus is that it is suboptimal with a dire need for improvement. In a study on the risk factors for dysphonia among aerobics instructors, Long et al. reported unfamiliarity with vocal hygiene in a large percentage of their study group, including subjects with and without voice problems (39% and 44%, respectively). The investigation included 54 health-fitness instructors who were asked to complete a 35-item questionnaire that included a section on voice symptoms and voice education [8]. In another study by Fontan et al. on voice problems and associated risk factors in sports fitness instructors, the results indicated that only 37% of the total group ($n = 320$) had received information on voice difficulties despite the fact that more than half the subjects had experienced voice symptoms. The authors also noted that 80% of sports fitness instructors reported their interest in learning how to prevent voice disorders [6]. Similarly, Rumbach et al. reported on the paucity of voice education and the need for better vocal training in their study on 38 fitness instructors diagnosed with voice disorders. Two-thirds of their study group were not satisfied with the level of support provided by the industry, and 7.82% did not receive any treatment despite the adverse effects voice disorders had on their emotional and social interactions [9]. Similarly, Buckley et al. reported limited knowledge about voice support in a group of 12 Australian elite football soccer coaches. Vocal health was a not a concept that was discussed frequently by the group despite the high occupational voice demand. Moreover, all subjects had experienced voice symptoms that were ignored and/or considered inevitable adverse events associated with their work. The data of that study were acquired using semi-structured interviews and a voice questionnaire [10]. In 2016, Fellman and Simberg investigated the prevalence and risk factors for voice problems in 109 coaches and reported that only 8.9% of the study group had received information on voice. Moreover, the information time was limited to less than 5 hours in 77.8% of those who had received voice education [11]. As in coaches and fitness instructors, the level of voice education and health awareness in athletes remains suboptimal. In a study of 75 aerobic participants, Heidel and Torgerson reported poor vocal hygiene and sleeping habits in their study group. The investigation was conducted using a questionnaire on medical/vocal history, water intake, and smoking [12]. Similarly, the adverse effect of androgenic anabolic steroid usage on voice remains underestimated in athletes. Increased awareness in regard to the possible adverse effects of these medications needs emphasis [13].

All the above confirms that voice education/health awareness is suboptimal in SOVU. Improvement in vocal hygiene and phonatory behavior in SOVU should be able to reduce the prevalence of phonatory disorders, as has been reported in other professional voice users [14, 15]. In 2010, Leppanen et al. studied the impact of vocal hygiene lecturing (3 hours) on voice and showed marked improvement in voice quality of female teachers after they had lectures. Additional treatment modalities that were offered to subgroups of teachers included laryngeal massage and voice training. The study included 90 subjects who were followed for 6 and 12 months [14]. In 2019, Porcaro et al. reported an increase in vocal hygiene engagement following enhanced voice education in 26 teachers who were assessed using a screening survey. Voice education consisted of an hour of education on voice hygiene, phonotraumatic behavior, and unhealthy vocal behavior [15]. Similar results were reported in 2014 by O'Neil and McMenamin in their study on voice use in professional soccer management. The authors noted the benefit of improving voice behavior/awareness as a means to prevent voice disorders [4].

In summary, voice education/health awareness in sports occupational voice users is limited. Given the well-known association between vocal hygiene/health awareness and voice complaints, athletes, coaches, and fitness instructors are at a high risk of having dysphonia. Development of voice educational programs should be effective in preventing phonotrauma and in reducing the prevalence of dysphonia in sports professional voice users, but confirmatory evidence in most sports occupations is lacking.

5.2.2 Dehydration and Fluid Loss

Dehydration and fluid loss are common among athletes [16–22]. In a study on fluid balance in six triathletes competing at the World Triathlon Grand Final, Logan-Sprenger reported a mean fluid loss of 2.15 L and a mean body mass loss of 3.3%. Three out of six triathletes in their study group were dehydrated at the end of the race despite fluid intake of 0.66 L per person [16]. Similarly, in a study by Rumbach on 38 fitness instructors, 71% complained of dryness in their throat that was partially ascribed to poor hydration and insufficient water intake [9]. The extent of dehydration in athletes varies with the type of sport and sport's environment [17–19]. Barnes et al. investigated the extent of fluid loss in relation to the type of activity in 1,303 athletes using whole-body sweating rate and Na+ loss as outcome measures. The highest fluid loss was reported in American football and in endurance sports [20]. Similarly, Sekiguchi et al. showed that the total distance covered during exercise is the best predictor of water loss. Ambient temperature and relative humidity strengthened the prediction provided by the total distance ($r2 = 0.302$). The study was conducted on 28 male soccer players whose percent body mass loss and state of hydration were gauged before and after training [21].

With a decrease in body fluids, muscle performance is undoubtedly affected. This is not surprising knowing that water constitutes 70–80% of body tissue and that water plays an integral role in the function of various systems in the body [23–25]. Judelson et al., in their study on the effect of hydration on muscle strength, power, and endurance, reported susceptibility of the neuromuscular system to fluid deficit and noted dehydration-induced decrease in maximal muscle performance [17]. Similarly, Barley et al. studied the impact of acute dehydration on neuromuscular function in combat sports athletes and reported impairment in muscle strength and endurance, as well as heightened fatigue perception among the participants. The authors used repeated knee extension exercises at 85% maximal voluntary isometric contraction (MVIC) as an outcome measure. Subjects were instructed to perform six MVIC (three as fast as possible and three as hard and fast as possible). The number of knee extensions decreased after dehydration, with an increased perception of fatigue [18].

Given that the phonatory apparatus is part of the musculoskeletal system, it is evident that dehydration-induced decrease in muscle performance and endurance affects phonation. This is consistent with the known adverse impact of dehydration on vocal folds' rheologic properties. In an investigation on the effect of hydration on vocal fold tissues, Chan and Tayama showed that dehydration leads to significant increase in vocal fold stiffness and viscosity, whereas rehydration leads to improvement in vocal fold viscoelastic shear properties. The study was conducted on five excised canine larynges that were incubated in solutions with different tonicity [26]. These results were confirmed by other clinical studies substantiating the unfavorable effect of dehydration on voice and the benefits of hydration. Verdolini et al. investigated the effect of hydration and dehydration on voice in 12 adults and reported an inverse relationship between the level of hydration and phonatory effort, particularly while performing high-pitched phonatory tasks [27]. In another study on six females with exudative lesions of the lamina propria (nodules/polyps), the same authors reported the therapeutic benefit of hydration on the clinical appearance and symptoms of affected patients [28]. Solomon et al. reported an increase in phonation threshold pressure (PTP) and phonatory effort in four women who were asked to read loudly for 2 hours. This increase was accompanied by abnormal laryngeal videostroboscopic changes, namely, spindle-shaped opening in three of the four subjects. The increase in phonatory effort and PTP at various conversational pitches was attenuated following systemic hydration [29]. Similar findings were reported by the same authors in another study conducted on four men. The results showed an increase in phonatory effort following prolonged phonation in all subjects, two of whom improved after hydration [30]. In 2001, Fisher et al. studied the impact of fluid removal on phonation and showed that 3–4% fluid volume reduction increases PTP. The fluid volume removal accounted for 31.6% of PTP variance and 40% of phonatory effort variance [31]. Hamdan et al. investigated the effect of fasting on voice in 28 female subjects and reported an increase in phonatory effort in 23 out of the 28 subjects. The most common voice symptoms while fasting were voice fatigue and deepening of the voice in 53.6% and 21.4% of the cases, respectively [32]. These self-reported symptoms were accompanied by a significant decrease in the mean maximum phonation time (15.97 seconds while non-fasting vs. 13.26 seconds while fasting) and by the presence of a posterior chink on laryngeal endoscopy in three subjects [32]. A similar study conducted on 26 male subjects also showed an increase in the phonatory effort in half the subjects. Moreover, there was a decrease in the habitual pitch that was ascribed to fluid loss and to the known inverse relation between mass and pitch [33] (Fig. 5.1).

In summary, dehydration in athletes is common despite fluid replacement. It is often unrecognized because most athletes rely on dark urine color as a sign of dehydration rather than changes in body mass index [22]. Poor skin rigor, tachycardia, headache, change in mental status, and impairment in cognitive performance should alert athletes and sports physicians to the possibility of dehydration. Phonatory symptoms may be added to the symptoms of dehydration in sports occupational voice users given the known adverse effect of fluid loss on muscle performance and on the rheologic properties of the vocal folds.

Fig. 5.1 A patient presenting with voice fatigue and intermittent change in voice quality. Vocal history is suggestive of dehydration and poor vocal hygiene. Telescopic laryngeal examination shows thick mucus at the free edge of the vocal folds

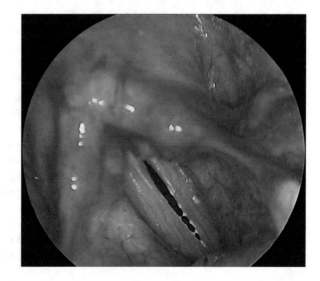

5.2.3   Asthma and Its Impact on Voice in Athletes

Athletes in general, and athletes of endurance sports in particular are more likely to be diagnosed with asthma or asthma-like symptoms in comparison to nonathletes in whom the prevalence of asthma does not exceed 10% according to a recent National Health and Examination Survey [34, 35]. In a review of 659 Olympic Italian athletes, Bonini et al. reported asthma and/or exercise-induced bronchoconstriction in 14.7% of the cases. Using four cross-sectional surveys, the authors noted an increase in the diagnosis of asthma along the course of 8 years [36]. Similarly, Lund, in his investigation on the prevalence and treatment of asthma in elite athletes, reported asthma-like symptoms and asthma in 55% and 14% of the cases, respectively. A higher prevalence was noted in endurance athletes who also had an increase in their airway neutrophils [37]. Similarly, Lennelöv et al. investigated the prevalence of self-reported asthma and self-reported wheezing in 87 skiers in comparison to a population-based reference group. The authors showed that both asthma and wheezing were more common in skiers in comparison to the reference group (23% vs. 12% and 25% vs. 14%, respectively) [38].

The high prevalence of asthma and asthma-like symptoms in athletes can be attributed to several factors. In a review on the causes of cough in athletes, Boulet et al. reported environmental exposures as main causes of asthma and respiratory tract infection. Additional causes of cough included rhinitis and upper airway cough syndrome [39]. Based on a review by Gleeson and Pyne, previous history of asthma and/or individual's predisposition to asthma was more common in high-performance athletes with respiratory illnesses, which in turn had substantial consequences on athletes' general health and performance [35]. Fields et al. reported that upper respiratory tract infection results in abnormal pulmonary function that can persist long after the infection subsides. Hence, diligent history taking and workup of athletes with recent history of upper respiratory tract infection and wheezing are crucial before resuming normal athletic activity [40]. Another individual risk factor for asthma is immune dysfunction with "breakdown in the homeostatic regulation of the mucosal immune system of the airways" as described by Colbey et al. [41]

In summary, asthma and asthma-like symptoms are very common in athletes. Given the importance of efficient breathing in phonation, athletes with history of asthma and/or wheezing are at high risk for developing dysphonia. The change in voice quality may be disease-induced as a result of impairment in expiratory flow and/or drug-induced secondary to the intake of steroid inhalers (Fig. 5.2). The reader can refer to the chapter on laryngeal manifestations of respiratory disorders in the book *Laryngeal Manifestations of Systemic Disease* for more information [42]. Nevertheless, given that many of the abovementioned studies did not prove asthma by pulmonary function testing with bronchodilator response or methacholine challenge, other diagnoses that can be confused with asthma should be considered in this population. Laryngopharyngeal reflux with aspiration is one example. Reflux is often aggravated by strenuous exercise activity, and aspiration of reflux can cause bronchoconstriction that can be mistaken easily from asthma.

Fig. 5.2 Pulmonary
function test showing
severe obstructive
pulmonary impairment
with significant response to
bronchodilator challenge

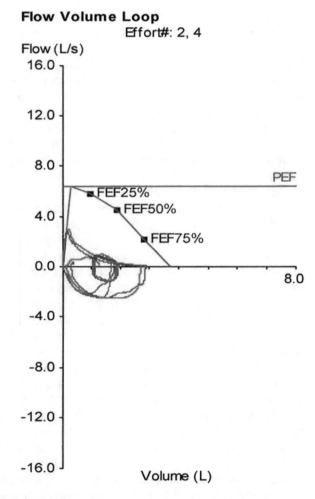

5.2.4 Gastroesophageal Reflux Disease in Athletes and Its Implication on Voice

Gastrointestinal symptoms are very common in athletes. The prevalence of these symptoms ranges between 30% and 70% and increases during high-performance endurance events [43]. Depending on the type of exercise and its intensity, gastrointestinal symptoms may be disquieting and disruptive to athletes' daily exercise. In a study by Hoffman on factors that affect completion of ultramarathon (161 km), nausea and vomiting were reported in 23% of the cases. These were considered among the most common reasons why athletes did not finish the race [44]. Gastrointestinal symptoms can be the result of various gastrointestinal disorders, the most common of which is gastroesophageal reflux disease (GERD). Other causes include gastrointestinal bleeding, ulceration, and inflammatory bowel disease [45–48]. In a review by Khodaee and Ansari on musculoskeletal injuries and illnesses of ultramarathoners, the authors described gastroesophageal reflux as common. Lower gastrointestinal symptoms such as abdominal cramps, diarrhea, and blood in stool were reported in 37–71% of cases. The authors advocated abstention from using nonsteroidal anti-inflammatory drugs to avoid gastrointestinal bleeding [49]. In a study by Collings et al. on the association between type of exercise and the prevalence of gastroesophageal reflux disease, the authors reported the highest frequency of heartburn and reflux in weight lifters in comparison to runners and cyclists. The study included ten athletes from different sports category, each with a positive history of exercise-induced heartburn. The subjects were evaluated using pH-metry while performing strenuous exercise at 65% and 85% of their maximal capacity. The authors identified a strong link between the type of exercise and reflux-related symptoms [50]. Similarly, in a survey on patients with GERD ($n = 100$), Jozkow et al. showed a weak but positive correlation between the number of gastroesophageal symptoms and physical activity. Physical activity was measured using the resting metabolic rate and minutes of performance during a period of 1 week. There was no association between pH-metric parameters and daily activity which was stratified in this study as low, moderate, or high [51].

The pathophysiology of GERD in athletes is multifaceted. Several theories have been postulated. These include mechanical factors such as the pressure gradient between the chest and abdomen, altered esophageal motility, changes in neuroendocrine level, and a decrease in splanchnic blood flow [43, 52]. The use of dynamic, constrained, or fluctuating body position in specific types of exercise is a main precipitating factor. Bitnar et al. investigated the impact of leg raising on esophageal pressure using high-resolution manometry in 58 patients with gastroesophageal reflux disease. They showed a significant increase in upper and lower esophageal sphincter pressures during leg raising in comparison to the resting position. The authors noted the strong link between diaphragmatic function and that of esophageal sphincter in athletes with GERD and who exhibited high intra-abdominal pressure during exercise [53]. In a study by Ravi et al. on the effect of exercise on esophageal function in 135 patients with esophageal disease, moderate exercise was considered a risk factor for reflux. The authors showed a decrease in esophageal wave amplitude during exercise in patients with diffuse esophageal spasm and nutcracker esophagus patients [54]. Nieuwenhoven et al. studied the gastrointestinal profile of symptomatic ($n = 10$) and asymptomatic athletes ($n = 10$), at rest and during exercise which included 90% of cycling and running at 70% of their maximal capacity. The results indicated that symptomatic athletes had more frequent and longer duration of reflux episodes during cycling than asymptomatic athletes. Moreover, they had higher intestinal permeability and longer oro-cecal transit time during running [55].

All the above confirms the high prevalence of GERD in athletes. Given that extra-esophageal manifestations are common in patients with GERD, particularly in patients with esophagitis, it is reasonable to conclude that athletes with GERD are likely to experience laryngopharyngeal symptoms, among which is dysphonia [56]. The pathophysiology of these symptoms include vagally mediated reflexes and/or the backflow of the refluxate material into the laryngeal inlet. Once the refluxate material reaches the laryngeal inlet, its harmful effect is unattenuated by the lack of cleating mechanisms including absence of mucosal peristalsis and saliva [57, 58]. The exposure of the gastric juice and aerosol to the laryngeal lining results in mucosal inflammation and an array of symptoms and signs. The most commonly reported are globus sensation, excessive throat clearing, cough, and change in voice quality. On laryngeal examination, patients may have mucosal edema, erythema, pseudosulcus vocalis, and interarytenoid pachydermia (Figs. 5.3 and 5.4). Less commonly encountered lesions are ulcerations in the vocal processes and/or granulomas (Fig. 5.5). LPRD is also a main culprit in the exacerbation of exudative lesions of the lamina propria, vocal fold mucosal changes, and the development of subglottic stenosis [59, 60]. The reader can refer to Chap. 4 of this book. The refluxate also can be aspirated causing pulmonary symptoms as discussed above. Laryngopharyngeal reflux also is associated with sleep disturbances which can be troublesome for athletes including voice professionals.

In summary, there is strong evidence in the literature to confirm the high prevalence of GERD in athletes. Given the linkage between GERD and laryngopharyngeal reflux disease (LPRD) and given the well-known effect of acidic and nonacidic reflux on the laryngopharyngeal mucosal lining and lumen, it is reasonable to conclude that the risk of voice disorders in athletes is significant. Although there are no studies in the literature comparing the prevalence of dysphonia in athletes with LPRD with those with no LPRD, a thorough workup of LPRD in athletes with dysphonia is mandatory in order to rule out laryngeal pathology. Treatment with antacids, H2 blockers, proton-pump inhibitors, lifestyle modifications and diet modifications, alginate, and sometimes anti-reflux surgery is highly recommended.

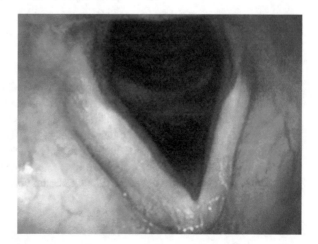

Fig. 5.3 A 48-year-old woman diagnosed with laryngopharyngeal reflux disease presenting with symptoms of globus sensation and throat clearing. Laryngeal examination showed edema of the lower lip of the vocal folds (pseudosulcus). Patient was on proton-pump inhibitors twice daily

Fig. 5.4 A 28-year-old female singer complaining of voice fatigue, loss of range, and voice breaks. Laryngeal examination showed edema of the left vocal fold extending to the subglottic region

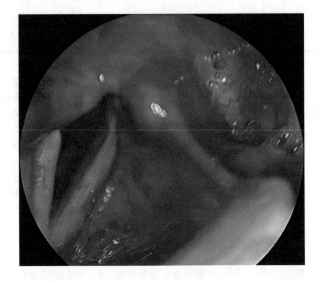

Fig. 5.5 A 53-year-old man with history of reflux disease presenting with foreign body sensation, throat clearing, and mild change in voice quality. Laryngeal examination showed right vocal process granuloma

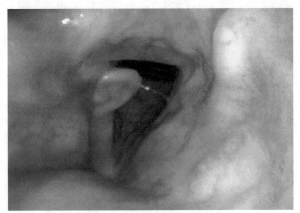

5.3   Environmental Risk Factors for Voice Disorders in Athletes

Environment-related risk factors are as important as individual-related risk factors in precipitating voice disorders among SOVU. These may elicit the development of vocal fold lesions or aggravate preexisting vocal fold pathology. Their compounding effect on vocal loading may be detrimental in SOVU with high voice demand. Environment-related risk factors include mainly allergens, ambient noise/poor working environment acoustics, extreme altitude, extreme temperature, and extreme humidity. A review of the impact of these factors on voice is presented.

5.3.1   Allergy in Sports Occupational Voice Users and Its Implications for Voice

Allergy is an inflammatory response to a foreign substance that can be either inhaled, ingested, or injected. As SOVU are frequently exposed to outdoor and indoor environmental allergens, the prevalence of symptomatic allergy in this population is high reaching up to 58.3% with marked variation among subgroups [36, 39, 61–70]. The disparity in prevalence is attributed to individual predisposing factors such as prior history of atopy and asthma and/or to anatomic variations. Another contributing factor to the wide range of prevalence is the type of diagnostic tests used in making the diagnosis. These include allergy skin testing, serology testing, structured interviews, and self-report questionnaires [39, 61] (Fig. 5.6 and Table 5.1). Allergy Questionnaire in Athletes referred to as AQUA is the questionnaire most commonly used to estimate the prevalence of allergy in athletes. The questionnaire consists of queries about social habits, duration, and intensity of training, as well as about the use of supplements and medications. A score greater than or equal to five has been shown to have a specificity and sensitivity of 97.1% and 58.3%, respectively [62]. In a study by Bonini et al. that included 128 professional soccer players, almost one out of two (46.8%) had positive skin testing [62]. In another study by the same authors on 659 Olympic athletes, the prevalence of rhinitis and skin allergy was 26.2% and 14.8%, respectively. The authors used skin-prick tests, pulmonary function tests, serum antibodies, cytokines, growth factors, and flow cytometry as diagnostic tests [36]. Similarly, Kurowski et al. reported symptoms of allergy using AQUA in 27% of 220 Olympic athletes. The diagnosis of allergic rhinitis was

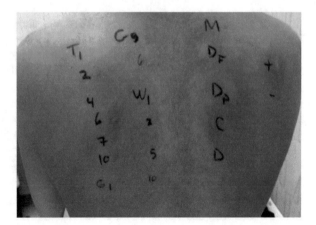

Fig. 5.6 Allergy skin testing for various allergens. Note the grading criteria where 0 stands for no reaction, 1+ for erythema less than 21 mm without wheal, 2+ for erythema more than 21 mm/ wheal less than 3 mm, 3+ for erythema 21 mm/wheal more than 3 mm without pseudopod, and 4+ for erythema and wheal with pseudopod (*T stands for tree, G stands for grass, W stands for weed, M stands for mold, Df stands for Dermatophagoides farinae, and Dp stands for D. pteronyssinus)

Table 5.1 Allergy skin testing sheet

Patient Name:								Patient Number:		
Date of Birth: ___/___/___ Age: ___ Medication:										
Last use of antihistamine (or other drug affecting histamine release): ___ days Testing Date: ___/___/___										
	Percutaneous			**Percutaneous**			**Percutaneous**		
	W/F (Wheal/Flare)			**W/F**			**W/F**		
Trees			**Weeds**			**Foods**		
1. Ash			1. Chenopodium			1. Egg		
2. Poplar			2. Pigweed			2. Milk		
3. Willow			3. Mugwort			3. Soybean		
4. Cypress			4. Plantain			4. Peanut		
5. Alder			5. Russian Thistle			5. Wheat		
6. Olive tree			6. Parietaria			6. Sesame seed		
7. Privet			7. Ragweed			7. Almond		
8. Eastern Oak mix			8. Nettle			8. Cashew		
9. Juniper mix			9. Dandelion			9. Hazelnut		
10. Birch mix			10. Weed mix			10. Walnut		
11. Cedar mountain			**Molds**			11. Shrimp		
12. Sycamore			1. Alternaria			12. Crab		
13. Pine mix			2. Penicillium mix			13. Clam		
Grasses			3. Aspergillus mix			14. Fish mix		
1. Bermuda			4. Mold mix 3					
2. Timothy			**Household inhalants**					
3. Ryegrass			1. D. farinae					
4. cereal			2. D. pteronyssinus					
4. grasses			3. Cockroach					
6. 7 grass mix			**Animals**					
Miscellaneous			1. Cat					
1			2. Dog					
2			3. Feather mix			**Controls**		
3						Saline		
4						Histamine		
5								

confirmed in 21% of the cases. The authors emphasized the underdiagnosis of allergy in athletes with respiratory symptoms [63]. In a survey by Surda et al. using a validated questionnaire, the authors reported rhinitis in elite and non-elite swimmers in 45% and 31% of cases, respectively, and in non-swimming athletes in 24% of cases [64]. Grace et al. investigated the prevalence of grass-pollen-related allergic rhinitis and conjunctivitis in 254 elite amateur Irish athletes and reported positive skin testing to at least one allergen in 27.1% of the cases. Among the most common allergens were grass pollen and house dust mite in 16.5% and 22%, respectively. All subjects had skin testing for six aeroallergens and had completed the AQUA [65]. Bougault et al. investigated the prevalence of allergies using skin testing in 85 soccer players and detected allergic disease in 33% of the cases. One out of two players (49%) had been sensitized to at least one respiratory allergen. The authors pointed to the underdiagnosis of allergy and exercise-induced bronchoconstriction in soccer players [66]. In a study by Alves et al. on the prevalence of exercise-induced rhinitis in 19 competitive swimmers and 13 professional runners, the authors reported an increase in symptoms of rhinitis in the former group. The most commonly described symptoms were nasal congestion, sneezing, and postnasal drip. Exercise-induced symptoms of rhinitis occurred mainly in nonatopic subjects. The decrease in peak inspiratory flow and the significant increase in post-nasal drip in that study supported the presence of what the authors referred to as "swimming-induced rhinitis" [67]. Perrotta et al. investigated the prevalence of allergy in 226 Italian bikers using AQUA and showed a prevalence of 47.8%. The majority of patients experienced symptoms of upper respiratory tract infections, particularly those whose training exceeded 3 hours per session [68]. Robson-Ansley et al. investigated the prevalence of allergy and upper respiratory tract symptoms using AQUA and serum level of immunoglobulin E in 208 runners of the London Marathon. The results showed that 40% had allergy and 47% had upper respiratory symptoms following the marathon. Moreover, there was an association between upper respiratory tract symptoms and a positive AQUA. AQUA was a significant predictor of upper respiratory tract symptoms [69]. In 2018, Teixeira et al. evaluated allergic symptoms and atopy in 59 elite endurance athletes and reported a prevalence of 54.2% and 57.6%, respectively. The studied group was evaluated using a validated allergy questionnaire and IgE levels. There was a notable lack of association between the presence of allergic symptoms and atopy in that study group [70]. The high prevalence of allergy in athletes is comparable to that observed in teachers, which is higher than that reported in the normal population [71–73]. In a study of 104 teachers by Lin et al., the respiratory health symptoms were mostly secondary to allergy and asthma and were attributed to poor working environment conditions and inappropriate ventilation system [71]. Similarly, in a study by Ohlsson et al. on the prevalence of voice symptoms in student teachers, the authors reported allergy as a main risk factor in addition to smoking, repeated throat infections, and voice-demanding hobbies. Seventeen percent of the study group had voice problems, and more than 25% of those had airborne allergens [72].

The high prevalence of allergy in athletes goes hand in hand with the high prevalence of nasal dysfunction and its associated adverse effect on athletes' physical performance [74–76]. Given the well-known nasal dysfunction associated with allergy and based on the unified airway concept by Krouse et al. [77], one can extrapolate that sports-related allergy is also a significant risk factor for dysphonia. An allergy-induced inflammatory reaction at one site of the airway may trigger a similar one at a different site. To that end, athletes with allergic rhinitis are more prone to develop voice disorders than those with no allergy. Using a questionnaire in 103 subjects, 49 of whom had been diagnosed with respiratory allergy, Simberg et al. showed a higher prevalence of dysphonia in patients with diagnosed respiratory allergies, particularly professional voice users, compared with nonallergic subjects [78]. Similarly, Randhawa et al. examined voice symptoms in 70 subjects undergoing allergy skin testing and reported the prevalence of these symptoms in 23.7% vs. only 7.8% in the control group [79]. Similarly, Turley et al. showed three times higher prevalence of voice symptoms in patients with nonallergic rhinitis and four times higher prevalence of voice symptoms in patients with allergic rhinitis in comparison to a control group. The study included 250 patients who were investigated using voice-related quality of life-validated questionnaires [80]. Interestingly, allergy is also more common in patients with dysphonia vs. patients with no dysphonia. Hamdan et al. proved that singers with voice complaints were more likely to have allergy than those with no voice complaint [81]. The study was conducted on 45 singers using a validated allergy questionnaire. Likewise, Altman et al. reported positive skin testing in almost one-third of patients with muscle tension dysphonia [82], and Brook et al. reported positive allergy testing in one out of two patients with globus sensation, hoarseness, and throat clearing [83]. Note that there was no control group in either studies.

The pathophysiology of dysphonia in athletes with allergy is multifaceted. Both mechanical factors and behavioral patterns are described in the literature. Trafficking of mucus either from the nose and sinuses downward or from the lungs upward is the most accepted explanation in affected patients [77, 84, 85] (Fig. 5.7). Other causes include local inflammatory laryngeal reaction [86–88]. Roth et al. showed that exposure of the vocal folds to an allergen results in voice dysfunction and in an increase in phonatory threshold pressure [86]. Similarly, Ansaranta et al. demonstrated the presence of laryngeal edematous and erythematous changes in patients with throat symptoms following histamine challenge [87]. These findings were substantiated by Belafsky et al. who also showed the presence of elevated eosinophil counts in the mucosal lining of the upper airway following exposure to iron soot and house mite allergens [88].

In summary, the prevalence of allergy in SOVU is high. Exposure to outdoor and/or indoor airborne allergens results in an array of upper respiratory symptoms. In view of the unified airway concept, affected patients are at a high risk of developing change in voice quality. The voice symptoms may be attributed to structural laryngeal changes or to dysfunction in laryngeal behavior. Proper workup of allergy in SOVU with upper airway symptoms cannot be overemphasized.

Fig. 5.7 Laryngeal examination of a patient with allergic rhinitis showing evidence of mucosal erythema, inflammation, and mucus strand between the vocal folds

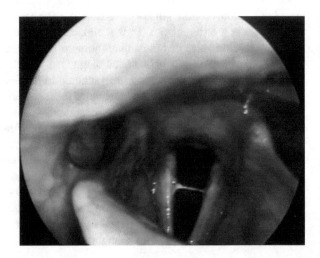

5.3.2 Background Noise and Poor Working Environment Acoustics

Sports occupational voice users are forced to vocalize in noisy environments. Athletic participants, spectators, cheerleaders, background music, and amplified announcers are mostly responsible for the background noise, pushing coaches, fitness instructors, and athletes to raise their voices in order to be heard. This vocal load increases in the presence of poor working environment acoustics. Numerous studies have shown that background noise and poor environment acoustics jeopardize phonation. Buckley et al. investigated vocal health and occupational voice use of 12 professional football coaches and showed that the background noise, the distance between coaches and their players, the need to phonate for prolonged period, and the room acoustics were serious occupational voice hazards [10]. The data analyzed were retrieved using a self-rating voice questionnaire and a semi-structured interview on their self-perception of vocal health. Similarly, O'Neil and McMenamin explored the day-to-day experiences of five soccer coaches and showed that the background noise of spectators, the distance between coaches and players, and the duration of the soccer match increased vocal loading as determined by their semi-structured interview. The authors emphasized the adverse impact of both environmental factors and psychosocial and personal factors on voice [4]. In 2015, Penteado et al. assessed the impact of stress and work environment on voice in 13 soccer coaches and 13 physical trainers. The authors reported that noise and acoustic problems aggravated voice disorders, often resulting in voice fatigue and alteration in voice quality [89]. In another study by Fellman and Simberg on vocal risk factors among soccer coaches, the authors reported loud background noise and reverberating environment among the most significant risk factors [11]. In a study by Rumbach on 38 fitness instructors with dysphonia, the authors highlighted that lack of sound amplification is a concern that often raised conflicts between fitness instructors and the management team, which sometimes led to withdrawal of instructors from the fitness industry [9].

All the above indicates that background noise and poor working environment acoustics are major threats to SOVU. This is not surprising given the well-known impact of noise as a pollutant. Noise is a hazard to our well-being. According to the World Health Organization, environmental noise can jeopardize the physical and emotional status of the human being. Noise has been incriminated in the pathogenesis of stress, irritability, alteration in mood and cognitive behavior, and nervousness [90]. Noise is also an acoustic hazard to phonation. An increase in background noise is frequently associated with high voice demand [91]. Numerous studies have confirmed the relation between environmental noise and vocal dose. The latter is a term used to quantify the exposure of the vocal folds to stress during contact acceleration or deceleration [92, 93]. It relates to the distance travelled by vocal folds' tissue particles, the energy dissipated during vocal fold contact, and the total phonation time. As such, prolonged phonation increases the risk of vocal fold injury, whereas pauses in phonation during speech enhance safety of the vocal folds [93].

With an increase in environmental noise, there is an increase in both voice intensity and vocal pitch. In a study by Guidini et al. on the correlation between classroom noise and teachers' voices, the authors reported an increase in teachers' voice intensity as the classroom noise increased. The teachers' voice intensity reached 68 dB, exceeding the average noise in the class by 7.48 Db [94]. Phadke et al. reported that 50% of teachers are forced to raise their voice in noisy classrooms. The sources of noise were road traffic, students' activities, and other classrooms [95]. Using self-report questionnaire, de Medeiros et al. found an association between high noise level and dysphonia in a study that included 2,103 teachers. Other environment- and work-related factors associated with dysphonia included poor ventilation and the need to perform intensive activities [96]. Similarly, Rabelo et al. investigated the influence of noise on vocal dose in 27 women using a voice questionnaire and auditory perceptual evaluation. The participants were evaluated under two conditions, in a classroom treated acoustically and in a classroom not treated acoustically. The results showed a significant increase in vocal dose, fundamental frequency, vocal intensity, and percentage of phonation with an increase in the background noise. Moreover, there was a significant increase in both fundamental frequency and intensity [97].

In summary, the literature confirms that noise is a significant threat that leads to compensatory increase in both vocal loudness and pitch. Sports occupational voice users performing in a noisy environment with poor acoustics are at higher risk of developing voice disorders in comparison to the normal population. The stress of communication is further accentuated in the current COVID pandemic. Wearing face masks is adding to the difficulty in verbalizing and being heard. Future studies investigating the correlation between sports environment acoustics and phonation are needed.

5.3.3   Altitude-Related Illnesses and Voice Disorders in Athletes

High altitude is one of many environment-related health risk factors [98]. The last decades have witnessed an upsurge in the number of high-altitude athletes such as hikers, mountain bikers, and cross-country skiers. Occasionally, mainstream athletic events such as the Olympics are held in cities at high altitude such as Mexico City. This upsurge has put high-altitude athletes, particularly those who ascent at a fast rate, at a significant risk for numerous health conditions. Altitude-associated health hazards can be stratified as acute or chronic [99–101]. The acute response to high altitude includes hyperventilation, tachycardia, and transient increase in blood pressure in attempt to compensate for the decrease in atmospheric oxygen. Other acute physiologic responses include an increase in renal bicarbonate excretion, diuresis, decrease in neurotransmitters synthesis, cerebral vasodilatation, and decrease in cognitive as well as sensory-motor function. In chronic altitude illnesses, patients develop compensatory increase in hemoglobin concentration, extreme polycythemia, cardiomyopathy, and pulmonary hypertension. These changes usually are addressed either pharmacologically or through training programs, the most important of which are live high-train high (LHTH), live low-train high (LLTH), and live high-train low (LHTL) [102, 103].

The acute and chronic physiologic responses to high altitude affect the physical performance of athletes. Given the neuromuscular structure of the larynx and vocal tract and their intricate association with body metabolic rate and respiratory support, voice is undoubtedly in jeopardy. Although there are no studies in the literature on voice changes in athletes at high altitude, one can fairly speculate that the cardiorespiratory and neuromuscular changes experienced at high altitude impact phonation adversely. Future studies in that regard are warranted.

High altitude is an environmental health risk factors. Athletes who train or compete at high altitude are subject to acute and chronic pathophysiologic changes that can affect their physical performance. The phonatory apparatus, similar to other systems in the body, is at risk of dysfunction leading to change in voice quality. Athletes, coaches, and sports mangers need to be aware of altitude-related phonatory adverse effects.

5.3.4 Temperature-Related Illnesses and Voice Disorders in Athletes

Similar to variations in altitude, variations in temperature effect on muscle function and athletic performance. Body temperature is one of the main indicators of health, and muscle temperature plays a role in regulating core temperature. There is a consensus that muscle contraction produces heat and that muscle contractility is affected by variation in body temperature. An increase in muscle temperature results in an increase in force development, contraction velocity, tetanic force, neural drive, and conduction velocity [104–108]. Moreover, an increase in temperature improves blood circulation within the muscle and improves metabolite clearance. Decrease in muscle temperature results in slower muscle contraction, a decrease in the sensibility of actomysion to calcium, and a decrease in nerve conduction velocity [109]. Additionally, a decrease in temperature promotes muscle glycolysis and accumulation of lactate [110]. Athletes training outdoors are very prone to temperature-related dysfunctions and illnesses, particularly athletes exposed to intensive training or physical activity in an environment with extreme temperature [110, 111].

Given the known effect of variations in temperature on muscle performance, athletes exposed to high or low temperature are at a significant risk of developing dysphonia. This can be attributed to impairment in laryngeal muscle function and/or changes in vocal fold rheologic properties. Future studies in that field are needed.

5.3.5   Humidity-Related Change in Voice Quality in Athletes

Athletes who exercise or compete in a low-humidity environment are at a significant risk of developing voice disorders. A low-humidity climate, similar to dehydration and high temperature, is thought of as a significant risk factor for dysphonia. In 2007, Tanner et al. investigated the effect of oral breathing of dry air with a relative humidity of less than 1% on voice, and they reported an increase in average phonatory threshold pressure by 0.5 cm H_2O [112]. Similarly, in 2016, the same authors reported an increase in self-reported effort and cepstral index of dysphonia following laryngeal drying with low-humidity air. The authors described an improvement after treatment with nebulized saline at different concentrations. Although the authors did not generalize the phonatory physiologic changes experienced following laryngeal desiccation, the authors noted the therapeutic effect of nebulized treatment [113]. These results were confirmed by similar studies on patients with Sjögren syndrome. Both acoustics and self-rating of voice severity improved by almost 20% following topical vocal fold hydration using nebulized isotonic saline [114]. This is in agreement with a previous study on indoor humidity and associated health effects. Wolkoff reported that elevated humidity improves symptoms of vocal fatigue and reduces the frequency of nasal symptoms, particularly in patients with obstructive sleep apnea [115].

All the above confirms that low humidity is an environmental challenge to phonation. This challenge increases in excessive heat conditions. Humidity plays a crucial role in dissipating exercise-induced heat. It is considered as the main cooling mechanisms when the ambient temperature exceeds 20 °C [116]. Athletes who perform in high-temperature and low-humidity weather are vulnerable to dysphonia as well as other effects of dehydration.

Humidity is another environmental challenge to athletes. Low humidity, particularly in high-temperature environments, may impact phonation. The phonatory apparatus, similar to other systems, is in jeopardy.

References

1. Rumbach AF, Maddox M, Hull M, Khidr A. Laryngeal symptoms in weightlifting athletes. J Voice. 2020;34(6):964.
2. Paluska SA, Lansford CD. Laryngeal trauma in sport. Curr Sports Med Rep. 2008;7(1):16–21.
3. Marcinow AM, Thompson J, Chiang T, Forrest LA, de Silva BW. Paradoxical vocal fold motion disorder in the elite athlete: experience at a Large Division I University. Laryngoscope. 2014;124(6):1425–30.
4. O'Neill J, McMenamin R. Voice use in professional soccer management. Logoped Phoniatr Vocol. 2014;39(4):169–78.
5. Gould D, Greenleaf C, Guinan D, Chung Y. A survey of US Olympic coaches: variables perceived to have influenced athlete performances and coach effectiveness. Sport Psychol. 2002;16(3):229–50.

6. Fontan L, Fraval M, Michon A, Déjean S, Welby-Gieusse M. Vocal problems in sports and fitness instructors: a study of prevalence, risk factors, and need for prevention in France. J Voice. 2017;31(2):261.e33–8.

7. Rumbach A, Khan A, Brown M, Eloff K, Poetschke A. Voice problems in the fitness industry: factors associated with chronic hoarseness. Int J Speech Lang Pathol. 2015;17(5):441–50.

8. Long J, Williford HN, Olson MS, Wolfe V. Voice problems and risk factors among aerobics instructors. J Voice. 1998;12(2):197–207.

9. Rumbach AF. Voice problems of group fitness instructors: diagnosis, treatment, perceived and experienced attitudes and expectations of the industry. J Voice. 2013;27(6):786.e1–9.

10. Buckley KL, O'Halloran PD, Oates JM. Occupational vocal health of elite sports coaches: an exploratory pilot study of football coaches. J Voice. 2015;29(4):476–83.

11. Fellman D, Simberg S. Prevalence and risk factors for voice problems among soccer coaches. J Voice. 2017;31(1):121.e9–15.

12. Heidel SE, Torgerson JK. Vocal problems among aerobic instructors and aerobic participants. J Commun Disord. 1993;26(3):179–91.

13. Pany S, Panigrahi SK, Rao EV, Patnaik L, Sahu T. Anabolic androgenic steroid abuse and their health impacts: a cross-sectional study among body builders in a city of Eastern India. Int J Prev Med. 2019;10:178.

14. Leppanen K, Ilomaki I, Laukkanen AM. One-year follow-up study of self-evaluated effects of voice massage, voice training, and voice hygiene lecture in female teachers. Logoped Phoniatr Vocol. 2010;35:13–8.

15. Porcaro CK, Howery S, Suhandron A, Gollery T, et al. Impact of vocal hygiene training on teachers' willingness to change vocal behaviors. J Voice. 2019; S0892-1997(19)30427-8.

16. Logan-Sprenger HM. Fluid balance and thermoregulatory responses of competitive triathletes. J Therm Biol. 2019;79:69–72.

17. Judelson DA, Maresh CM, Anderson JM, et al. Hydration and muscular performance. Sports Med. 2007;37(10):907–21.

18. Barley OR, Chapman DW, Blazevich AJ, Abbiss CR. Acute dehydration impairs endurance without modulating neuromuscular function. Front Physiol. 2018;9:1562.

19. Costa RJ, Hoffman MD, Stellingwerff T. Considerations for ultra-endurance activities: part 1-nutrition. Res Sports Med. 2019;27(2):166–81.

20. Barnes KA, Anderson ML, Stofan JR, et al. Normative data for sweating rate, sweat sodium concentration, and sweat sodium loss in athletes: an update and analysis by sport. J Sports Sci. 2019;37(20):2356–66.

21. Sekiguchi Y, Adams WM, Curtis RM, Benjamin CL, Casa DJ. Factors influencing hydration status during a National Collegiate Athletics Association Division 1 Soccer Preseason. J Sci Med Sport. 2019;22(6):624–8.

22. Love TD, Baker DF, Healey P, Black KE. Measured and perceived indices of fluid balance in professional athletes. The use and impact of hydration assessment strategies. Eur J Sport Sci. 2018;18(3):349–56.

23. Jones LC, Cleary MA, Lopez RM, Zuri RE, Lopez R. Active dehydration impairs upper and lower body anaerobic muscular power. J Strength Cond Res. 2008;22(2):455–63.

24. Kovacs MS. A review of fluid and hydration in competitive tennis. Int J Sports Physiol Perform. 2008;3(4):413–23.

25. Riebl SK, Davy BM. The hydration equation: update on water balance and cognitive performance. ACSMs Health Fit J. 2013;17(6):21–8.

26. Chan RW, Tayama N. Biomechanical effects of hydration in vocal fold tissues. Otolaryngol Head Neck Surg. 2002;126(5):528–37.

27. Verdolini K, Titze IR, Fennel A. Dependence of phonatory effort on hydration level. J Speech Hear Res. 1994;37(5):1001–7.

28. Verdolini-Marston K, Sandage M, Titze I. Effect of hydration treatment on laryngeal nodules and polyps and related voice measures. J Voice. 1994;8:30–47.

29. Solomon NP, DiMattia MS. Effects of a vocally fatiguing task and systemic hydration on phonation threshold pressure. J Voice. 2000;14(3):341–62.
30. Solomon NP, Glaze LE, Arnold RR, van Mersbergen M. Effects of a vocally fatiguing task and systemic hydration on men's voices. J Voice. 2003;17(1):31–46.
31. Fisher KV, Ligon J, Sobecks JL, Roxe DM. Phonatory effects of body fluid removal. J Speech Lang Hear Res. 2001;44(2):354–67.
32. Hamdan AL, Sibai A, Rameh C. Effect of fasting on voice in women. J Voice. 2007;21(4):495–501.
33. Hamdan AL, Ashkar J, Sibai A, Oubari D, Husseini ST. Effect of fasting on voice in males. Am J Otolaryngol. 2011;32(2):124–9.
34. Akinbami LJ, Rossen LM, Fakhouri TH, Fryar CD. Asthma prevalence trends by weight status among US children aged 2–19 years, 1988–2014. Pediatr Obes. 2018;13(6):393–6.
35. Gleeson M, Pyne DB. Respiratory inflammation and infections in high-performance athletes. Immunol Cell Biol. 2016;94(2):124–31.
36. Bonini M, Gramiccioni C, Fioretti D, et al. Asthma, allergy and the Olympics: a 12-year survey in elite athletes. Curr Opin Allergy Clin Immunol. 2015;15(2):184–92.
37. Lund TK. Asthma in elite athletes: how do we manage asthma-like symptoms and asthma in elite athletes? Clin Respir J. 2009;3(2):123.
38. Lennelöv E, Irewall T, Naumburg E, Lindberg A, Stenfors N. The prevalence of asthma and respiratory symptoms among cross-country skiers in early adolescence. Can Respir J. 2019;2019:1514353.
39. Boulet LP, Turmel J, Irwin RS, et al. Cough in the athlete: CHEST guideline and expert panel report. Chest. 2017;151(2):441–54.
40. Fields KB, Thekkekandam TJ, Neal S. Wheezing after respiratory tract infection in athletes. Curr Sports Med Rep. 2012;11(2):85–9.
41. Colbey C, Cox AJ, Pyne DB, Zhang P, Cripps AW, West NP. Upper respiratory symptoms, gut health and mucosal immunity in athletes. Sports Med. 2018;48(1):65–77.
42. Hamdan AL. Laryngeal manifestations of respiratory disorders. In: Hamdan AL, Sataloff RT, Hawkshaw MJ. Laryngeal manifestations of systemic diseases. San Diego: Plural Publishing; 2018. p. 159–82.
43. Waterman JJ, Kapur R. Upper gastrointestinal issues in athletes. Curr Sports Med Rep. 2012;11(2):99–104.
44. Hoffman MD. Performance trends in 161-km ultramarathons. Int J Sports Med. 2010;31(01):31–7.
45. Paluska SA. Current concepts: recognition and management of common activity-related gastrointestinal disorders. Phys Sports Med. 2009;37(1):54–63.
46. Simons SM, Kennedy RG. Gastrointestinal problems in runners. Curr Sports Med Rep. 2004;3(2):112–6.
47. Leggit JC. Evaluation and treatment of GERD and upper GI complaints in athletes. Curr Sports Med Rep. 2011;10(2):109–14.
48. Singh AM, McGregor RS. Differential diagnosis of chest symptoms in the athlete. Clin Rev Allergy Immunol. 2005;29(2):87–96.
49. Khodaee M, Ansari M. Common ultramarathon injuries and illnesses: race day management. Curr Sports Med Rep. 2012;11(6):290–7.
50. Collings KL, Pratt PF, Rodriguez-Stanley S, Bemben M, Miner PB. Esophageal reflux in conditioned runners, cyclists, and weightlifters. Med Sci Sports Exerc. 2003;35(5):730–5.
51. Jozkow P, Wasko-Czopnik D, Dunajska K, Medras M, Paradowski L. The relationship between gastroesophageal reflux disease and the level of physical activity. Swiss Med Wkly. 2007;137(3334):465–70.
52. Jozkow P, Wasko-Czopnik D, Medras M, Paradowski L. Gastroesophageal reflux disease and physical activity. Sports Med. 2006;36(5):385–91.

53. Bitnar P, Stovicek J, Andel R, et al. Leg raise increases pressure in lower and upper esophageal sphincter among patients with gastroesophageal reflux disease. J Bodyw Mov Ther. 2016;20(3):518–24.
54. Ravi N, Stuart RC, Byrne PJ, Reynolds JV. Effect of physical exercise on esophageal motility in patients with esophageal disease. Dis Esophagus. 2005;18(6):374–7.
55. van Nieuwenhoven MA, Brouns F, Brummer RJ. Gastrointestinal profile of symptomatic athletes at rest and during physical exercise. Eur J Appl Physiol. 2004;91(4):429–34.
56. Jaspersen D, Kulig M, Labenz J, et al. Prevalence of extraesophageal manifestations in gastroesophageal reflux disease: an analysis based on the ProGERD study. Aliment Pharmacol Ther. 2003;17(12):1515–20.
57. Koufman JA. Laryngopharyngeal reflux 2002: a new paradigm of airway disease. Ear Nose Throat J. 2002;81(9 Suppl 2):2–6.
58. Koufman JA. Laryngopharyngeal reflux is different from classic gastroesophageal reflux disease. Ear Nose Throat J. 2002;81(9 Suppl 2):7–9.
59. Sataloff RT, Castell DO, Katz PO, Sataloff DM, Hawkshaw MJ. Reflux and other gastroenterologic conditions that may affect the voice. In: Sataloff RT. Professional voice: the science and art of clinical care. 4th ed. San Diego: Plural Publishing; 2017. p. 907–98.
60. Lechien JR, Saussez S, Harmegnies B, Finck C, Burns JA. Laryngopharyngeal reflux and voice disorders: a multifactorial model of etiology and pathophysiology. J Voice. 2017;31(6):733–52.
61. Del Giacco SR, Carlsen KH, Du Toit G. Allergy and sports in children. Pediatr Allergy Immunol. 2012;23(1):11–20.
62. Bonini M, Braido F, Baiardini I, et al. AQUA©: allergy questionnaire for athletes. Development and validation. Med Sci Sports Exerc. 2009;41(5):1034–41.
63. Kurowski M, Jurczyk J, Krysztofiak H, Kowalski ML. Exercise-induced respiratory symptoms and allergy in elite athletes: allergy and asthma in polish Olympic athletes (A2POLO) project within GA2LEN initiative. Clin Respir J. 2016;10(2):231–8.
64. Surda P, Putala M, Siarnik P, Walker A, Bernic A, Fokkens W. Rhinitis and its impact on quality of life in swimmers. Allergy. 2018;73(5):1022–31.
65. Grace M, Hunt D, Hourihane JO. The prevalence of grass pollen-related allergic rhinoconjunctivitis in Elite Amateur Irish Athletes. Ir Med J. 2016;109(8):448.
66. Bougault V, Drouard F, Legall F, Dupont G, Wallaert B. Allergies and exercise-induced bronchoconstriction in a youth academy and reserve professional soccer team. Clin J Sport Med. 2017;27(5):450–6.
67. Alves A, Martins C, Delgado L, Fonseca J, Moreira A. Exercise-induced rhinitis in competitive swimmers. Am J Rhinol Allergy. 2010;24(5):e114–7.
68. Perrotta F, Simeon V, Bonini M, et al. Evaluation of allergic diseases, symptom control, and relation to infections in a Group of Italian Elite Mountain Bikers. Clin J Sport Med. 2020;30(5):465–9.
69. Robson-Ansley P, Howatson G, Tallent J, et al. Prevalence of allergy and upper respiratory tract symptoms in runners of the London marathon. Med Sci Sports Exerc. 2012;44(6):999–1004.
70. Teixeira RN, dos Santos Leite G, Bonini M, et al. Atopy in elite endurance athletes. Clin J Sport Med. 2018;28(3):268–71.
71. Lin S, Lawrence WR, Lin Z, Francois M, Neamtiu IA, Lin Q, Csobod E, Gurzau ES. Teacher respiratory health symptoms in relation to school and home environment. Int Arch Occup Environ Health. 2017;90(8):725–39.
72. Ohlsson AC, Andersson EM, Södersten M, Simberg S, Barregård L. Prevalence of voice symptoms and risk factors in teacher students. J Voice. 2012;26(5):629–34.
73. Ebert CS, Pillsbury HC. Epidemiology of allergy. Otolaryngol Clin North Am. 2011;44(3):537–48.
74. Walker AC, Surda P, Rossiter M, Little SA. Nasal disease and quality of life in athletes. J Laryngol Otol. 2018;132(9):812–5.

75. Salem L, Dao VA, Shah-Hosseini K, Mester J, Mösges R, Vent J. Impaired sports performance of athletes suffering from pollen-induced allergic rhinitis: a cross-sectional, observational survey in German athletes. J Sports Med Phys Fitness. 2019;59(4):686–92.
76. Tokodi M, Csábi E, Kiricsi Á, et al. The effect of nasal provocation with a single-dose allergen on the physical and cognitive performance of patients with ragweed allergy. Physiol Int. 2017;104(4):334–43.
77. Krouse JH, Altman KW. Rhinogenic laryngitis, cough, and the unified airway. Otolaryngol Clin North Am. 2010;43(1):111–21.
78. Simberg S, Sala E, Tuomainen J, Rönnemaa AM. Vocal symptoms and allergy–a pilot study. J Voice. 2009;23(1):136–9.
79. Randhawa PS, Nouraei S, Mansuri S, Rubin JS. Allergic laryngitis as a cause of dysphonia: a preliminary report. Logoped Phoniatr Vocol. 2010;35(4):169–74.
80. Turley R, Cohen SM, Becker A, Ebert CS Jr. Role of rhinitis in laryngitis: another dimension of the unified airway. Ann Otol Rhinol Laryngol. 2011;120(8):505–10.
81. Hamdan AL, Sibai A, Youssef M, Deeb R, Zaitoun F. The use of a screening questionnaire to determine the incidence of allergic rhinitis in singers with dysphonia. Arch Otolaryngol Head Neck Surg. 2006;132(5):547–9.
82. Altman KW, Atkinson C, Lazarus C. Current and emerging concepts in muscle tension dysphonia: a 30-month review. J Voice. 2005;19(2):261–7.
83. Brook CD, Platt MP, Reese S, Noordzij JP. Utility of allergy testing in patients with chronic laryngopharyngeal symptoms: is it allergic laryngitis? Otolaryngol Head Neck Surg. 2016;154(1):41–5.
84. Grossman J. One airway, one disease. Chest. 1997;111(2):11S–6S.
85. Dworkin-Valenti JP, Sugihara E, Stern N, Naumann I, Bathula S, Amjad E. Laryngeal inflammation. Ann Otol Rhinol. 2015;2:1058–66.
86. Roth DF, Abbott KV, Carroll TL, Ferguson BJ. Evidence for primary laryngeal inhalant allergy: a randomized, double-blinded crossover study. Int Forum Allergy Rhinol. 2013;3(1):10–8.
87. Ansaranta M, Geneid A, Kauppi P, Malmberg LP, Vilkman E. Laryngeal mucosal reaction during bronchial histamine challenge test visualized by videolaryngostroboscopy. J Voice. 2017;31(4):470–5.
88. Belafsky PC, Peake J, Smiley-Jewell SM, Verma SP, Dworkin-Valenti J, Pinkerton KE. Soot and house dust mite allergen cause eosinophilic laryngitis in an animal model. Laryngoscope. 2016;126(1):108–12.
89. Penteado RZ, Silva NB, Montebello MI. Voice, stress, work and quality of life of soccer coaches and physical trainers. Codas. 2015;27(6):588–97.
90. Berglund B, Lindvall, T, Schwela DH; World Health Organization Occupational and Environmental Health Team. Guidelines for community noise. London: World Health Organization. Published April, 1999. Accessed 1 Oct 2020. https://apps.who.int/iris/handle/10665/66217.
91. Cutiva LC, Burdorf A. Effects of noise and acoustics in schools on vocal health in teachers. Noise Health. 2015;17:17–22.
92. Svec JG, Popolo PS, Titze IR. Measurement of vocal doses in speech: experimental procedure and signal processing. Logoped Phoniatr Vocol. 2003;28:181–92.
93. Titze IR, Svec JG, Popolo PS. Vocal dose measures: quantifying accumulated vibration exposure in vocal fold tissues. J Speech Lang Hear Res. 2003;46:919–32.
94. Fernanda Guidini R, Bertoncello F, Zanchetta S, Suzigan Dragone ML. Correlations between classroom environmental noise and teachers' voice. Revista da Sociedade Brasileira de Fonoaudiologia. 2012;17(4):398–404.
95. Phadke KV, Abo-Hasseba A, Švec JG, Geneid A. Influence of noise resulting from the location and conditions of classrooms and schools in Upper Egypt on teachers' voices. J Voice. 2019;33(5):802–e1.

96. de Medeiros AM, Barreto SM, Assunção AÁ. Voice disorders (dysphonia) in public school female teachers working in Belo Horizonte: prevalence and associated factors. J Voice. 2008;22(6):676–87.

97. Rabelo AT, Santos JN, Souza BO, Gama AC, de Castro Magalhães M. The influence of noise on the vocal dose in women. J Voice. 2019;33(2):214–9.

98. Huey RB, Eguskitza X. Limits to human performance: elevated risks on high mountains. J Exp Biol. 2001;204(Pt 18):3115–9.

99. Bergeron MF, Bahr R, Bartsch P, et al. International Olympic Committee consensus statement on thermoregulatory and altitude challenges for high-level athletes. Br J Sports Med. 2012;46:770–9.

100. Fulco CS, Beidleman BA, Muza SR. Effectiveness of preacclimatization strategies for high-altitude exposure. Exerc Sport Sci Rev. 2013;41:55–63.

101. Hackett PH, Roach RC. High-altitude illness. N Engl J Med. 2001;345:107–14.

102. Wilber RL, Stray-Gundersen J, Levine BD. Effect of hypoxic "dose" on physiological responses and sea-level performance. Med Sci Sports Exerc. 2007;39:1590–9.

103. Koehle MS, Cheng I, Sporer B. Canadian Academy of Sport and Exercise Medicine position statement: athletes at high altitude. Clin J Sport Med. 2014;24:120–7.

104. Racinais S, Oksa J. Temperature and neuromuscular function. Scand J Med Sci Sports. 2010;20(Suppl 3):1–18.

105. Oksa J, Rintamäki H, Mäkinen T, Martikkala V, Rusko H. EMG-activity and muscular performance of lower leg during stretch-shortening cycle after cooling. Acta Physiol Scand. 1996;157:1–8.

106. Bàràny M. ATPase activity of myosin correlated with speed of muscle shortening. J Gen Physiol. 1967;50:197–218.

107. Segal SS, Faulkner JA, White TP. Skeletal muscle fatigue in vitro is temperature dependent. J Appl Physiol. 1986;61:660–5.

108. Stephenson DG, Williams DA. Calcium-activated force responses in fast- and slow-twitch skinned muscle fibers of the rat at different temperatures. J Physiol. 1981;317:281–302.

109. Bigland-Ritchie B, Donovan EF, Roussos CS. Conduction velocity and EMG power spectrum changes in fatigue of sustained maximal efforts. J Appl Physiol. 1981;51:1300–5.

110. Blomstrand E, Bergh U, Essen-Gustavsson B, Ekblom B. Influence of low muscle temperature on muscle metabolism during intense dynamic exercise. Acta Physiol Scand. 1984;120:229–36.

111. Khodaee M, Ansari M. Common ultramarathon injuries and illnesses: race day management. Am Coll Sports Med. 2012;11(6):290–7.

112. Tanner K, Roy N, Merrill RM, Elstad M. The effects of three nebulized osmotic agents in the dry larynx. J Speech Lang Hear Res. 2007;50(3):635–46.

113. Tanner K, Fujiki RB, Dromey C, Merrill RM, Robb W, Kendall KA, Hopkin JA, Channell RW, Sivasankar MP. Laryngeal desiccation challenge and nebulized isotonic saline in healthy male singers and nonsingers: effects on acoustic, aerodynamic, and self-perceived effort and dryness measures. J Voice. 2016;30(6):670–6.

114. Tanner K, Nissen SL, Merrill RM, Miner A, Channell RW, Miller KL, Elstad M, Kendall KA, Roy N. Nebulized isotonic saline improves voice production in Sjögren's syndrome. Laryngoscope. 2015;125(10):2333–40.

115. Wolkoff P. Indoor air humidity, air quality, and health–an overview. Int J Hyg Environ Health. 2018;221(3):376–90.

116. Coris EE, Ramirez AM, Van Durme DJ. Heat illness in athletes. Sports Med. 2004;34(1):9–16.

Chapter 6
Voice Disorders in Coaches and Fitness Instructors: Prevalence and Pathophysiology

6.1 Introduction

The lifetime occurrence of voice disorders in the general population is 3–9%, with a point prevalence of 0.98% [1]. The prevalence varies with age, gender, and type of occupation [1–3]. Adult females are more likely to complain of voice disorders than adult males, and elderly people are more prone to voice changes than younger people [2, 3]. In professional voice users who rely heavily on their voice to make a living, the prevalence of dysphonia increases markedly [4–7]. In a large review by Williams which combined two study groups, one from the United States and one from Sweden, the author reported singing and teaching as being among the professions with the highest risk for voice disorders [5]. In another study by Roy et al., the authors noted a higher lifetime prevalence of dysphonia in teachers in comparison to non-teachers (57.7% vs. 28.8%, respectively). The study included 1243 teachers who had been evaluated using a voice disorder questionnaire [6]. Similarly, Cutiva et al. in their systemic review of voice disorders in teachers and non-teachers demonstrated a higher prevalence of dysphonia in teachers. The authors highlighted the etiologic role of work-related factors in the pathogenesis of dysphonia [7]. Martins et al. reported prolonged phonation, poor classroom facilities, and environmental noise as being significant risk factors for dysphonia [8].

Fitness instructors and coaches, similar to professional voice users of other disciplines with high voice demands, are also at a higher risk of developing voice disorders in comparison to the general population. Many of the voice ergonomic risk factors reported in the working environment of teachers, such as poor air quality, noise, stress, and, lack of sound amplifiers, also are described in the working environment of sports-occupational voice users (SOVU) [9–11]. Coaches and fitness instructors often engage in highly demanding voice tasks while performing strenuous exercise. The need to project their voice and communicate in a noisy environment (indoor and/or outdoor) with poor acoustic properties is a day-to-day challenge.

Voice overload may be in the form of prolonged phonation, voicing at a distance, or using pitch and/or loudness out of the individual's comfortable voice range. In a study by Fellman and Simberg, the authors noted that intense voice overload is a common problem that leads to abstention from coaching once a year in 3.7% of cases [12]. In a study by Penteado et al. of 13 soccer coaches and 13 physical trainers, the authors highlighted the voice complaints of participants associated with poor voice care and the stressful working conditions [13]. Coaches and fitness instructors are also under considerable stress and emotional pressure that can affect their voice. Voice is a barometer for one's emotions and psychological equilibrium [14]. In a study by Kelley on stress and burnout of 131 male and 118 female collegiate head baseball and football coaches, the author reported a significant level of emotional exhaustion and a low-to-moderate extent of depersonalization that were predictive of burnout [15]. Similarly, in a review of 12 elite coaches, Thelwell et al. found that coaches perceived themselves as less effective when stressed in comparison to when they are not stressed, which in turn affected their coaching quality and the performance of their teams [16]. The study was conducted using a semistructured interview that looked at stress signals and the impact of stress on coaches and athletes.

This chapter reviews the prevalence of voice disorders in coaches and fitness instructors, with a thorough discussion of the pathophysiology of dysphonia in this group of SOVU. The association between body kinetics and laryngeal behavior is stressed, and the pathogenic role of mouth breathing, lower airway disease, and body fatigue/stress in the development of voice disorders is thoroughly reviewed.

6.2   Prevalence of Voice Disorders in Coaches and Fitness Instructors

Voice complaints in coaches and fitness instructors have spiked with the upsurge in sports activities over the last three to four decades. Similar to professional voice users in other industries, this subgroup of SOVU with high voice demands is at high risk for developing voice disorders. The increased predisposition to dysphonia stems from individual and environmental risk factors. Because of these challenges, laryngeal dysfunction may occur leading to a large array of voice symptoms. In 1993, Heidel and Torgerson reported hoarseness in 55% of female aerobics instructors after having had started instructing. Moreover, 58% of the study group ($n = 50$) reported loss of their voice while instructing or participating in aerobics [17]. Long et al. studied the prevalence of voice problems in 54 aerobics (50 females and 4 males) instructors and reported partial or complete aphonia in 44% of cases. Notably, the voice symptoms were experienced during or following the instruction classes, although a large percentage also had experienced throat discomfort and tension at the start of their career as instructors [18]. In 2002, Wolfe et al. investigated the impact of 30 min of exercise on voice in three female aerobics instructors with voice symptoms and three without voice symptoms. Although there were no significant changes in the perturbation parameters and electroglottographic (EGG) parameters after exercise, aerobics instructors with voice symptoms had an increase in jitter, a decrease in harmonic-to-noise ratio, and an increase in fundamental frequency. These acoustic findings were attributed to excessive laryngeal tension. The authors also noted that using a loud voice for a prolonged period was a precipitating factor for dysphonia [19]. It is worth noting that the study included only six participants and that future investigations on the immediate- and short-term effect of exercise on voice parameters are warranted. Similarly, Newman and Kersner reported the prevalence of voice problems in 52% of female aerobics instructors using a self-completion questionnaire survey. The prevalence of voice problems was associated with the number of teaching hours per week and the amount of stress experienced by the instructor. Instructors who taught more than 10 h per week or had been teaching for more than 6 years were more likely to have voice problems than those who taught less than 10 h per week or had been teaching for 6 years. The authors emphasized the importance of voice training as a preventive measure for dysphonia in this group of occupational voice users whose quality of life was affected adversely by voice dysfunction [20]. Rumbach conducted a study looking at the prevalence of voice disorders in 361 fitness instructors (280 females, 81 males) and reported chronic hoarseness in 39.6%. Strained voice and contracted vocal range were experienced by less than one-third of the subjects [21]. In another study of five male soccer coaches, O'Neil and McMenamin described voice strain with a feeling of tightness in the throat as the most common voice symptom that often was associated with an intermittent change in voice quality and/or aphonia [22]. Additionally, one out of the five subjects in their study group had reported chest tightness that was ascribed to musculoskeletal tension. In 2015, Buckley et al., in their pilot study of occupational voice health of elite sports coaches, reported voice symptoms and sensation of voice fatigue and straining in all their study participants ($n = 12$). The voice symptoms were attributed partially to the percent phonation time (19%) which was moderate and very comparable to that reported in teachers and call center workers (17% and 15%, respectively) [23]. In 2016, in a study by Fontan et al. of 320 sports and fitness instructors, approximately half the subjects (55%) reported difficulties, mainly sore throat and loss of voice. The mean voice handicap index (VHI) of the study group was 12.9, ranging between 0 and 80, with lower means being described in males in comparison to females (10.3 vs. 14.9, respectively) [24]. In 2017, Fellman and Simberg investigated voice health risk factors of 109 soccer coaches and reported two or more voice symptoms in 28.4% of the cases. The most commonly reported voice-related symptoms were throat clearing while talking and hoarseness in 30.3% and 23% of the cases, respectively. The voice symptoms questionnaire included questions such as "voice becomes strained or tires, voice becomes low or hoarse, voice breaks while talking, difficulty in being heard, throat clearing or coughing while talking, and sensation of pain or lump in the throat" [12]. It is important to note that the questionnaire was not a validated questionnaire but the questions were taken from previous investigations on voice problems.

The high prevalence of voice symptoms and phonatory complaints in coaches and fitness instructors has been substantiated by abnormal acoustic and aerodynamic measurements, similar to those that have been reported in other professional voice users such as teachers [25]. In a study by Buckley et al., elite football coaches with voice symptoms had higher-than-normal fundamental frequency (F0) and voice intensity (150 Hz; SD, 30 Hz; and 83.67 Db SPL, respectively). Unfortunately, there was no control group in that study. The authors attributed the findings to phonotrauma and possible vocal fold structural changes [23]. In 2009, Grillo and Fugowski conducted a longitudinal study on the impact of physical education training on voice in seven female teachers using both objective and subjective measures. At the start of the semester, all teachers rated their voice as clear, whereas at the end of the semester, three of the seven reported hoarseness, and six reported voice fatigue. At the middle and end of the semester, there was an increase in the means of F0, shimmer (%), and absolute jitter. The increase in these acoustic parameters was attributed to aberrant vocal fold vibration as a result of high voice demand. Similarly, using repetition of /pi/, the authors found an increase in the mean flow rate and subglottic pressure in the middle of the semester and a decrease in the mean flow rate at the end of the semester. The increase in subglottic pressure and mean flow rate was attributed to incomplete closure of the vocal folds and to compensatory and/or adaptive laryngeal behaviors [26]. In 2016, Dallaston and Rumbach investigated the self-perception of voice quality and the acoustic parameters of six female group fitness instructors before and immediately after 1 h of training. Three of the six instructors reported acute auditory-perceptual and/or sensory changes commensurate with an increase of their VHI scores. There was also a significant increase in both voice intensity and fundamental frequency, which was ascribed to the excessive laryngeal tension following voice loading. The role of excessive tension in increasing the fundamental frequency was substantiated by the inability of the participants following exercise to match the lowest pitch they had before exercise. The authors noted that the acoustic changes were subtle and within the normal range [27]. The linkage between the acoustic and aerodynamic parameters in coaches and fitness instructors with voice disorders supported the results of numerous investigations establishing the interrelationship between subglottic pressure, fundamental frequency, and voice intensity, as well as neuromuscular control of laryngeal function [28, 29].

In summary, the prevalence of voice disorders in coaches and fitness instructors is higher than that reported in the normal population. The voice complaints often are associated with alterations in many acoustic and aerodynamic measurements. These alterations can be attributed to excessive laryngeal tension associated with voice abuse/misuse and the high voice demand. Notably, many of these studies were conducted on small groups of participants. Nevertheless, similar to what have been reported in teachers on the favorable impact of voice hygiene training [30, 31], one can speculate that improvement in voice hygiene awareness and voice training may be beneficial in reducing the prevalence of voice disorders in coaches and fitness instructors. Future studies in SOVU are warranted.

6.3 Pathophysiology of Voice Disorders in Coaches and Fitness Instructors

The etiology of dysphonia in coaches and fitness instructors is multifaceted. Dysphonia can be secondary to functional, structural, and/or neurologic laryngeal disorders. A thorough discussion of laryngeal anatomy and physiology is presented in Chap. 1 and on the diagnosis and treatment of common voice disorders in Chap. 4. In this section, the authors review the pathophysiology of voice disorders in coaches and fitness instructors, with emphasis on the linkage between body kinetics and laryngeal behavior, the effect of mouth breathing on vocal fold vibration, and the adverse effect of exercise-induced bronchoconstriction and body fatigue on voice.

6.3.1 Body Kinetics Behavior and Laryngeal Function

The association between body kinetics behavior and laryngeal function is well known. In 1931, Negus described laryngeal "air trapping" during strenuous exercise as a form of laryngeal hyperfunction that improves musculoskeletal performance (Fig. 6.1) [32]. The trapping of the airflow by the valve-shaped human larynx, similar to that of arboreal animals, allows fixation of the chest wall with subsequent enhancement of performance during physical activity. Similar exercise-induced laryngeal patterns were reported subsequently by many authors. In 2000, Naito and Niimi investigated the laryngeal function of three volunteers who performed various forearm exercises. The authors noted closure of the larynx at the beginning of maximum effort exercise and a 20% decrease in the power of the upper limbs when the larynx was not closed (Fig. 6.2) [33]. Koblick reported hardening of the glottic

Fig. 6.1 Fiber-optic laryngeal examination during "air trapping." (Note the sphincter-like closure of the supraglottic and glottic structures)

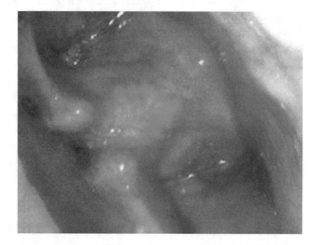

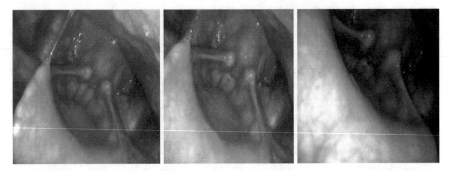

Fig. 6.2 Fiber-optic laryngeal examination showing the supraglottic configuration during arm weight lifting at the start (*left*), 10 s later (*middle*), and 20 s later (*right*)

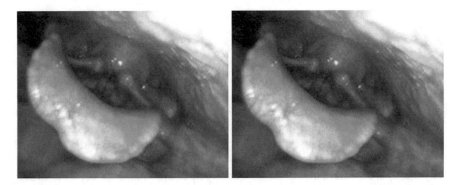

Fig. 6.3 Fiber-optic laryngeal examination showing the supraglottic configuration at the modal register at rest (*left*) and during arm weight lifting (*right*). (Note the difference in the anteroposterior dimension, i.e., the distance between the petiole and inter-arytenoid surface)

attack during phonation when physical activity was performed simultaneously. There was also increased difficulty in speech and inhibition of voice loudness and intensity. The study was conducted on aerobics instructors who were asked to perform speech tasks while exercising [34]. Similar results were reported by Orlikoff who showed an increase in laryngeal resistance and contact quotient during weight lifting. The study was conducted using electroglottography on 20 subjects who were asked to sustain phonation at a comfortable pitch and loudness and to repeat the syllable /pi/ while having their arms stretched and holding weight [35]. Arm weight lifting while performing a glissando at a comfortable pitch and loudness also can result in decreased voice range associated with limited stretching or shortening of the vocal folds (author's observation (ALH)) (Figs. 6.3 and 6.4) The strong linkage between laryngeal behavior and body kinetics has helped in the development of voice therapy exercises to treat glottic insufficiency. Pulling and pushing exercises, in addition to other forms of isometric exercises, have been advocated in the treatment of various laryngeal movement disorders. The rationale behind these exercises is to increase muscle tone and subsequently help improve voice efficiency. The

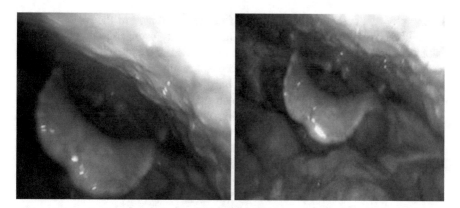

Fig. 6.4 Fiber-optic laryngeal examination showing supraglottic configuration at the low register at rest (*left*) and during arm weight lifting (*right*). (Note the marked shortening in the anteroposterior dimension, i.e., the distance between the petiole and inter-arytenoid surface)

techniques and benefits were described by Sataloff et al. [36, 37] and in a study by Yamaguchi et al. on three cases of glottic incompetence [38].

The information above highlights that physical activity and strain can lead to an increase in contact pressure between the vocal folds, similar to what happens during voice loading. With an increase in voice intensity and/or pitch, there is an increase in adductor contact pressure with forceful closure of the vocal folds [39–41]. In a study by Jiang and Titze on vocal fold intraglottal pressure, the authors noted that the mid-membranous portion of the vocal folds is the most vulnerable part during phonation. The impact pressure is associated with the subglottic pressure and the extent of vocal fold adduction [41]. Similarly, vocal fold intravascular pressure depends on the rate and amplitude of vocal fold vibration during a glottic cycle. Based on a study by Czerwonka et al., with voice loading, the pressure may exceed 20 cm H_2O leading to fluid leakage with subsequent inflammation and formation of vocal fold masses [42]. These findings concur those of Casper in their investigation on the effect of excessive vocalization on vocal fold morphology and function of 42 drill sergeants during the course of 6 days. Using laryngeal videostroboscopic examination, the authors demonstrated the presence of vocal fold edematous and erythematous changes with a decrease in mucosal waves [43]. Drill sergeants may be included in the category fitness instructors. Similarly, Stemple et al. studied ten female subjects who were asked to read loudly for 2 h. The authors showed an anterior and posterior glottic chink in half the subjects following testing that had not been present at baseline. Moreover, there was a significant increase in the mean fundamental frequency (204 ± 29 Hz pretesting vs. 223 ± 25 post-testing) [44]. Primov-Fever et al. investigated the impact of physical effort on voice in 14 physical education students. The voice was recorded at rest, during exercise (mild, moderate, and severe), and after exercise. The authors showed a significant increase in fundamental frequency from 138.02 Hz to 193.62 Hz at high-intensity exercise. Similarly, there was a significant increase in jitter (0.33 vs. 1.12) and shimmer (2.31 vs. 5.57) during physical activity. The increase in F0 was attributed to the increase in the overall body tension that occurs during high-intensity exercise [45]. This conclusion was supported by the increase in the blood level of lactate with the increase in exercise intensity. The authors also pointed to the importance of forced phonation often observed as a compensatory behavior to counteract the increase in aerodynamic forces during breathing [45]. Hillman et al., in their experimental study of 15 patients with vocal hyperfunction, highlighted the high collision forces and high velocity of vocal fold closure. The authors also stressed the pathogenic role of these collision forces in inducing vocal fold trauma [46]. Body kinetic-induced vocal fold behavior also can lead to extrinsic laryngeal muscle tension which in turn also might be associated with the harsh glottic attack, thus eliciting a self-perpetuating cycle of laryngeal hyperfunction. This is not surprising given the intricate contribution of extrinsic laryngeal muscles to voice production and their role in modulating voice efficiency [47–49].

In summary, body kinetic function is linked to laryngeal behavior. Intense physical activity can lead to an increase in laryngeal muscle tension and forceful adduction of the vocal folds. As in cases of grunting associated with strenuous physical performance, supraglottic constriction also is often observed [50–52]. Coaches and fitness instructors who exhibit laryngeal hyperfunctional behavior are at a high risk of developing voice disorders. Inefficient voice production and voice symptoms may prevail. Future investigations on the association between body hyperkinetic treatment exercises and voice improvement are needed.

6.3.2 Mouth Breathing and Voice Disorders

Vocal fold dryness is a major contributor to dysphonia. The dryness can be due to systemic dehydration, as discussed in Chap. 5 in the section on individual vocal health risk factors, or due to local dehydration secondary to mouth breathing. Mouth breathing is common in athletes, coaches, and fitness instructors as a means to maximizing ventilation and oxygenation. In a study by Ramonatxo et al. on mouth occlusion pressure and breathing pattern while performing incremental exercise tests, the authors showed differences in ventilation rate as the exercise load increased. The study was conducted on eight normal subjects who performed arm and leg exercises with a stepwise increase in the power output (25 watts for arms exercise and 50 watts for leg exercise) until exhaustion [53]. Similarly, Morton et al. compared nose breathing with mouth breathing alone and mouth and nose breathing in 20 healthy subjects and reported a reduction in breathing rate, tidal volume, and FE02 in nasal breathing alone. Their results substantiated the important role of mouth breathing in improving ventilation and oxygenation [54].

The adverse impact of mouth breathing and inhalation of dry air on phonation is well-known. Jiang et al. investigated the effect of dry air exposure on phonatory threshold pressure (PTP) and showed an increase of PTP (10.0 cm H_2O before and 15.0 cm H_2O after), with an increase in the average airflow and a decrease in the acoustic output. This in vitro study conducted on 17 excised canine larynges also showed that rehydration can restore the efficiency of vocal fold vibration. Rehydrating dehydrated larynges by bathing them in normal saline resulted in a decrease in the PTP [55]. Similarly, Sivasankar and Fisher investigated the effect of mouth breathing (air with 20% humidity) on voice in ten female students and showed an increase in PTP at a comfortable pitch. This increase was perceived as an increase in vocal effort in six of the ten subjects. On the other hand, nasal breathing was shown to reduce PTP and to decrease the phonatory effort in seven of ten subjects [56]. Their results are in agreement with those of Hernler et al. in 1997. The authors demonstrated an increase in perturbation parameters following inhalation of dry air for 10 min. The investigation was conducted on eight subjects who were asked to inhale dry air vs. standard and humidified air. The authors also noted the high sensitivity of the vocal folds to air humidity [57].

Respiratory rate is also important, along with mouth breathing and humidity of the air. Respiratory rate is associated strongly with the intensity of physical exercise. Many decades ago, Otis and Clark showed that that an increase in the rate of ventilation, commonly observed during exercise, can lead to an increase in voice intensity and pitch. The increase in voice intensity and pitch was attributed hypothetically to an increase in subglottic pressure. Interestingly, there were marked changes in speech and articulation noted by the authors as alterations in phrasing with a decrease in the number of letters or numbers voiced per breath. However, the time required for a given speech task remained the same [58]. In another study by Primov-Fever et al. on the impact of physical effort on voice, the authors showed a significant increase in the fundamental frequency and perturbation parameters during intense physical activity. The increase was attributed partially to the increase in airflow during expiration, which is a common physiologic phenomenon that occurs in parallel with a decrease in exhalation time. The authors alluded to the important role of breathing in maintaining voice stability which, when compromised, can lead to voice dysfunction [45]. In 2004, Rotstein et al. investigated the difficulties in speech production during an incremental running task. The authors found a significant association between various cardiopulmonary measurements and the perceived difficulty in speech production [59]. The increase in laryngeal effort during exercise also was demonstrated by Sandage et al. in 2013 in their study on voice function during resting breathing vs. high-intensity exercise. The authors showed an increase in perceived phonatory effort and PTP following 8 min of submaximal exercise. Of significance also was the decrease in the pharyngeal temperature following the test, which may have contributed to the increase in phonatory effort [60].

The increase in phonatory effort and the high prevalence of voice symptoms following mouth breathing and/or increase in ventilation rate can be attributed to alterations in the consistency and thickness of the vocal fold mucus layer. This layer, often referred to as the sol layer [56], is responsible for the regulation of ionic influx into and out of the vocal folds. Thinning of this layer leads to an increase in mucus adhesion, thus making the separation of the vocal folds during vibration harder. As a result, the adhesion between the vocal folds during a glottic cycle increases leading to an increase in phonatory effort and PTP [61–63]. In 1998, Finkelhor et al.

studied the effect of increased vocal fold viscosity on vocal fold range of oscillation and showed that dehydration increases PTP. The study was conducted on excised larynges that were exposed to various osmotic solutions with the purpose of inducing dehydration and rehydration by shifting fluids in and out of the vocal folds [63]. Numerous authors have reported various vocal fold mucus characteristics in patients with voice disorders. Using laryngeal videostroboscopic examination, Hsiao et al. showed a higher prevalence of uneven mucus layer in patients with laryngeal tension-fatigue syndrome in comparison to those without voice disorders [64]. Bonilha et al. showed that patients with hyperfunctional voice disorders have different mucus characteristics than patients with hypo-functional voice disorders [65]. Similarly, Hsiung, in his study of 160 patients with vocal nodules, found different locations of the mucus on the vocal folds. These were attributed to increased mucus viscosity and alteration in vocal fold aerodynamic and mechanical forces [66].

In summary, mouth breathing leads to alteration in the vocal fold mucus layer with a subsequent decrease in its volume and/or increase in its viscosity. Coaches and fitness instructors who rely on mouth breathing in addition to nasal breathing during coaching are subject to change in voice quality and to an increase in phonatory effort. The recent increase in the usage of face masks may cause alterations in the temperature and humidity of inhaled air. Future studies on the effect of these alterations on voice are needed.

6.3.3   Exercise-Induced Bronchoconstriction

Exercise-induced bronchoconstriction can play a pathogenic role in the development of voice disorders. Although it is more commonly reported in athletes [67–70], coaches and fitness instructors who also inhale large volumes of dry cold air while coaching are also susceptible to this respiratory condition. Its prevalence varies with the duration of physical activity, its intensity, and type, with a higher prevalence being reported in endurance sports in comparison to non-endurance sports. It also is associated with the ventilation rate which may exceed 200 liters/minute depending on the type of athletic activity [71, 72]. The pathophysiology of exercise-induced bronchoconstriction is not clear. It is thought to be the result of transient narrowing of the airway following strenuous physical activity. Airway drying also might be involved as it can be with exercise-induced asthma. Injury to the airway epithelial lining that fails to repair adequately and impairment in neuro-modulation of bronchial activity also have been suggested in the pathophysiology of exercise-induced bronchoconstriction [73]. Similar to asthma, environmental risk factors such as excessive cold or hot air, inhalation of allergens, and dehydration are thought to exacerbate exercise-induced respiratory symptoms [74]. Based on a review by Cosca and Navazio, high altitude, allergy and extremely cold temperature are important risk factors for bronchoconstriction that need to be considered in the assessment of patients with respiratory illnesses [75]. A discussion on the vocal health risk factors can be found in Chap. 5.

In summary, exercise-induced bronchoconstriction, although under-recognized in coaches and fitness instructors, may contribute to the pathogenesis of dysphonia in this subgroup of SOVU. The lack of breath support may lead to hyperfunctional voice disorders and various laryngeal symptoms. Hyperfunction is well recognized as a common compensatory strategy in people with impaired breath support which undermines the power source of the voice. Proper identification and treatment of exercise-induced bronchoconstriction in coaches and fitness instructors with voice disorders are important.

6.3.4 Body Fatigue/Stress and Dysphonia

Body fatigue is a physiologic or psychological reaction to a workload imposed on the body. The symptoms commonly reported include decrease in physical endurance and/or muscular function, which may adversely impact daily activity and production. When these symptoms become persistent or last for more than 6 months, the term chronic fatigue syndrome is often used [76, 77]. Many authors have investigated body fatigue with emphasis on both its peripheral and central components. Peripheral fatigue refers to impairment in function at the neuromuscular junction level, whereas central fatigue refers to a reduction in motor unit recruitment and coordination. Both peripheral and central body fatigue may affect phonation negatively, particularly in coaches and fitness instructors whose physical fitness is linked intricately to voice performance. The decrease in neural control and coordination in patients with central fatigue can jeopardize voice stability, as voice requires adequate complex motor cortex input. Laryngeal muscles may exhibit cellular changes similar to those reported in the musculoskeletal structures of patients with peripheral fatigue [78–83].

Patients with body fatigue also may experience alterations in oxygen supply and/ or extraction, which often leads to a high dependence on anaerobic resources. Anaerobic energy supply can result in the accumulation of lactic acid and other metabolites. The implications for these metabolic alterations on body function in subjects with body fatigue do not spare the phonatory apparatus. Nanjundeswaran et al. investigated the metabolic mechanisms of voice fatigue in three groups of women, 12 with voice fatigue and various degrees of voice training, 12 with normal voice and no voice training and whose cardiovascular systems were unconditioned, and 10 who were vocally healthy and vocally untrained and whose cardiovascular systems were trained. The authors showed that in the voice fatigue group, both aerobic and anaerobic resources were relied upon for oxygen consumption [84]. Increased tissue strain is another suggested cause of voice fatigue that should not be disregarded. The increased voice loudness and pitch in coaches and fitness instructors can result in excessive tensile and collision stresses, leading to deformation of the nonmuscular components of the vocal folds with consequent damage to the vocal fold mucosa and lamina propria [85, 86]. Additional inherent risk factors for voice disorders in coaches and fitness instructors are sleep deprivation and stress. In

2016, Fontan et al. reported that sleep duration correlated negatively with VHI ($R = -0.19$; the less the sleep, the higher the VHI) [24]. Similarly, Fellman and Simberg showed a significant association between stress and voice symptoms. Coaching-induced stress and feeling fatigued were described in almost one-third of the cases (32.1% and 28.4%, respectively). Hence, the connection between voice symptoms and psycho-emotional risk factors also needs to be emphasized [12].

The phonatory output of coaches and fitness instructors with body fatigue and stress is in jeopardy. Voice symptoms may vary from voice fatigue and loss of power to aphonia. The pathophysiology of dysphonia includes neuromuscular fatigue, central fatigue, and strain associated with alteration in vocal fold tissue properties. Other causes of dysphonia that should not be underestimated include respiratory muscle fatigue and dehydration.

References

1. Ramig LO, Verdolini K. Treatment efficacy: voice disorders. J Speech Lang Hear Res. 1998;41(1):S101–16.
2. Roy N, Merrill RM, Gray SD, Smith EM. Voice disorders in the general population: prevalence, risk factors, and occupational impact. Laryngoscope. 2005;115(11):1988–95.
3. Martins RH, Benito Pessin AB, Nassib DJ, Branco A, Rodrigues SA, Matheus SM. Aging voice and the laryngeal muscle atrophy. Laryngoscope. 2015;125(11):2518–21.
4. Verdolini K, Ramig LO. Occupational risks for voice problems. Logoped Phoniatr Vocol. 2001;1;26(1):37–46.
5. Williams NR. Occupational groups at risk of voice disorders: a review of the literature. Occup Med. 2003;53(7):456–60.
6. Roy N, Merrill RM, Thibeault S, Parsa RA, Gray SD, Smith EM. Prevalence of voice disorders in teachers and the general population. J Speech Lang Hear Res. 2004;47(2):281–93.
7. Cutiva LC, Vogel I, Burdorf A. Voice disorders in teachers and their associations with work-related factors: a systematic review. J Comm Disord. 2013;46(2):143–55.
8. Martins RH, Pereira ER, Hidalgo CB, Tavares EL. Voice disorders in teachers. A review. J Voice. 2014;28(6):716–24.
9. Rantala LM, Hakala SJ, Holmqvist S, Sala E. Connections between voice ergonomic risk factors and voice symptoms, voice handicap, and respiratory tract diseases. Voice. 2012;26(6):819–e13.
10. Simberg S, Santtila P, Soveri A, Varjonen M, Sala E, Sandnabba NK. Exploring genetic and environmental effects in dysphonia: a twin study. J Speech Lang Hear Res. 2009;52(1):153–63.
11. Smith E, Lemke J, Taylor M, Kirchner HL, Hoffman H. Frequency of voice problems among teachers and other occupations. J Voice. 1998;12(4):480–8.
12. Fellman D, Simberg S. Prevalence and risk factors for voice problems among soccer coaches. J Voice. 2017;31(1):121.e9–121.e15.
13. Penteado RZ, Silva NB, Montebello MI. Voice, stress, work and quality of life of soccer coaches and physical trainers. InCod. 2015;27(6):588–97.
14. Seifert E. Stress and distress in non-organic voice disorder. Swiss Med Wkly. 2005;135(27-28):387–97.
15. Kelley BC. A model of stress and burnout in collegiate coaches: Effects of gender and time of season. Res Q Exerc Sport. 1994;65(1):48–58.
16. Thelwell RC, Wagstaff CR, Chapman MT, Kenttä G. Examining coaches' perceptions of how their stress influences the coach–athlete relationship. J Sports Sci. 2017;35(19):1928–39.

17. Heidel SE, Torgerson JK. Vocal problems among aerobic instructors and aerobic participants. J Commun Disord. 1993;26(3):179–91.
18. Long J, Williford HN, Olson MS, Wolfe V. Voice problems and risk factors among aerobics instructors. J Voice. 1998;12(2):197–207.
19. Wolfe V, Long J, Youngblood HC, Williford H, Olson MS. Vocal parameters of aerobic instructors with and without voice problems. J Voice. 2002;16:52–60.
20. Newman C, Mrumbac K. Voice problems of aerobics instructors: implications for preventative training. Logoped Phoniatr Vocol. 1998;23(4):177–80.
21. Rumbach A, Khan A, Brown M, Eloff K, Poetschke A. Voice problems in the fitness industry: Factors associated with chronic hoarseness. Int J Speech Lang Pathol. 2015;17(5):441–50.
22. O'Neill J, McMenamin R. Voice use in professional soccer management. Logoped Phoniatr Vocol. 2014;39(4):169–78.
23. Buckley KL, O'Halloran PD, Oates JM. Occupational vocal health of elite sports coaches: An exploratory pilot study of football coaches. J Voice. 2015;29(4):476–83.
24. Fontan L, Fraval M, Michon A, Déjean S, Welby-Gieusse M. Vocal problems in sports and fitness instructors: a study of prevalence, risk factors, and need for prevention in France. J Voice. 2017;31(2):261.e33–8.
25. Niebudek-Bogusz E, Kotyło P, Śliwińska-Kowalska M. Evaluation of voice acoustic parameters related to the vocal-loading test in professionally active teachers with dysphonia. Int J Occup Med Environ Health. 2007;20(1):25–30.
26. Grillo EU, Fugowski J. Voice characteristics of female physical education student teachers. J Voice. 2011;25(3):e149–57.
27. Dallaston K, Rumbach AF. Vocal performance of group fitness instructors before and after instruction: Changes in acoustic measures and self-ratings. J Voice. 2016;30(1):127–e1.
28. Plant RL, Younger RM. The interrelationship of subglottic air pressure, fundamental frequency, and vocal intensity during speech. J Voice. 2000;14(2):170–7.
29. Chhetri DK, Park SJ. Interactions of subglottal pressure and neuromuscular activation on fundamental frequency and intensity. Laryngoscope. 2016;126(5):1123–30.
30. Porcaro CK, Howery S, Suhandron A, Gollery TP, Connie K, et al. Impact of vocal hygiene training on teachers' willingness to change vocal behaviors. J Voice. 2019;S0892-1997(19):30427–8.
31. Leppanen K, Ilomaki I, Laukkanen AM. One-year follow-up study of self-evaluated effects of voice massage, voice training, and voice hygiene lecture in female teachers. Logoped Phoniatr Vocol. 2010;35:13–8.
32. Negus VE. The mechanism of the Larynx. St Louis: CV Mosby; 1931.
33. Naito A, Niimi S. The larynx during exercise. Laryngoscope. 2000;110(7):1147–50.
34. Koblick HM. 2002. Effects of simultaneous exercise and speech tasks on the perception of effort and vocal measures in aerobic instructors. (Doctoral dissertation, University of Central Florida, 2002).
35. Orlikoff RF. Voice production during a weightlifting and support task. Folia Phoniatr Logop. 2008;60(4):188–94.
36. Rose B, Horman M, Sataloff RT. Voice therapy. In: Sataloff RT. Professional voice: The science and art of clinical care. 4th ed. San Diego: Plural Publishing; 2017. p. 1171–95.
37. Raphael BN, Sataloff RT. Increasing vocal effectiveness. In: Sataloff RT. Professional voice: The science and art of clinical care. 4th ed. San Diego: Plural Publishing; 2017. p. 1201–13.
38. Yamaguchi H, Yotsukura Y, Sata H, et al. Pushing exercise program to correct glottal incompetence. J Voice. 1993;7:250–6.
39. Yamana T, Kitajima K. Laryngeal closure pressure during phonation in humans. J Voice. 2000;14(1):1–7.
40. Hess MM, Verdolini K, Bierhals W, Mansmann U, Gross M. Endolaryngeal contact pressures. J Voice. 1998;1;12(1):50–67.
41. Jiang JJ, Titze IR. Measurement of vocal fold intraglottal pressure and impact stress. J Voice. 1994;8(2):132–44.

42. Czerwonka L, Jiang JJ, Tao C. Vocal nodules and edema may be due to vibration-induced rises in capillary pressure. The Laryngoscope. 2008;118(4):748–52.
43. Casper J. The effects of excessive vocalization on acoustic and videostroboscopic measures of vocal Fold Condition. J Voice. 1999;13(2):294.
44. Stemple JC, Stanley J, Lee L. Objective measures of voice production in normal subjects following prolonged voice use. J Voice. 1995;1;9(2):127–33.
45. Primov-Fever A, Lidor R, Meckel Y, Amir O. The effect of physical effort on voice characteristics. Folia Phoniatrica et Logopaedica. 2013;65(6):288–93.
46. Hillman RE, Holmberg EB, Perkell JS, Walsh M, Vaughan C. Objective assessment of vocal hyperfunction: An experimental framework and initial results. J Speech Lang Hear Res. 1989;32(2):373–92.
47. Konrad HR, Rattenborg CC, Kain ML, Barton MD, Logan WJ, Holaday DA. Opening and closing mechanisms of the larynx. Otolaryngol Head Neck Surg. 1984;92(4):402–5.
48. Vilkman E, Sonninen A, Hurme P, Körkkö P. External laryngeal frame function in voice production revisited: a review. J Voice. 1996;10(1):78–92.
49. Angsuwarangsee T, Morrison M. Extrinsic laryngeal muscular tension in patients with voice disorders. J Voice. 2002;16(3):333–43.
50. Welch AS, Tschampl M. Something to shout about: a simple, quick performance enhancement technique improved strength in both experts and novices. J App Sport Psychol. 2012;24(4):418–28.
51. Rumbach AF, Maddox M, Hull M, Khidr A. Laryngeal symptoms in weightlifting athletes. J Voice. 2020;34(6):964.
52. Davis KM, Sandage MJ, Plexico L, Pascoe DD. The perception of benefit of vocalization on sport performance when producing maximum effort. J Voice. 2016;30(5):639–e11.
53. Ramonatxo M, Prioux J, Prefaut C. Differences in mouth occlusion pressure and breathing pattern between arm and leg incremental exercise. Acta Physiol Scand. 1996;158(4):333–41.
54. Morton AR, King K, Papalia S, Goodman C, Turley KR, Wilmore JH. Comparison of maximal oxygen consumption with oral and nasal breathing. Aust Sci Med Sport. 1995;27(3):51–5.
55. Jiang J, Verdolini K, Jennie NG, Aquino B, Hanson D. Effects of dehydration on phonation in excised canine larynges. Ann Otol Rhinol Laryngol. 2000;109(6):568–75.
56. Sivasankar M, Fisher KV. Oral breathing increases Pth and vocal effort by superficial drying of vocal fold mucosa. J Voice. 2002;16(2):172–81.
57. Hemler RJ, Wieneke GH, Dejonckere PH. The effect of relative humidity of inhaled air on acoustic parameters of voice in normal subjects. J Voice. 1997;11(3):295–300.
58. Otis AB, Clark RG. Ventilatory implications of phonation and phonatory implications of ventilation. Ann NY Acad Sci. 1968;155(1):122–8.
59. Rotstein A, Meckel Y, Inbar O. Perceived speech difficulty during exercise and its relation to exercise intensity and physiological responses. Eur J Appl Physiol. 2004;92(4–5):431–6.
60. Sandage MJ, Connor NP, Pascoe DD. Voice function differences following resting breathing versus submaximal exercise. J Voice. 2013;27(5):572–8.
61. Verdolini-Marston K, Sandage M, Titze I. Effect of hydration treatment on laryngeal nodules and polyps and related voice measures. J Voice. 1994;8:30–47.
62. Verdolini K, Titze IR, Fennel A. Dependence of phonatory effort on hydration level. J Speech Hear Res. 1994;37(5):1001–7.
63. Finkelhor BK, Titze IR, Durham PL. The effect of viscosity changes in the vocal folds on the range of oscillation. J Voice. 1988;1(4):320–5.
64. Hsiao TY, Liu CM, Lin KN. Videostrobolaryngoscopy of mucus layer during vocal fold vibration in patients with laryngeal tension-fatigue syndrome. Ann Otol Rhinol Laryngol. 2002;111(6):537–41.
65. Bonilha HS, White L, Kuckhahn K, Gerlach TT, Deliyski DD. Vocal fold mucus aggregation in persons with voice disorders. J Comm Disord. 2012;45(4):304–11.
66. Hsiung MW. Videolaryngostroboscopic observation of mucus layer during vocal cord vibration in patients with vocal nodules before and after surgery. Acta Otolaryngol. 2004;124(2):186–91.

67. Turcotte H, Langdeau JB, Thibault G, Boulet LP. Prevalence of respiratory symptoms in an athlete population. Respir Med. 2003;97(8):955–63.
68. Boulet LP, Turmel J. Cough in exercise and athletes. Pulm Pharmacol Ther. 2019;55:67–74.
69. Kurowski M, Jurczyk J, Krysztofiak H, Kowalski ML. Exercise-induced respiratory symptoms and allergy in elite athletes: Allergy and Asthma in Polish Olympic Athletes (A2POLO) project within GA2LEN initiative. Clin Respir J. 2016;10(2):231–8.
70. Durmic T, Lazovic B, Djelic M, et al. Sport-specific influences on respiratory patterns in elite athletes. J Brasileiro Pneumol. 2015;41(6):516–22.
71. Bonini M, Silvers W. Exercise-induced bronchoconstriction: background, prevalence, and sport considerations. Immunol Allergy Clin. 2018;38(2):205–14.
72. Haahtela T, Malmberg P, Moreira A. Mechanisms of asthma in Olympic athletes–practical implications. Allergy. 2008;63(6):685–94.
73. Couto M, Kurowski M, Moreira A, et al. Mechanisms of exercise-induced bronchoconstriction in athletes: current perspectives and future challenges. Allergy. 2018;73(1):8–16.
74. Carlsen KH. Mechanisms of asthma development in elite athletes. Breathe. 2012;8(4):278–84.
75. Cosca D, Navazio F. Common problems in endurance athletes. Am Fam Phys. 2007;76(2):237–44.
76. Carriker CR. Components of Fatigue: Mind and Body. J Strength Cond Res. 2017;31(11):3170–6.
77. Fukuda K, Straus SE, Hickie I, Sharpe MC, Dobbins JG, Komaroff A. The chronic fatigue syndrome: a comprehensive approach to its definition and study. Ann Int Med. 1994;121(12):953–9.
78. Enoka RM, Stuart DG. Neurobiology of muscle fatigue. J Appl Physiol. 1992;72:1631–48.
79. Fitts RH. Cellular mechanisms of muscle fatigue. Physiol Rev. 1994;74:49–94.
80. Gandevia SC, Enoka RM, McComas AJ, et al. Neurobiology of muscle fatigue. Advances and issues. Adv Exp Med Biol. 1995;384:515–25.
81. Noakes TD, St Clair Gibson A, Lambert EV. From catastrophe to complexity: a novel model of integrative central neural regulation of effort and fatigue during exercise in humans. Br J Sports Med. 2004;38:511–4.
82. Davis MP, Walsh D. Mechanisms of fatigue. J Support Oncol. 2010;8:164–74.
83. Gandevia SC. Spinal and supraspinal factors in human muscle fatigue. Physiol Rev. 2001;81:1725–89.
84. Nanjundeswaran C, VanSwearingen J, Abbott KV. Metabolic mechanisms of vocal fatigue. J Voice. 2017;31(3):378–e1.
85. Solomon NP. Vocal fatigue and its relation to vocal hyperfunction. Int J Speech Lang Pathol. 2008;10(4):254–66.
86. Titze IR. Mechanical stress in phonation. J Voice. 1994;8(2):99–105.

Chapter 7
Sports-Related Musculoskeletal Injuries in Athletes: Implications for Voice

7.1 Prevalence of Musculoskeletal Injuries in Athletes

Musculoskeletal injuries occur when the body is unable to dissipate force-induced stress during exercise [1]. Based on the International Olympic Committee, sports injury is defined as "a new or recurring musculoskeletal complaint incurred during competition or trauma that requires medical attention, regardless of the potential absence from competition or training" [2]. The musculoskeletal injury can be either acute as in a single insult to healthy tissues, subacute as in repetitive microtrauma with inadequate recovery, or chronic when subsequent degenerative changes develop over time [3–5]. Injuries that occur at the previously injured sites or injuries linked to a previous acute insult also are considered subacute and may often lead to chronic changes. Both the intensity and volume of force-induced stresses incurred during exercise contribute to the extent of injury to soft tissues and skeletal structures. In a systematic review on burnout in youth sports, DiFiori et al. stressed the complexity of overuse injuries in highly committed athletes with no specification to their level of professionalism. The authors highlighted their long-term adverse effect on health and their impact on the ability of athletes to participate in competitive games [4]. In a study by Yang et al. on the epidemiology of overuse and acute injuries among 573 competitive collegiate athletes, the authors noted an overall injury rate of 6.31 per 1000 athletic exposures (practice and games). The rate of acute injuries was higher than that of overuse injuries, with a rate ratio of 2.34 [5].

Despite advocating numerous preventive strategies such as warm-up exercises, enhanced nutrition, and psychological intervention, musculoskeletal injuries are still common in athletes [6]. Any breakdown in the kinetic chain responsible for mobilizing or stabilizing a body part during exercise, be it in training or in competition, can lead to injury. Based on a large review of the terminology for muscle injuries used in sports, Mueller-Wohlfahrt et al. classified muscle injuries into four categories: type 1 is a functional muscle disorder that is exertion related, type 2 is a neuromuscular functional disorder, type 3 involves a partial tear, and type 4 involves a total tear. Notably in types 3 and 4, the injury is evident macroscopically, whereas in types 1 and 2 the injury is not visible to the naked eye [7]. Notwithstanding the severity of injuries to soft tissues, bones also are at risk of injury. Almekinders and Engle emphasized the importance of repetitive physical stress as a cause of stress fractures to weight-bearing bones, particularly in ultra-endurance sports. The most common presenting symptom in these cases is pain at the site of the stress fracture that often is misdiagnosed [8].

The rate of injury to soft tissues and bones varies with the stress load on the musculoskeletal system. In a review of 1,053,370 college sports-related injuries, the rate was higher during practice than during competition, although the severity of injuries was higher during competitive games than during training [9]. Similarly, Pfirrmann et al., in their systematic review of injury incidences in professional adult and elite youth soccer players, reported a higher prevalence of training injuries in young players in comparison to professionals. However, the overall injury rate (training and matches) was higher during matches than during training. The authors reiterated that the level of competitiveness is an important determinant of injury rate [10]. This is in agreement with the review of Eckard who also found an association between the training load and the rate of injuries in athletes [11].

An important determinant of the musculoskeletal injury rate is the type of sport. Exercise-induced stress varies across different types of sports. Soligard et al. analyzed the rate of injuries and illnesses in the Olympic winter games in 2014 and reported the highest rates in skiing, snowboard slope style, and snowboard cross. As a result of these injuries, almost two out of five injured athletes had to abstain from participating in competition [12]. Kerr ZY et al. analyzed the rate of injuries among student athletes in 25 NCAA championship sports and reported the highest overall injury rate among male wrestlers (13.1 per 1000) and the highest competition injury rate in men's football [9]. The types of sports also are known to affect the sites of musculoskeletal injuries. Abrams et al. reviewed the epidemiology of musculoskeletal injuries in tennis players and reported ankle sprains as the most frequent acute injury to the lower extremities. Lateral epicondylitis and shoulder pain were reported as chronic overuse injuries, particularly in high-level players [13]. Pieter et al. reviewed injuries during competition in Taekwondo and reported the lower extremities followed by the head and neck as the most common site of injury in men (44.5% and 29.6%, respectively) (Fig. 7.1). The prevalence rate of head and neck injuries was higher than that reported in other kinds of sports such as soccer or American football. Contusions constituted the majority of head injuries in both genders and were attributed to deficiencies in the blocking skills of athletes [14]. Lopes et al. reviewed running-related musculoskeletal injuries and reported medial tibial stress syndrome and Achilles tendinopathy as the most frequent injuries, reaching a prevalence rate of 9.5%. In ultramarathon runners, the patellofemoral syndrome (characterized by anterior knee pain secondary to increased stress on the patella and femur) is reported commonly and ranges in prevalence from 7.4% to 15.6% [15]. Schoffl et al. reported on the prevalence of finger and shoulder injuries in rock climbing and noted long biceps tendon ruptures and shoulder dislocation as the most commonly

Fig. 7.1 Knee X-ray of a
26-year-old woman with a
separated transverse
mid-patellar fracture with
associated knee joint
effusion

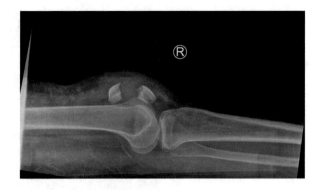

diagnosed injuries in this sport [16]. Jacobs et al. screened 19 articles on musculo-skeletal injuries in dancers and found that the lower extremities, back, and hip were the most frequent sites of injury. The authors suggested the need to increase preventive measures and to enhance the diagnosis and treatment of musculoskeletal injuries in dancers [17]. Weinstein et al. reviewed common injuries in winter sports and reported a high prevalence of upper extremity injuries in snowboarding and a high prevalence of lower extremities injuries in skiing. The authors highlighted the need for early diagnosis of these injuries and the development of preventive strategies [18]. Keogh and Winwood reviewed the epidemiology of injuries in weight-training sports and found that the lower back, shoulder, and knee were the ost common sites of injury (Fig. 7.2). Other commonly reported anatomic sites were the elbow and wrist. The highest rate of injury was in Highland games and Strongman games (7.5 per 1000 h and 4.5–6.1 injuries per 1000 h, respectively) [19].

In addition to the type of sport, there are also individual factors that affect the rate of musculoskeletal injuries. These include age, gender, and degree of professionalism. There is growing evidence in the literature to support the consensus that participation of adolescents at an early stage in life has led to a substantial increase in the prevalence of musculoskeletal injuries in young people [49]. Age-related variations in soft tissue structures, such as collagen fibers' mechanical properties and extracellular matrix constituents, can explain the disparity in the rate of injury and in the recovery rate across the different age groups. Patel et al. reviewed the important role of adolescent growth and development in understanding sports-related musculoskeletal injuries and suggested age-related modulation in recovery [20]. Gender is also a variable to consider in the assessment of musculoskeletal injuries in athletes. Sexual dimorphism plays an important role in either increasing or decreasing the risk of injury among athletes. Clearly et al. reported a higher frequency of concussion and anterior cruciate ligament injury in females compared to males. The authors pointed to the female athlete triad (low energy level, menstrual dysfunction, low density of mineral bone) and to the increasing pressure imposed on young female athletes [21]. Pieter et al., in their review of the literature on Taekwondo competition, reported differences in the site of injuries in women vs. men. Lower extremities injuries were more common in women in comparison to men (53.1% vs. 44.5%, respectively), whereas head and neck injuries were more

Fig. 7.2 Left knee magnetic resonance imaging (MRI) of a 24 year-old man with transverse fracture of the anterior aspect of the tibial plateau

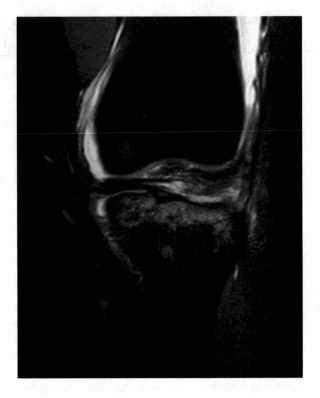

common in men in comparison to women (29.6% vs. 15.2%, respectively). The authors alluded to the need to develop preventive strategies and improve surveillance during competition [14]. Similarly, Yang et al. noted that although men had a higher rate of acute injuries, women were more prone to overuse injuries. The authors highlighted the need for future studies to clarify sexual dimorphism in sports musculoskeletal injuries [5]. Professionalism also plays a role in the prevalence of musculoskeletal injuries. In their review of the impact of professionalism on the rate of musculoskeletal injuries in adults and elite youth soccer players, Pfirmrmann et al. showed that training injuries were more common in youth players in comparison to professionals [10].

In addition to the above, the psychological condition of the athlete is an important variable to consider in analyzing sports-related injuries. Jacobs et al. reviewed some of the factors responsible for musculoskeletal injuries in dancers and reiterated the importance of psychological and psychosocial issues in the development of body injuries, especially the coping strategies used once injuries have been sustained. The authors also emphasized the importance of body fatigue in the exacerbation of muscle and tendon strains. The impact of psychological stress is substantiated further in athletes with a history of previous muscle or tendon injury and in athletes who had witnessed similar injuries happening to their partners [17].

In summary, the prevalence rate and site of musculoskeletal injuries vary among athletes considerably. The type of sports and the amount of stress imposed in competition and training contribute substantially to the occurrence of these injuries. Age, gender, and psychological stress also need to be considered in the interpretation of sports injuries.

7.2 Pathophysiology of Dysphonia in Athletes with Musculoskeletal Injuries

All body structures are involved in voice production. Sports-related musculoskeletal injuries can jeopardize phonation either directly or indirectly. In addition to laryngeal trauma which is the topic of another chapter in this book, sports-related musculoskeletal injuries can cause change in voice quality by promoting tension to structures adjacent to the larynx, by causing neuromuscular dysfunction and neural impairment, or by impairing muscular and aerodynamic support (the power source of the voice). Incurred pain and stress during the event of injury or along the course of its management also may jeopardize phonation.

7.2.1 Postural Imbalance in Sports-Related Musculoskeletal Injuries and Its Impact on Voice

An aligned posture is an asset for a speaker or singer. In addition to its favorable role in breathing, an aligned posture allows the free movement of the laryngeal structures with minimal tension, thus increasing voice efficiency [22]. In one study by Franco et al., patients with dysphonia were found to have a higher kyphosis index and thoracic length curvature in comparison to subjects with no dysphonia. The investigation included 74 adults whose sagittal plane photographs were analyzed for posture [23]. Patients with deviant posture and/or abnormal head position may be more prone to voice problems than subjects with normal posture and/or head position. Gilman and Jhones investigated the impact of head position and body stance on the self-perception of voice effort in 46 healthy adults with no voice problems. The results showed that exaggerated backward and forward head position while sitting precipitated an increase in self-perceived phonatory effort, as did standing with knees locked or "soft." The authors noted that an abnormal stance or head position is a significant risk factor for voice [24]. This probably occurs in sports that commonly involve body positions that are not ideal for phonation. Knight et al. showed that neck extension improves the singing power ratio, fundamental frequency amplitude, and low-frequency partials. The participants of their study group were asked to sustain three vowels at three different pitches while the head and neck assumed four different positions [25]. Rantala et al. studied the association between working postures and voice in 30 teachers. The results showed that the use of 3 un-ergonomic postures or more was associated with voice symptoms, namely, voice breaks and an increase in sound pressure level. The authors alluded to the benefit of tailoring the working environment to accommodate better the voice needs of teachers [26]. Longo et al. investigated the impact of body posture on singing in 17 professional singers who performed with and without an instrument [27]. The authors showed that shoulder and back posture had an impact on the performer's voice. Singers who sang while playing the guitar had an increase in noise and a decrease in singers' formant. In that study, voice analysis was conducted using the multidimensional voice program. Similarly, Kooijman et al. reported a significant correlation between tension/posture score and dysphonia in 25 female teachers whose posture and laryngeal tension were assessed by professional speech therapists [28]. The voice outcome measures included the Voice Handicap Index (VHI) and the Dysphonia Severity Index. Notably, posterior weight-bearing and increased sterno-cleidomastoid muscle (SCM)/geniohyoid muscle tonicity were significant predictors of an elevated VHI score in the study group [28].

The data above supports a strong association between posture and voice disorders. Sports-related musculoskeletal injuries often lead to abnormal postures and imbalance. Postural changes or malalignment in the head/neck position following sports injuries can jeopardize free laryngeal movement, alter the vocal tract, and cause an increase in resistance to phonation. Athletes with musculoskeletal injuries may develop excessive muscle tension within their laryngeal structures and/or in their articulatory apparatus as a result of postural imbalance or misalignment in the head/neck position. Baroody et al. reported the adverse impact of upper and middle cervical extension on the anatomic location of the styloid process and mastoid process, as well as its adverse effect on the movement of the sternohyoid and stylohyoid muscles [30]. As a result, affected patients may suffer from increased voice effort and contracted voice range. Future laryngeal electromyographic studies in athletes with postural imbalance and dysphonia vs. those without dysphonia are warranted. A deviant posture secondary to a musculoskeletal injury may also put the athletic performer in an awkward stance. The effect of this problem on a singer who struggles with balancing his or her posture while performing is well known, and the problem also may impair athletic performance. This is particularly true in athletes with spine and pelvic fractures. The position of the pelvis is critical for optimal breath support. Anterior or posterior hip over-projection following a hip fracture can cause a malalignment in posture with adverse impact on breath support. Similarly, athletes with injury to the vertebral column also may suffer from muscular imbalance that is a threat to their voice [29].

Given the strong linkage between voice and posture, it is reasonable to speculate that comprehensive treatment of voice disorders in athletes with dysphonia, which routinely includes improving body stance, also may enhance athletic support indirectly by correcting errors in posture. Bruno et al. demonstrated that the amount of body sway decreases following voice rehabilitation in subjects with voice disorders [31]. Similarly, in the study by Nacci et al. on the impact of speech therapy/rehabilitation on posture in 40 patients with hyperfunctional dysphonia, the authors showed improvement in all posture-graphic parameters. The results confirmed the strong association between proprioceptive awareness and postural performance [32].

In summary, postural imbalance secondary to musculoskeletal injuries can affect voice. The impact is mediated via an increase in laryngeal muscle tension and resistance and decrease in efficiency of the support system (power source). Treatment of dysphonia in athletes with deviant postures improves their body proprioception and posture. Similarly, one can speculate that treatment of postural imbalance in athletes may help reduce the rate of voice disorders, and improvement of posture through voice training might enhance athletic performance. This statement remains hypothetical and needs further investigation.

7.2.2 Impairment in Breathing Following Musculoskeletal Injuries and Its Impact on Voice

Musculoskeletal injuries to most parts of the body may affect breathing. The extent of breathing impairment depends on the degree of injury and the anatomic site involved. Numerous authors highlighted the importance of breathing as a power source in phonation [30, 33, 34]. Compromised breathing following musculoskeletal injuries in athletes not only affects the support for voice production but also the ability of the speaker to modulate his or her voice pitch and loudness. For example, trauma to the back may jeopardize breathing by interfering with thoracic expansion during contraction of the diaphragm, the largest muscle involved in inspiration. Similarly, musculoskeletal injuries to the chest wall can be detrimental to inspiration and expiration. The chest wall is also crucial in "air trapping," a physiologic mechanism that allows us to perform high intensity physical tasks [33]. As such, athletes with restricted mobility of their chest wall following musculoskeletal injuries may suffer from inability to project their voice and/or sustain prolonged phonation. Professional voice users may complain of restricted voice volume and range. Similarly, injuries to the abdominal wall put the phonatory apparatus in jeopardy. Sataloff et al. advocated abstention from vocally demanding tasks until the abdominal support for voice production is restored to normal [34]. This is particularly true in professional voice users who rely heavily on breath support to initiate vocal fold oscillation and to modulate voice pitch and loudness. The adverse impact of impaired breathing following musculoskeletal injuries to the chest wall and abdomen is not limited to the power supply but also extends to the larynx. Low lung volume is associated with a high-positioned larynx and hyperfunctional laryngeal behavior. The voice of injured athletes may suffer not only from restricted modulation in pitch and loudness but also from drastic change. The harsh glottal attack and increased contact pressure between the vocal folds, as a result of the hyperfunctional laryngeal behavior in patients with high-positioned larynx, can predispose to structural vocal fold alterations that should not be ignored [30, 34]. Another cause of breathing impairment in athletes is trauma-induced pneumothorax. Spontaneous pneumothorax, though rare, has been reported in weightlifters and has been

Fig. 7.3 Chest X-ray of a
21-year-old man showing
right pneumothorax

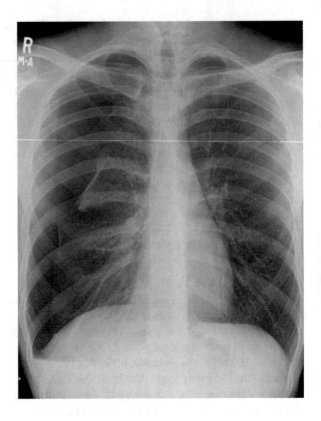

attributed to improper breathing technique [35]. Soundappan et al. described three cases of sports-related pneumothorax in children following blunt trauma to the chest. The authors highlighted the subtlety of the clinical presentation in these patients, more so in those with high fitness level. Tension pneumothorax may remain unrecognized until hemodynamic complications arise (Fig. 7.3) [36].

Given the key role of breathing in phonation, injuries to the respiratory muscles and their skeletal support may have adverse effect on voice. Trauma-induced musculoskeletal injuries with subsequent respiratory dysfunction may be detrimental to athletes who need to vocalize while performing strenuous exercise and to phonation outside the athletic environment. As most vocal fold injuries occur in association with insufficient respiratory muscle support, it is easy to understand athletes with breathing impairment following musculoskeletal injuries are at high risk of developing voice problems.

7.2.3 Sports-Related Musculoskeletal Injuries to the Upper Extremities and Their Impact on Voice

Sports-related musculoskeletal injuries to the upper extremities vary in severity and longevity. Demertzis et al. divided upper extremity neuromuscular injuries into direct and indirect injuries. Direct injuries include soft tissues contusions and lacerations, whereas indirect injuries include strains, exertion compartment syndrome, delayed-onset muscle soreness, and peripheral nerve injuries [37]. Both direct and indirect injuries to the upper extremities impact phonation by virtue of their proximity to the cervical muscles and larynx. The proximity of the laryngeal framework to the upper extremities predisposes the extrinsic laryngeal muscles to pain sensation and compensatory muscle behavior in response to upper extremity injuries. Such muscle activity and asymmetry can lead to dysphonia. For example, excessive tension in the injured arms may be transmitted to the external laryngeal muscles and subsequently to the internal laryngeal muscles. The excessive muscle tension can lead to compensatory hyperfunctional laryngeal behavior with subsequent muscle tension dysphonia [28–30]. Examples of athletes at risk are professional tennis players who experience shoulder pain and recreational tennis players who commonly complain of tennis elbow [13]. Other examples of athletes at risk are heavy rock climbers, weightlifters [16, 19], and, to a lesser extent, runners who may sustain injuries to the upper extremities by falling. Notably, all athletes are at risk during competitive games and strenuous activity.

In summary, musculoskeletal injuries to the upper extremities may affect phonation by causing excessive asymmetric tension in the laryngeal muscles. This may lead to hyperfunctional voice disorders and subsequently vocal fold structural changes. Future research on the prevalence of dysphonia in athletes with upper extremity injuries is encouraged.

7.2.4 Pain in Sports-Related Musculoskeletal Injuries and Its Impact on Voice

Pain is a personal experience that may occur in the presence or absence of physical injury. It is influenced by several factors: biochemical, physiologic, cognitive, and affective [38]. Psychosocial influences such as a strong athletic identity, a competitive mind-set, and a history of physical injury are also substantial contributors to pain perception. The etiology of pain is multidimensional and includes nociceptive pain inferring to sensitization of nociceptors by inflammatory mediators, ischemic pain resulting from insufficient blood supply and/or oxygenation to tissues, and neuropathic pain secondary to injury to neural structures. Central sensitization and affective pain are equally important in the interpretation and management of injured athletes [38–40]. Affective pain is exemplified best in athletes with previous musculoskeletal injuries and in those who had witnessed similar injuries during competition.

When present, pain has negative consequences on the functional ability of the athlete as well as his or her quality of life. Many systems may be affected, including the phonatory system. This is not surprising given the strong link between musculo-skeletal pain and high voice demand [41–46]. The prevalence of musculoskeletal pain is significantly higher in patients with excessive voice load, such as teachers. The musculoskeletal sites most commonly affected are the neck, larynx, shoulders, chest, and back. Chiu and Lam investigated the prevalence and risk factors of neck pain in 3100 schoolteachers and reported workload, head-down posture, and psy-chological stress as the main precipitating factors [45]. Similarly, Alsiddiky et al. reported teaching level, vitamin D deficiency, and the presence of chronic illnesses as common factors contributing to neck pain that occurred in up to 11.3% of their study group [46]. Da Silva et al. conducted a study on musculoskeletal pain in teachers with and without voice disorders and reported more "common" pain at the back of the neck, shoulder, and temporal region in the dysphonia group in compari-son to the non-dysphonia group. Moreover, the pain was more intense in the back of the neck and in the larynx in the dysphonia group in comparison to the non-dysphonia group (31.09 vs. 26.62, and 25.90 vs. 17.18, respectively). Notably, the difference in the intensity of the pain between the two groups was not significant. However, in the dysphonia group, there was a significant correlation between the weekly workload and the frequency and intensity of pain in the laryngeal region. The information on weekly load was derived from a questionnaire on the amount of hours per week spent with students [47]. Similarly, Ramos et al. investigated the prevalence of musculoskeletal pain in 37 patients with dysphonia in comparison to 37 patients without dysphonia using the Voice-Related Quality of Life Questionnaire and the Musculoskeletal Pain Questionnaire. The results indicated a higher fre-quency and intensity of pain in the larynx and a higher frequency of pain in the submandibular region and anterior aspect of the neck, in the dysphonia group in comparison to the non-dysphonia group [48]. Given that the phonatory apparatus is part of the musculoskeletal system, one can extrapolate that athletes with sports-related musculoskeletal pain might be at a higher risk of having dysphonia than those with no pain, although the association between pain and dysphonia has been established but which causes which remains unproven. This probably is particularly true in athletes with pain and tension in the neck and musculoskeletal structures adjacent to the larynx. Morrison et al. associated functional laryngeal voice disor-ders to excessive laryngeal muscular tension and an abnormally high-positioned larynx [50]. Based on the review of mechanical stress in phonation, Titze reported that contractile stress of the laryngeal muscles, in addition to the tensile and aerody-namic stresses, affects the collision force between the vocal folds that is responsible for vocal fold damage [51].

The athletic voice is also in jeopardy during the course of pain management. The use of corticosteroid medications and other anti-inflammatory drugs may increase the risk of dysphonia by aggravating gastroesophageal reflux disease and increasing the risk of vocal fold hemorrhage. The effect of gastroesophageal reflux disease on the larynx is well known. Commonly reported symptoms include globus pharyngeus, throat clearing, and cough in addition to dysphonia [52]. Athletes with musculoskeletal injuries and who are on nonsteroidal anti-inflammatory drugs (NSAID or steroids) need to be aware of the adverse effect of treatment on reflux and the laryngopharyngeal complex.

In summary, pain is a major contributor to dysphonia in athletes. Its impact is multidimensional. Injury-related pain in structures adjacent to the larynx may lead to excessive tension in the laryngeal muscles with subsequent muscle tension dysphonia. Pain may also have an indirect effect on voice via its affective and/or central component. The intake of steroids or nonsteroidal anti-inflammatory medications should also alert the treating physician to laryngopharyngeal reflux disease as a contributing factor to dysphonia and to the risk of vocal fold hemorrhage. Treatment and rehabilitation strategies with the least intake of medications should be advocated.

7.2.5 Stress and Post-Traumatic Stress Disorders (PTSD) in Athletes: Implications for Voice

Stress disorders are not uncommon in athletes, particularly in those whose safety has been jeopardized. The stress may be acute, as in acute stress disorder lasting up to 1 month, or chronic, as in post-traumatic stress disorders (PTSD). The estimated prevalence of acute stress disorder is in the range of 23–45%, with young athletes being at a higher risk than old athletes. Interestingly, one out of two patients with acute stress disorder may develop PTSD later [53]. Based on a review by Aron et al., the prevalence rate of PTSD in elite athletes may reach 25%. Among the precipitating factors is history of sports injury and/or abusive behavior within the team [54]. In rare instances, athletes may experience stress-related trauma even by watching violent events and/or trauma to their team members. Exposure of athletes to trauma video footage can induce exaggerated stress reactions, fear, and anxiety [55]. Of similar importance is prior history of sexual trauma or assault [56]. Timpka et al. investigated the association between suicidal thoughts and previous history of physical abuse or sexual assault in 192 athletes and reported suicidal ideation in women and men in 17.4% and 14.2%, respectively. Among the factors associated with suicidal thoughts were low sense of coherence, sexual abuse, and behavioral disengagement [57].

The symptoms of stress-related disorders in athletes with musculoskeletal injuries may vary with the intensity of the insult, its frequency, and timing. Although stress-related complaints usually are reported within the first few days following injury, athletes with musculoskeletal injuries may present with stress symptoms much later. According to the Diagnostic and Statistical Manual of Mental Disorders (DSM), stress-related disorders are classified into four categories. The first category is intrusion and includes recurrent memories and flashbacks of the event that often are associated with nightmares and intense distress following the recollection of the traumatic event. The second category is negative mood/cognition and is character-ized by negative trauma-related emotions with distorted beliefs and inability to recall events as they happened. The third category is dissociative and is character-ized by derealization, decreased awareness, and decreased emotional response. The fourth category is categorized by hypervigilance and aggressiveness [58]. In a study on the prevalence of PTSD symptoms among young athletes with anterior cruciate ligament rupture, Padaki et al. reported symptoms of avoidance, intrusion, and hyperarousal in 87.5%, 83.3%, and 75% of cases, respectively [59]. Moreover, age and gender were significant determinants of the prevalence of these symptoms, with higher prevalence rates being reported in female athletes in comparison to male athletes [59]. In another study, Shuer et al. reported high scores on the intrusion subscale in injured athletes, similar to the scores reported in subjects who had expe-rienced natural disasters. Moreover, the scores of athletes on the subscale of avoid-ance and denial were higher than those who had experienced natural disasters. The study was conducted on 280 athletes, 42% of whom had been diagnosed with a chronic injury. The authors emphasized the need for psychiatric intervention early in the treatment of athletes with acute injury in order to circumvent the associated post-traumatic stress sequel [60]. Similarly, in a cross-sectional study by Gkikopoulos et al. of 52 athletes, the authors showed a significant correlation between athletes' psychology and the outcome of medical therapy, physiotherapy, and absenteeism following injury [61].

All the above highlights the significance and various degrees of mental stress that follow physical injury or sexual assault in athletes. Given the well-known auto-nomic, endocrine, and cardiorespiratory effects of stress on voice, and the strong link between the phonatory system and rest of the body, it is clear that the voices of athletes with stress disorders are in jeopardy. Numerous studies have confirmed the adverse effect of stress on voice. Holmqvist et al. reported the correlation between 6 voice symptoms and 4 stress symptoms in their study of 1728 subjects. Lump sensation in the throat or muscle tension, a voice-related symptom, was associated with all the stress symptoms investigated. The authors emphasized on the patho-genic role of stress in patients with voice disorders and the need to acknowledge stress as a voice risk factor [62]. Van Lierde et al. studied the impact of stress on the female voice by asking 54 female subjects to read a paragraph under normal and stressful conditions. The authors showed that stress resulted in a breathy and strained voice, commensurate with a decrease in voice quality and intensity. The need to consider stress in the workup of functional dysphonia was emphasized by the authors [63]. Larrouy-Mastri and Moromme investigated the effect of stress on the singing accuracy in two groups of student singers, a first year group and a second year group. Using a self-reported questionnaire on anxiety and objective measure-ments of sung performance, the authors showed that stress had a dual effect. The impact was positive on the first year students group but negative on the second year students group when the challenge increased. The authors also noted the significant correlation between voice accuracy and the intensity of cognitive symptoms [64].

Similarly, the predictive value of acoustic analysis in detecting stressful situa-tions has been reported. In a review of voice indices of stress, Giddens et al.

described the fundamental frequency (F0) as the most frequently reported acoustic index of stress. The authors highlighted the impact of gender and intersubject differences in the interpretation of acoustic parameters of stress [65]. Protopapas and Lieberman reported a correlation between the level of stress and the mean as well as maximum, F0, and hypothesized the dominant effect of formant frequency structure on the F0 effect [66]. The phonatory consequences of sports-related stress and other psychological sequel are easy to understand in the context of substantial information available on the psychology of voice disorders, as summarized by Rozen et al. [67]

In summary, assessment of mental well-being is as important as the physical well-being in the workup of dysphonia in athletes with musculoskeletal injuries. Stress and stress-related disorders impact the phonatory system commonly. Early recognition is crucial to optimal management of these patients. In the absence of adequate psychological defenses, psychological distress may deter effectiveness of and adherence to rehabilitation therapy [68]. Management of injured athletes must be comprehensive and multidisciplinary.

References

1. Igolnikov I, Gallagher RM, Hainline B. Sport-related injury and pain classification. Handb Clin Neurol. 2018;158:423–30.
2. Engebretsen L, Soligard T, Steffen K, et al. Sports injuries and illnesses during the London summer Olympic games 2012. Br J Sports Med. 2013;47(7):407–14.
3. Paterno MV, Taylor-Haas JA, Myer GD, Hewett TE. Prevention of overuse sports injuries in the young athlete. Orthop Clin North Am. 2013;44(4):553–64.
4. DiFiori JP, Benjamin HJ, Brenner JS, et al. Overuse injuries and burnout in youth sports: a position statement from the American Medical Society for Sports Medicine. Br J Sports Med. 2014;48(4):287–8.
5. Yang J, Tibbetts AS, Covassin T, Cheng G, Nayar S, Heiden E. Epidemiology of overuse and acute injuries among competitive collegiate athletes. J Athl Train. 2012;47(2):198–204.
6. Smyth EA, Newman P, Waddington G, Weissensteiner JR, Drew MK. Injury prevention strategies specific to pre-elite athletes competing in Olympic and professional sports—a systematic review. J Sci Med Sport. 2019;22(8):887–901.
7. Mueller-Wohlfahrt HW, Haensel L, Mithoefer K, et al. Terminology and classification of muscle injuries in sport: the Munich consensus statement. Br J Sports Med. 2013;47(6):342–50.
8. Almekinders LC, Engle CR. Common and uncommon injuries in ultra-endurance sports. Sports Med Arthrosc Rev. 2019;27(1):25–30.
9. Kerr ZY, Marshall SW, Dompier TP, Corlette J, Klossner DA, Gilchrist J. College sports-related injuries—United States, 2009–10 through 2013–14 academic years. MMWR Morb Mortal Wkly Rep. 2015;64(48):1330–6.
10. Pfirrmann D, Herbst M, Ingelfinger P, Simon P, Tug S. Analysis of injury incidences in male professional adult and elite youth soccer players: a systematic review. J Athl Train. 2016;51(5):410–24.
11. Eckard TG, Padua DA, Hearn DW, Pexa BS, Frank BS. The relationship between training load and injury in athletes: a systematic review. Sports Med. 2018;48(8):1929–61.
12. Soligard T, Steffen K, Palmer-Green D, et al. Sports injuries and illnesses in the Sochi 2014 Olympic winter games. Br J Sports Med. 2015;49(7):441–7.

13. Abrams GD, Renstrom PA, Safran MR. Epidemiology of musculoskeletal injury in the tennis player. Br J Sports Med. 2012;46(7):492–8.
14. Pieter W, Fife GP, O'Sullivan DM. Competition injuries in taekwondo: a literature review and suggestions for prevention and surveillance. Br J Sports Med. 2012;46(7):485–91.
15. Lopes AD, Hespanhol LC, Yeung SS, Costa LO. What are the main running-related musculoskeletal injuries? Sports Med. 2012;42(10):891–905.
16. Schöffl V, Simon M, Lutter C. Finger and shoulder injuries in rock climbing. Orthopade. 2019;48(12):1005–12.
17. Jacobs CL, Hincapié CA, Cassidy JD. Musculoskeletal injuries and pain in dancers: a systematic review update. J Dance Med Sci. 2012;16(2):74–84.
18. Weinstein S, Khodaee M, VanBaak K. Common skiing and snowboarding injuries. Curr Sports Med Rep. 2019;18(11):394–400.
19. Keogh JW, Winwood PW. The epidemiology of injuries across the weight-training sports. Sports Med. 2017;47(3):497–501.
20. Patel DR, Yamasaki A, Brown K. Epidemiology of sports-related musculoskeletal injuries in young athletes in United States. Transl Pediatr. 2017;6(3):160–6.
21. Cleary S, Chi V, Feinstein R. Female athletes: managing risk and maximizing benefit. Curr Opin Pediatr. 2018;30(6):874–82.
22. Cardoso R, Lumini-Oliveira J, Meneses RF. Associations between posture, voice, and dysphonia: a systematic review. J Voice. 2019;33(1):124.e1–124.e12.
23. Franco D, Martins F, Andrea M, Fragoso I, Carrão L, Teles J. Is the sagittal postural alignment different in normal and dysphonic adult speakers? J Voice. 2014;28(4):523.e1–8.
24. Gilman M, Johns MM. The effect of head position and/or stance on the self-perception of phonatory effort. J Voice. 2017;31(1):131.e1–4.
25. Knight EJ, Austin SF. The effect of head flexion/extension on acoustic measures of singing voice quality. J Voice. 2019;S0892-1997(19):30117–1.
26. Rantala L, Sala E, Kankare E. Teachers' working postures and their effects on the voice. Folia Phoniatr Logop. 2018;70(1):24–36.
27. Longo L, Di Stadio A, Ralli M, et al. Voice parameter changes in professional musician-singers singing with and without an instrument: the effect of body posture. Folia Phoniatr Logop. 2020;72(4):309–15.
28. Kooijman PG, De Jong FI, Oudes MJ, Huinck W, Van Acht H, Graamans K. Muscular tension and body posture in relation to voice handicap and voice quality in teachers with persistent voice complaints. Folia Phoniatr Logop. 2005;57(3):134–47.
29. Rubin JS, Blake E, Mathieson L, Kanana H. The effects of posture on voice. In: Sataloff RT. Professional voice. The science and art of clinical care. 4th ed. San Diego: Plural Publishing; 2017. p. 1309–18.
30. Baroody MM, Sataloff RT, Caroll LM. The singing voice specialist. In: Sataloff RT. Professional voice. The science and art of clinical care. 4th ed. San Diego: Plural Publishing; 2017. p. 1231–50.
31. Bruno E, De Padova A, Napolitano B, et al. Voice disorders and posturography: variables to define the success of rehabilitative treatment. J Voice. 2009;23(1):71–5.
32. Nacci A, Fattori B, Mancini V, et al. Posturographic analysis in patients with dysfunctional dysphonia before and after speech therapy/rehabilitation treatment. Acta Otorhinolaryngol Ital. 2012;32(2):115–21.
33. Negus VE. The mechanism of the larynx. St Louis: CV Mosby; 1931.
34. Sataloff RT. Bodily injuries and their effects on the voice. In: Sataloff RT. Professional voice: the science and art of clinical care. 4th ed. San Diego: Plural Publishing; 2017. p. 1003–5.
35. Marnejon T, Sarac S, Cropp AJ. Spontaneous pneumothorax in weightlifters. J Sports Med Phys Fit. 1995;35(2):124–6.
36. Soundappan SV, Holland AJ, Browne G. Sports-related pneumothorax in children. Pediatr Emerg Care. 2005;21(4):259–60.

37. Demertzis JL, Rubin DA. Upper extremity neuromuscular injuries in athletes. Semin Musculoskelet Radiol. 2012;16(4):316–30.
38. Hainline B, Turner JA, Caneiro JP, Stewart M, Moseley GL. Pain in elite athletes—neurophysiological, biomechanical and psychosocial considerations: a narrative review. Br J Sports Med. 2017;51(17):1259–64.
39. Kosek E, Cohen M, Baron R, et al. Do we need a third mechanistic descriptor for chronic pain states? Pain. 2016;157(7):1382–6.
40. Gamsa A. Is emotional disturbance a precipitator or a consequence of chronic pain? Pain. 1990;42(2):183–95.
41. Chong EY, Chan AH. Subjective health complaints of teachers from primary and secondary schools in Hong Kong. Int J Occup Saf Ergon. 2010;16(1):23–39.
42. Cardoso JP, Araújo TM, Carvalho FM, Oliveira NF, Reis EJ. Psychosocial work-related factors and musculoskeletal pain among schoolteachers. Cad Saude Publica. 2011;27(8):1498–506.
43. Cardoso JP, Ribeiro ID, Araújo TM, Carvalho FM, Reis EJ. Prevalence of musculoskeletal pain among teachers. Rev Brasde Epidemiol. 2009;12:604–14.
44. Ng YM, Voo P, Maakip I. Psychosocial factors, depression, and musculoskeletal disorders among teachers. BMC Public Health. 2019;19(1):234.
45. Chiu TT, Lam PK. The prevalence of and risk factors for neck pain and upper limb pain among secondary school teachers in Hong Kong. J Occup Rehabil. 2007;17(1):19–32.
46. Alsiddiky A, Algethami H, Ahmed E, Tokhtah H, Aldouhad J. The prevalence of musculoskeletal pain & its associated factors among female Saudi school teachers. Pak J Med Sci. 2014;30(6):1191–6.
47. Da Silva Vitor J, Siqueira LT, Ribeiro VV, Ramos JS, Brasolotto AG, Silverio KC. Musculoskeletal pain and occupational variables in teachers with voice disorders and in those with healthy voices—a pilot study. J Voice. 2017;31(4):518.e7–518.e13.
48. Ramos AC, Floro RL, Ribeiro VV, Brasolotto AG, Silverio KC. Musculoskeletal pain and voice-related quality of life in dysphonic and non-dysphonic subjects. J Voice. 2018;32(3):307–13.
49. Patel DR, Nelson TL. Sports injuries in adolescents. Med Clin North Am. 2000;84(4):983–1007.
50. Morrison MD, Rammage LA. Muscle misuse voice disorders: description and classification. Acta Otolaryngol. 1993;113(3):428–34.
51. Titze IR. Mechanical stress in phonation. J Voice. 1994;8(2):99–105.
52. Lechien JR, Mouawad F, Barillari MR, et al. Treatment of laryngopharyngeal reflux disease: a systematic review. World J Clin Cases. 2019;7(19):2995–3011.
53. Wismen T, Foster K, Curtis K. Mental health following traumatic physical injury: an integrative literature review. Injury. 2013;44(11):1383–90.
54. Aron CM, Harvey S, Hainline B, Hitchcock ME, Reardon CL. Post-traumatic stress disorder (PTSD) and other trauma-related mental disorders in elite athletes: a narrative review. Br J Sports Med. 2019;53(12):779–84.
55. Appaneal RN, Perna FM, Larkin KT. Psychophysiological response to severe sport injury among competitive male athletes: a preliminary investigation. J Clin Sport Psychol. 2007;1(1):68–88.
56. Leahy T, Pretty G, Tenenbaum G. A contextualized investigation of traumatic correlates of childhood sexual abuse in Australian athletes. Int J Sport Exerc Psychol. 2008;6(4):366–84.
57. Timpka T, Spreco A, Dahlstrom O, et al. Suicidal thoughts (ideation) among elite athletics (track and field) athletes: associations with sports participation, psychological resourcefulness and having been a victim of sexual and/or physical abuse. Br J Sports Med. 2021;55:198–205.
58. Regier DA, Kuhl EA, Kupfer DJ. The DSM-5: classification and criteria changes. World Psychiatry. 2013;12(2):92–8.
59. Padaki AS, Noticewala MS, Levine WN, Ahmad CS, Popkin MK, Popkin CA. Prevalence of posttraumatic stress disorder symptoms among young athletes after anterior cruciate ligament rupture. Orthop J Sports Med. 2018;6(7):2325967118787159.

60. Shuer ML, Dietrich MS. Psychological effects of chronic injury in elite athletes. West J Med. 1997;166(2):104–9.
61. Gkikopoulos G, Chronopoulou C, Christakou A. Examining re-injury worry, confidence and attention after a sport musculoskeletal injury. J Sports Med Phys Fitness. 2019;60(3):428–34.
62. Holmqvist S, Santtila P, Lindström E, Sala E, Simberg S. The association between possible stress markers and vocal symptoms. J Voice. 2013;27(6):787.e1–787.e10.
63. Van Lierde K, Van Heule S, De Ley S, Mertens E, Claeys S. Effect of psychological stress on female vocal quality. Folia Phoniatr Logop. 2009;61(2):105–11.
64. Larrouy-Maestri P, Morsomme D. The effects of stress on singing voice accuracy. J Voice. 2014;28(1):52–8.
65. Giddens CL, Barron KW, Byrd-Craven J, Clark KF, Winter AS. Vocal indices of stress: a review. J Voice. 2013;27(3):390.e21–9.
66. Protopapas A, Lieberman P. Fundamental frequency of phonation and perceived emotional stress. J Acoust Soc Am. 1997;101(4):2267–77.
67. Rosen DC, Sataloff JB, Sataloff RT. Psychology of Voice Disorders, Second Edition. San Diego: Plural Publishing; 2020; p. 1–417.
68. Brewer BW, Van Raalte JL, Cornelius AE, et al. Psychological factors, rehabilitation adherence, and rehabilitation outcome after anterior cruciate ligament reconstruction. Rehabil Psychol. 2000;45(1):20.

Chapter 8
Exercise-Induced Laryngeal Obstruction (EILO) in Athletes

8.1 Prevalence

Vocal fold dysfunction refers to abnormal adduction of the vocal folds during inspiration leading to respiratory symptoms such as dyspnea, cough, and stridor. The term was described initially by Patterson et al. in 1974 who suggested a nonorganic etiology of this condition [1]. In 1983, Christopher et al. described five patients with paroxysms of breathing difficulties and extra-thoracic airway obstruction who had been misdiagnosed with and treated for asthma. The respiratory symptoms were characterized by intermittent noisy breathing and wheezing, associated with adduction of the true and false vocal folds during inspiration [2]. The authors stressed the role of psychological factors in the etiology of this laryngeal behavior and the need for early diagnosis. Since the inception of the term "vocal cord dysfunction," 40 additional descriptive terms have been reported in the literature, depicting similar conditions of paroxysms of shortness of breath and dyspnea induced by a variety of triggers. These terms include paradoxical vocal fold movement disorders, hysteric croup, fictitious asthma, irritable larynx, and laryngeal hyperresponsiveness, among many others [2]. The terms paradoxical vocal fold motion disorder (PVFMD) and paradoxical vocal fold movement (PVFM) are used mostly by otolaryngologists, whereas the term vocal fold dysfunction (VFD) or vocal cord dysfunction (VCD) is used mostly by pulmonologists and allergists [3]. In 2013, an international task force was assembled to solve the heterogeneity in the nomenclature of vocal fold dysfunction. The European Society of Otolaryngology in collaboration with the American College of surgeons has recommended to the term "induced laryngeal obstruction" (ILO) to describe the onset of intermittent airway symptoms following exposure to a trigger and complete regression of these symptoms following cessation of exposure to the trigger [4]. The acronym "ILO" was stratified further into subcategories based on the type of trigger reported by the patient. These include

© The Author(s), under exclusive license to Springer Nature Switzerland AG 2021
A.-L. Hamdan et al., *Voice Disorders in Athletes, Coaches and other Sports Professionals*, https://doi.org/10.1007/978-3-030-69831-7_8

cough, perfume, other environmental irritants, hyperventilation, and exercise, among other environmental irritants.

In athletes, the onset of laryngeal obstructive symptoms following exercise is referred to as exercise-induced laryngeal obstruction (EILO). This entity is induced primarily by hyperventilation and physical activity, unlike other types of vocal fold dysfunction triggered by non-exercise stimuli. The link between obstructive laryngeal behavior and exercise was highlighted as early as 1984 by Lakin et al. in a case report of a female athlete with a 10-year history of exercise-induced wheezing, nonresponsive to anti-asthmatic medications. Her inspiratory stridor was associated with collapse of the posterior aspect of aryepiglottic folds during inspiration and flattening of the inspiratory phase of the flow-volume loop. The authors stressed the abnormal supraglottic laryngeal behavior not commonly seen in patients with paradoxical vocal fold movement disorders and highlighted the role of physical conditioning in the management of this entity [5].

The prevalence of EILO is hard to delineate from the literature given the heterogeneity in the terms used to describe this and related entities. Nieleon et al. reviewed the prevalence of EILO in a cohort of 91 athletes with suspected asthma and reported a prevalence of 35%. The diagnosis was confirmed using continuous laryngoscopic examination during exercise [6]. In another study by Rundell and Spiering which included 370 elite athletes, the authors reported inspiratory stridor in 5.1% of the cases, with a high predominance in females (18 females vs. 1 male). The authors highlighted the underdiagnosis of vocal fold dysfunction in athletes with exercise-induced bronchoconstriction [7]. The disparity in the prevalence of EILO is ascribed primarily to the variations in the study groups, terms used to describe symptoms of induced laryngeal obstruction, and diagnostic tests used to investigate affected patients.

Exercise-induced laryngeal obstruction has gained a lot of attention over the last few decades because of its adverse impact on quality of life and the unnecessary usage of medical resources (emergency room visits, use of steroid medications, and others) to treat this condition [8, 9]. Impairment in exercise tolerance while training and/or competing can be detrimental physically and psychologically. Patients may experience a high level of anxiety, stress, poor control of their physical condition and breathing, and withdrawal from sports and daily activities [9]. This chapter reviews the clinical presentation of EILO in athletes. The terms EILO, exercise PVFMD, PVFM, and VFD are quoted as reported by the authors who are referenced. The pathophysiology and associated comorbidities are reviewed. The diagnostic workup and up-to-date treatment modalities are stressed.

8.1.1   Clinical Presentation: Symptoms and Findings

Clinical assessment of EILO in athletes can be very challenging. Similar to other medical conditions, the workup includes a detailed medical history and physical examination. Questions about the nature of the airway symptoms, their onset and duration, and associated comorbidities are asked. The most commonly reported symptoms in affected athletes are shortness of breath, stridor, cough, throat/chest discomfort, difficulty swallowing, and change in voice quality [10–14]. In a review of the diagnostic criteria of vocal fold dysfunction by Morris et al., dyspnea, wheezing, and stridor were the most commonly reported symptoms in 73%, 36%, and 28% of cases, respectively. Other reported symptoms included chest tightness, throat tightness, and cough in 25%, 22%, and 12% of cases, respectively. Dysphonia was reported in only 12% of the study group. Notably, the review was not limited to athletes with EILO and included psychogenic vocal cord dysfunction (VFD), irritant-associated VFD, and other types of VFD [10]. In a study by Chiang et al. of 104 patients with exercise-induced PVFMD, dyspnea and dysphonia (hoarseness and/or weak voice) were the most commonly reported symptoms in 99% and 60% of cases, respectively. Other reported symptoms included cough and dysphagia in 38% and 22% of cases, respectively [11]. Note that the 104 patients were selected from a cohort of 758 patients with confirmed PVCMD. The authors did not specify whether the participants were athletes [11]. Similarly, Marcinow et al., in their review of 46 athletes diagnosed with PVFMD, reported chest tightness, cough, and throat tightness in 57%, 22%, and 41% of cases, respectively. All patients had shortness of breath, and almost half the patients had noisy breathing. Only 15% had a change in voice quality [12].

The presence of airway obstructive symptoms during or following exercise in athletes is not a clinical discriminator between EILO and lower airway diseases. In a study by Nielsen et al. that included 88 athletes, one-third (35%) of whom diagnosed with EILO, inspiratory stridor did not differentiate between EILO and asthma. Moreover, almost two-thirds of those diagnosed with EILO were on asthma medications, although many of those were determined to have been misdiagnosed, and asthma medications were stopped. [6] AL-Alwan et al. in their review of the clinical presentation of vocal fold dysfunction in athletes noted several clinical diagnostic criteria that helped physicians differentiate vocal fold dysfunction from exercise-induced bronchoconstriction (EIB). These included inspiratory stridor, interruption of the airway symptoms by panting, and most importantly spontaneous regression of these symptoms after exercise [13]. In a review of inspiratory stridor in elite athletes, Rundell and Spiering identified the spontaneous resolution of symptoms only a few minutes after cessation of physical activity, unlike exercise-induced bronchoconstriction [7].

Laryngeal examination is mandatory in the workup of athletes with EILO. Based on the report of Morris et al. on the diagnostic criteria of vocal fold dysfunction, inspiratory adduction of the anterior two-thirds of the vocal folds with a posterior diamond-shaped chink is observed typically on laryngeal endoscopy (Fig. 8.1). Note that at least 50% closure of the vocal folds during inspiration must be seen to make the diagnosis [10]. The authors stressed that abnormal laryngeal behavior is not confined to the glottis. Supraglottic constriction at the level of the false vocal folds and aryepiglottic folds also may be observed. [4] Powell et al. in their study on paradoxical vocal fold dysfunction in juveniles reported abnormally positioned epiglottis, anteroposterior constriction, and medialization of the false vocal folds in 36%,

41%, and 45% of the cases, respectively. Fifty-five percent showed an abnormal adductory movement of the true vocal folds during asymptomatic respiration [14]. The laryngeal examination is also paramount in excluding other laryngeal lesions and in diagnosing preexisting or subsequent vocal fold structural changes. In a study by Chiang et al., flexible laryngeal examination revealed edema posteriorly in 89% of cases and laryngeal lesions such as nodules, polyps, granuloma, and ulcerations in almost one out of four patients with exercise-induced PVFMD. Interestingly, 7% had evidence of abnormal vocal fold mobility [11]. Similarly, in a study by Marcinow et al. of 46 elite athletes, 11% had abnormal laryngeal findings, namely, vocal folds polypoid lesions and ulcerations [12].

Failure to observe abnormal laryngeal behavior in between the attacks has prompted the use of provocative laryngeal endoscopic examination, often referred to as post-exertion flexible laryngoscopy (FL). The rationale of the provocative laryngeal endoscopy is to allow visualization of vocal fold adduction following provocation in an attempt to simulate an attack of inspiratory stridor. In EILO, examples of triggers commonly used include rapid deep breathing, speaking tasks such as rapid counting, or the use of a treadmill, bike, or stair climber. According to the consensus of the international task force on inducible laryngeal obstruction, the location of the laryngeal obstruction, the onset time, and the duration of symptoms are diagnostic clinical indicators of EILO [3]. The diagnostic criteria used in the study by Chiang et al. included the presence of at least two episodes of inappropriate vocal fold adduction during ten respiratory cycles in patients with no known cause of upper airway obstruction. Additionally, they stated that normal vocal fold mobility at some point during the laryngeal examination must be observed [11]. In

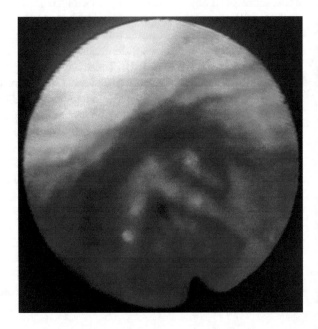

Fig. 8.1 Laryngeal endoscopic view of a female patient during an attack of paradoxical vocal fold movement. Note the adduction of the vocal folds during inspiration and the diamond-shaped opening posteriorly

that study, post-exertion flexible laryngoscopy was shown to increase the sensitivity of diagnosing exercise-induced PVFMD. Approximately 48% of 104 patients with exercise-induced PVFMD had evidence of PVFMD on FL at rest, whereas 89% had evidence of PVFMD during the post-exertion laryngoscopy. Notably, 78% of patients without evidence of PVFMD on initial assessment were diagnosed with exercise PVFMD following exertion [11].

The false-positive interpretation of flexible laryngoscopy (FL) in patients with laryngeal dysfunction and strong gag reflex and the fast resolution of paradoxical vocal fold adduction in provocative laryngeal endoscopic examination lead to a new diagnostic modality for EILO. Continuous laryngoscopic evaluation has emerged as a more sensitive alternative to diagnose laryngeal dysfunction in athletes. Continuous laryngoscopy (CL) allows continuous visualization of the glottis and supraglottic structures throughout the challenge rather than just during a brief period following exertion [5, 15–20]. The widespread use of CL led to a change in the understanding of the laryngeal behavior of athletes suspected of having EILO. By providing immediate feedback, numerous studies using continuous laryngoscopic evaluation asserted that EILO is not confined to adductory movement of the vocal folds. The inward collapse of the supraglottic structures often precedes the paroxysm of vocal fold closure. Tervonen et al. reported abnormal laryngeal findings on flexible laryngoscopy with a bicycle ergometry test in 9 of 25 patients suspected of having exercise-induced vocal fold dysfunction. The diagnostic signs included supraglottic collapse in addition to vocal fold adduction while patients were having inspiratory stridor [15]. In a study of four females with history of stridor and dyspnea during exercise, Heimdal et al. showed evidence of medial motion of the dorsal part of the aryepiglottic folds and adduction of the true vocal folds in all patients. The laryngeal evaluation was performed continuously while patients exercised on a treadmill until exhaustion. Notably, only 2 of 12 control subjects exhibited mild medial rotation of the aryepiglottic folds during inspiration [16]. Christensen et al. described a software diagnostic tool that measures the laryngeal inlet and its cross-sectional area during inspiration using CL. The study conducted on 97 patients showed the utility of this test in differentiating between exercise-induced vocal fold dysfunction and exercise-induced laryngomalacia, with a positive predictive value of 0.79 [17]. Olin et al. stressed the importance of CL in allowing visualization of the laryngeal structures at different levels of the individual's working capacity. Its added value is most helpful in patients whose symptoms appear at peak-work capacity and resolve rapidly afterward, thus prohibiting visualization of the adduction and collapse of the true and false vocal folds shortly following peak-effort exercise [18]. Similarly, Maat et al. reported a positive correlation between CL exercise video scoring and symptom scores. The study was conducted on 100 patients who ran on a treadmill and had their laryngeal video recordings evaluated by two independent laryngologists [19]. Walsted et al. extended further the application of CL in the evaluation of respiratory symptoms in athletes. Their report was the first to describe the use of this diagnostic technique in a swimming environment [20].

Pulmonary function testing is also key in differentiating EILO from lower airway diseases, particularly asthma. Complete assessment of the flow-volume loop is mandatory. The typical finding is a truncation of the inspiratory phase of the flow-volume loop, a sign that is indicative of extra-thoracic obstruction. Other significant findings include reduction in the ratio of maximal inspiratory to maximal expiratory flow at 50% capacity and "an abnormally high ratio of forced inspiratory flow at 25% vital capacity to forced inspiratory flow at 75% vital capacity." [13] In a large study of 105 active duty military patients with exertion-induced dyspnea, Morris et al. showed that the methacholine challenging test and spirometry were diagnostic in 41% and 16% of cases, respectively. A positive methacholine challenge supports a diagnosis of asthma, whereas a negative test suggests the diagnosis of other entities such as EILO. The authors advocated the routine use of these tests in the evaluation of patients with history of exercise-induced respiratory symptoms [21]. However, in another study by the same authors, pulmonary function testing had little value in differentiating between patients with vocal fold dysfunction and those without. The investigation carried on 52 subjects, 40 with exertion dyspnea and 12 with no respiratory symptoms, showed abnormal flow-volume loops in 20% of patients with exertion dyspnea and diagnosed with VFD in comparison to 14% in those with exertion dyspnea and no VFD. Notably, in the VFD subgroup, 60% had a positive methacholine test, though the decrease in FEV1/FVC was less in comparison to those not diagnosed with VFD [22]. Note that these findings do not question the diagnostic yield of methacholine challenge test but rather highlight the high prevalence of asthma in patients with VFD in comparison to patients with no VFD, which is in agreement with a study by Newman et al. who also reported asthma in 53 of 95 patients diagnosed with VFD [23]. Hence, the methacholine challenging test should be interpreted cautiously.

Although the clinical triad of dyspnea, adductory movement of the vocal folds, and truncation of the inspiratory phase of flow-volume loop is commonly used in the diagnosis of EILO, its diagnostic specificity is not perfect in patients with exercise-induced laryngeal stridor. Olin et al. described five cases of exertional dyspnea with inspiratory stridor in whom 70–86% glottic opening and normal flow-volume loop were noted. The authors challenged the conventional diagnostic criteria of PVFMD asserting the need to witness closure of the vocal folds during inspiration and blunting of the inspiratory phase of the flow-volume loop. The authors ascribed audible stridor in these patients associated with increased intrathoracic pressure during inspiration, to a compensatory behavior needed to maintain normal airflow across the increased glottic resistance associated with mild adduction of the vocal folds [24]. This explanation remains hypothetical with no scientific proof. The authors argued that glottic narrowing in isolation does not always cause audible stridor; rather, a combination of increased airflow and glottic adduction is needed. That being stated, it is evident that many patients with VFMD and normal or wide glottic aperture are underdiagnosed. Moreover, given the difficulty of laryngeal examination during exercise, and the short duration of abnormal laryngeal behavior in affected patients, direct visualization of glottic closure is not always easy to document.

Laryngeal electromyography (LEMG) also is useful in diagnosing EILO. Affected patients display an increase in recruitment in the adductor muscles during inspiration consistent with the adduction of the vocal folds seen on endoscopy. LEMG also can assist in differentiating between the various etiologies of laryngeal dysfunction, namely, psychogenic vs. reflux-induced vs. respiratory dystonia [25]. In patients with respiratory dystonia, the increase in aberrant recruitment often can be seen not only during inspiration but throughout the glottic cycle, and paradoxical adductor activation often is present even when the patient is asymptomatic. In psychogenic dysphonia or PVFM, there often is simultaneous, fairly asymmetric activation of abductor and adductor muscles. Further information on the clinical application of laryngeal EMG in patients with laryngeal movement disorders is a vailable in Chap. 25 of Professional Voice: the Science of Art and Clinical Care [25].

In summary, EILO occurs primarily in athletes following exercise and is characterized by intermitted dyspnea and stridor associated with vocal fold adduction. Vocal fold behavior among patients varies from mild adduction to complete adduction during inspiration. Additional findings such as collapse of supraglottic tissues may be observed. EILO is diagnosed best with provocative or continuous laryngoscopy. Spirometry invariably shows evidence of extra-thoracic obstruction with a negative methacholine challenge test. It is important to note that EILO rarely responds to anti-asthmatic medications. EILO may be accompanied by dysphonia, and the dysphonia may last far longer than the paradoxical adduction.

8.2 Pathophysiology

The pathophysiology of EILO in athletes is not well understood. Five pathophysiologic mechanisms have been discussed thoroughly in the literature in the context of exercise and non-exercise-induced laryngeal obstruction. These include mechanical factors, laryngeal hypersensitivity, psychogenic predisposition, autonomic nervous system dysfunction, and excessive laryngeal tension, respiratory dystonia, and laryngopharyngeal reflux disease.

8.2.1 Mechanical Factors

The patency of the laryngeal lumen during inspiration depends on the respiratory behavior, the mobility of the vocal folds, and the rigidity of the laryngeal structures (cartilages, muscles, ligaments, and mucosal folds). Based on the Bernoulli principle, when the airflow velocity within the laryngeal lumen increases, there is an increase in the inward-pulling forces [26]. In cases of heavy breathing, the intense pulling forces can lead to collapse of the luminal wall with subsequent airway occlusion. Hence, the increase in minute ventilation commonly observed in athletes during their peak physical activity can predispose to inspiratory collapse of the laryngeal structures. The narrower the laryngeal inlet, the higher the airflow resistance, and the more turbulent the airflow. With an increase in airflow turbulence, there is an increase in the collision of air molecules against its surrounding structures, leading to vibration and audible stridor.

The mechanical factor hypothesis is supported by the fact that EILO occurs predominantly in adolescent athletes whose laryngeal apertures are narrower than those of adults [14]. The reduced laryngeal size and inlet in young athletes compared to adult athletes has been demonstrated by numerous studies [27, 28]. In a study by Wysocki et al. on pubertal laryngeal growth, the authors showed that the younger the individual, the narrower the larynx. The study conducted on adults ($n = 20$) and children larynges ($n = 34$) showed a positive correlation between most anatomic parameters and age [27]. Similarly, Hocevar-Boltezar et al., in their study of 54 subjects of different age groups, highlighted the disproportionate growth of different components of the respiratory tract and alluded to the pathogenic role of this disproportionate growth in laryngeal obstruction. The preponderance of exercise-induced laryngeal symptoms in females supports further the mechanical factor hypothesis given the gender difference in laryngeal proportions, opening, and size of vocal folds [28].

In summary, EILO in athletes can be attributed in some cases to the inward-pulling forces on the supraglottic and glottic structures during inspiration. In peak physical activity and hyperventilation, this inward pull is intensified and can lead to severe or complete collapse of the airway. The differential growth of laryngeal structures and the sexual dimorphism observed at puberty support the mechanical factor theory. In addition, even mild collapse can be symptomatic in athletes due to alteration in the aerodynamic behavior in the supraglottic region.

8.2.2   Laryngeal Hypersensitivity

There is consensus in the literature that laryngeal hypersensitivity accentuates vocal fold adduction as a protective laryngeal behavior. It is considered as a laryngeal maladaptation that results in dysfunction and an array of syndromes such as chronic cough, muscle tension dysphonia, and paradoxical vocal fold movement [29]. Rapid high-volume bursts of ventilation through the mouth result in fast penetration of non-humidified cool air into the upper airway with subsequent drying and irritation of the vocal folds. This repeated exposure of the laryngeal mucosa to cold air and environmental irritants can lead to laryngeal sensory stimulation and paradoxical vocal fold motion, in isolation or combination with lower airway diseases such as asthma [30, 34].

The pathogenic role of laryngeal hypersensitivity in EILO is seen mostly in athletes exposed to cold air in indoor ice arenas and air polluted fields and stadiums. In a study by Rundell and Spiering that included 370 athletes with a history of inspiratory stridor, the prevalence of vocal cord dysfunction was notably higher in outdoor athletes in comparison to indoor athletes (8.3% vs. 2.5%, respectively) [7]. The overall prevalence of vocal fold dysfunction was around 5.1%, half of whom also had exercise-induced bronchospasm. In a study by Vertigan et al. in 2018 on the laryngeal behavior in patients with chronic refractory cough, a phenotype of cough hypersensitivity syndrome, cough frequency was 16.5/h in patients with vocal fold dysfunction. Paradoxical vocal fold movement during inspiration increased to 67% following odor challenge in comparison to 47% at rest. The authors stressed the pathogenic role of laryngeal dysfunction in patients with refractory cough and the abnormal laryngeal behavior in cases of laryngeal hypersensitivity [32]. The same authors compared laryngeal sensitivity in patients with PVFM, MTD, chronic refractory cough, and globus and showed significant impairment in all subgroups. The authors emphasized the overlap in the clinical features of these entities and the need to have a common treatment strategy for laryngeal hypersensitivity in afflicted patients [33]. These findings are in agreement with the study by Ryan et al. who showed improvement in paradoxical vocal fold movement and extra-thoracic airway hyperresponsiveness following treatment of chronic cough. The investigation included two groups of patients with cough, those with and those without PVFM based on laryngeal examination [34].

In summary, laryngeal hypersensitivity can play a pathogenic role in EILO. It is considered as an upregulation in the intensity and frequency of the adductor laryngeal reflex as a protective mechanism [31]. Laryngeal hypersensitivity may present as a clinical spectrum that can include excessive laryngeal muscle tension and chronic cough. Control of the triggering factors may help reduce the frequency and intensity of airway symptoms. Environmental stimuli should be investigated in both indoor and outdoor arenas.

8.2.3 Psychogenic Disorders

The pathogenic role of psychogenic disorders in patients with EILO is still an issue of ongoing debate in the literature. The interest stems from the known disturbances in respiration in patients with panic attack, anxiety, and pain. Wilhelm et al. reported chronic hypocapnia and evidence of respiratory dysregulation in patients with functional disorders and chronic pain [35]. Numerous studies indicate a higher prevalence of EILO in athletes during competition vs. training and in those who are under pressure in comparison to those who are not [35–39]. Based on a study by McFadden and Zawadski on vocal fold dysfunction masquerading as "choking" during athletic activities, the authors reported that athletes who felt the need for utmost performance and who participated in competitive sports were more likely to develop EILO. The authors used the term psychogenic vocal cord dysfunction to stress the functional component in this subgroup of patients [36]. Similarly, Powell et al. in 2007 speculated that stress and personality disorders are important triggers of laryngeal obstruction. In their study of 12 adolescent patients with acute onset of inspiratory stridor and lack of any chemical or biological stimulus, the authors concluded that psychogenic illness is a cause of vocal fold dysfunction [37]. In a study by Forrest et al. of 117 patients diagnosed with PVFM, 47 of whom underwent psychological evaluation using the Minnesota Multiphasic Personality Inventory and the

Life Experiences Survey, the authors demonstrated the presence of a conversion disorder in 20% of their study group, and 4.3% were proven to be malingerers [38]. However, stress-related disorders can be the sequelae of EILO and failure of treatment, rather than the cause, and a diagnosis of psychogenic EILO should be based on positive evidence and only after other etiologies have been ruled out.

In summary, psychological disorders can predispose to EILO with a high prevalence of conversion disorders being reported in athletes under pressure. Competition and behavioral predisposition also may precipitate the symptoms of upper airway obstruction. Notably, stress-related disorders in EILO may well be the sequel of this condition rather than the precursors or cause.

8.2.4   Autonomic Nervous System Dysfunction

Breathing requires the coordinated activity of motor neurons centrally. It is controlled primarily by a well-localized interneuron population, the Dbx1-derived pre-Botzinger complex, which is held responsible for the rhythmic inspiratory movement. The inspiratory-expiratory phase transition is influenced by short-term synaptic depression in these neurons [40]. Although the autonomic nervous system is involved mostly in controlling respiratory rate and expiratory time, numerous authors have found that a subpopulation of the Dbx-derived neurons connects to the hypoglossal nucleus in the medulla and plays a role in maintaining the patency of the airway. It also has been shown that this subset of premotor neurons is actively engaged in breathing and project to XII motor neurons which in turn contain motor neurons that contribute to the patency of the airway. As such, dysfunction in this network can contribute to breathing disorders such as sleep apnea [40–42].

The autonomic nervous system (ANS) also plays a crucial role in laryngeal behavior [43]. This is based on the well-known sympathetic and parasympathetic innervation of the laryngeal structures and the laryngeal response following ANS activation seen in stage fright. Voice breaks and changes in voice pitch and loudness are described typically, and they are accompanied by systemic symptoms such as dizziness and dry mouth [43–45]. Similarly, patients with functional voice disorders frequently exhibit neurovegetative symptoms. Demmink-Geertman and Dejonckere in their prospective study of 184 patients with nonorganic voice disorders and 126 controls reported a high prevalence of neurovegetative symptoms in patients with voice-related complaints. Moreover, the prevalence of neurovegetative symptoms decreased with a decrease in voice complaints after therapy [46]. In 2013, Helou et al. showed that increased activation of the autonomic nervous system in the body is associated with increased activity of the intrinsic laryngeal muscles, as well. Using a cold pressor as a stimulus to the whole body autonomic nervous system, the authors showed an increase in muscle activity of the cricothyroid, thyroarytenoid, and cricoarytenoid muscles that persisted even after attenuation of the cardiovascular response. The authors alluded to the linkage of laryngeal behavior to stress and emotional stimuli [47].

In summary, the autonomic nervous system is linked to laryngeal behavior. Increased activity of the autonomic nervous system in response to psychological, emotional, and physical stressors may lead to increased laryngeal responsiveness with resultant hyperactivity and possible obstruction. Research in that field is needed to investigate this hypothesis further.

8.2.5 Increased Laryngeal Tension

It is well known that the anatomic position of the larynx is linked to its function. The vertical position of the larynx in association with breathing and phonation has been the subject of thorough investigation in the literature [48–50]. A low-positioned larynx, commonly observed in subjects who rely on abdominal breathing, facilitates the adduction of the vocal folds during phonation. Opening of the glottis is eased by the downward pull of the trachea associated with diaphragmatic contraction during inspiration. A high-positioned larynx in patients with poor breathing support is associated with hard glottal attacks and hyperfunctional laryngeal behavior. Athletes who are accustomed to chest or clavicular breathing routinely experience excessive tension in the cervical and extrinsic laryngeal muscles, often leading to a high-positioned larynx. This unfavorable position of the larynx not only shortens the length of the vocal tract but also may limit abduction of the vocal folds and compromise the patency of the laryngeal lumen. Using a multichannel electroglottograph, Iwarson and Sundberg showed an association between high lung volume and low-positioned larynx which in turn correlated with voice pitch. The study was conducted on 29 subjects who were asked to phonate at different pitches, loudnesses, and lung volumes [49]. The inhalation mode of breathing and the impact of body posture on the position of the larynx were emphasized by the authors.

The studies above support the strong link between laryngeal muscle tension and laryngeal narrowing, a major limitation to exercise performance [51]. Vertigan et al. investigated respiratory function in 15 patients diagnosed with muscle tension dysphonia (MTD) in comparison to 15 healthy subjects. Using flexible laryngeal examination, the authors showed a higher prevalence of abnormal glottic closure in patients with MTD vs. controls. Moreover, using pulmonary function testing, the study group demonstrated a decrease in FIF-5O after provocation with nebulized hypertonic saline. The authors emphasized the subclinical aberrant vocal fold behavior during inspiration in patients with muscle tension dysphonia [52]. These results are in agreement with other studies by the same authors highlighting the commonalities in the etiologies of MTD and PVFMD, particularly laryngeal hypersensitivity, and the presence of paradoxical vocal fold behavior in patients diagnosed with muscle tension dysphonia. The authors also stressed the improvement in PVFM following treatment of refractory cough [32].

In summary, there is strong linkage between laryngeal tension and laryngeal airway obstruction. Excessive laryngeal muscle tension may be a pathogenic factor in patients with EILO. More research in this field is needed.

8.2.6   Respiratory Dystonia

Respiratory dystonia is a form of laryngeal dystonia that affects primarily breathing. Similar to other forms of dystonia, such as spasmodic dysphonia, respiratory dystonia is characterized by involuntary contraction of the laryngeal adductor muscles. Affected patients suffer from adduction of the vocal folds during inspiration or throughout the respiratory cycle. Unlike spasmodic dysphonia that affects phonation, respiratory dystonia affects breathing and presents with inspiratory stridor and shortness of breath. Phonatory disturbances are often not present [53]. Respiratory dystonia is one of the causes of EILO. Based on the experience of the author (RTS), respiratory dystonia is the main cause of EILO, particularly in patients with no psychopathology background and/or history of reflux disease. Electromyography of the adductor muscles typically shows signs of increased recruitment even at rest, and thus it is helpful in differentiating respiratory dystonia from psychogenic causes, reflux-induced laryngeal spasm, and other etiologies. The author of this manuscript (RTS) has previously described eight patients with adductor laryngeal breathing dystonia, six of whom were idiopathic, and four of whom had other types of dystonia. All patients had inspiratory stridor and adduction of the vocal folds during inspiration [53].

In summary, respiratory dystonia is a form of dystonia that affects the laryngeal adductor muscles. The clinical picture varies and represents a spectrum of airway obstructive symptoms. EILO is a common presentation of respiratory. Laryngeal electromyography is useful in diagnosing respiratory dystonia and in differentiating it from other etiologies of EILO such as psychogenic causes and laryngopharyngeal reflux diseases.

8.2.7   Laryngopharyngeal Reflux Disease

An important etiology of EILO is laryngopharyngeal reflux (LPR) disease. LPR is characterized by backflow of the gastric content into the laryngeal inlet and pharynx. The most common underlying mechanism is dysfunction in upper esophageal sphincters with or without esophageal dysmotility. The lack of peristalsis and buffering mechanisms in the pharynx and larynx allows the refluxate material to induce mucosal damage leading to an array of symptoms. These include cough, globus sensation, throat clearing, change in voice quality, dysphagia, and laryngospasm that can cause EILO and be mistaken for psychogenic or dystonic PVFMD. The reflux-induced laryngeal dysfunction is either vagally mediated or attributed to mechanical factors, namely, direct aspiration of the reflux material into the airway. A more detailed description of the clinical presentation and pathophysiology of LPR as a voice risk factor is available in Chap. 5 of this book. The prevalence of LPR and GERD in athletes with EILO is reviewed in the section below on LPR as a comorbid disease in patients with laryngeal dysfunction.

8.3 Associated Comorbidities

Limitation in breathing during exercise has multiple etiologies. These include structural laryngeal lesions, respiratory muscle fatigue with peripheral vasoconstriction, large alveolar-arterial oxygen pressure difference leading to arterial hypoxemia, extra-thoracic obstruction such as ILO, and other causes such as paresis and paralysis [51]. Exercise-induced or non-exercise-induced ILO is associated with comorbidities that compound the frequency and intensity of attacks or mask their presence. These include asthma, exercise-induced asthma and exercise-induced bronchoconstriction, psychological and personality disorders, gastroesophageal/laryngopharyngeal reflux disease, and neurogenic laryngeal movement disorders. Less frequently encountered causes include fibromyalgia, rheumatoid arthritis and other autoimmune diseases, and other disorders.

8.3.1 Asthma, Exercise-Induced Asthma, and Exercise-Induced Bronchoconstriction: Implications for EILO in Athletes

Exercise-induced respiratory symptoms are common in athletes and remain underdiagnosed. [54] Often, these are ascribed to asthma and/or exercise-induced asthma (EIA), and the prevalence of which in athletes is 55% and 70%, respectively [54, 55]. In 2016, Kurowski et al. investigated the prevalence of allergy and asthma in 220 Polish professional Olympic athletes using an allergy questionnaire, allergy skin prick testing, spirometry, and methacholine challenge test. Exercise-induced asthma and asthma occurred in 28.4% and 11.3% of cases, respectively [56]. Salem et al. studied 636 athletes and reported asthma in 30.2% of the cases, although half the affected subjects (47.6%) were on immunotherapy [57]. Perrotta et al. reported poorly controlled asthma in one out of five elite mountain bikers. Allergy was present in 47.8% of the total group, and those with allergy had more frequent respiratory tract infections. The authors advocated screening programs for early detection of allergy and asthma symptoms in athletes [58].

The prevalence of asthma is known to be significantly higher in athletes with laryngeal dysfunction in comparison to athletes with no laryngeal dysfunction. In a study by Chiang et al. of 104 patients with exercise-induced PVFMD, asthma and allergies were comorbid diseases in 42% of cases [11]. In another study by Marcinow et al. that included 46 athletes with PVFMD, asthma was second to environmental allergies in occurrence with a prevalence of 46% and 39%, respectively. Notably, the prevalence of allergies was higher in athletes with paradoxical vocal fold movement disorders in comparison to nonathletes with PVFMD [12]. Similarly, Newman et al. reported concurrent history of asthma in 56% of a study group ($n = 95$) diagnosed with PVFM and who were on anti-asthmatic medications [23]. EILO is also more prevalent in asthmatics. In a study by Christensen et al. on the prevalence of

EILO in the general public, the authors reported a higher rate in patients with airway hyperresponsiveness in comparison to those with no airway hyperresponsiveness (26.1% vs. 7.5% of cases, respectively). The participants between the ages of 14 and 24 years were evaluated using a questionnaire, methacholine challenge, and continuous laryngoscopic examination [59].

Exercise-induced respiratory symptoms also can result from exercise-induced bronchoconstriction (EIB). Exercise-induced bronchoconstriction is a common lower airway condition that interferes with athletes' ability to compete. It is defined "transient airway narrowing that occurs during or following exercise." [60] Its prevalence is in the range of 10–20% in the normal population and increases markedly in asthmatics and athletes [61, 62]. Based on a study by Levai et al. on the susceptibility of athletes to provocative environmental factors, the authors reported EIB in 44.8% of subjects. The study group included 44 swimmers who were evaluated using a respiratory symptom questionnaire and spirometry [63]. Bougault et al. investigated EIB in soccer players and reported a prevalence of 16%. The study was conducted on youth soccer players and professional soccer players using spirometry and a eucapnic voluntary hyperpnea test. Skin sensitization to five allergens or more was predictive of EIB. [64]

Similarities in the clinical presentation of asthma, EIA, EIB, and EILO often have led to the misdiagnosis and mismanagement of affected patients. The commonality in the clinical presentation is attributed partially to the commonality in precipitating factors. These include high-minute ventilation and environmental stressors such as cold air, chlorinated swimming water, contaminated air, and inhaled pollutants. The presenting symptoms of dyspnea, chest tightness reported by athletes with asthma, EIA, and/or EIB can mimic symptoms of laryngeal dysfunction and lead to a delay in diagnosis of up to 10 years at least. [65] Hence, the importance of diligent history taking and sophisticated physical examination in athletes with respiratory symptoms cannot be overemphasized. Unlike EILO where symptoms occur primarily during exercise and are audible to the patient and others, EIB and asthma symptoms occurs toward the end of exercise, and the audible sounds of breathing are rarely noted by surrounding peers and coaches [2, 23, 66]. Moreover, the respiratory symptoms need 30–60 min to resolve and are not improved by distraction or panting as observed in patients with EILO [13]. Physical examination and auscultation of the chest and neck checking for wheezing, murmur, and persistent stridor usually guide the physician toward the diagnosis of lower airway disease [6]. Other important discriminators between EILO, EIB, and asthma are failure to improve on conventional anti-asthma medications and truncation or flattening of the inspiratory loop while the patient is symptomatic. Similarly, provocative testing may not be diagnostic, and a negative methacholine challenge test does not guarantee or rule out laryngeal dysfunction [10–13]. In a study by Rundell on inspiratory stridor in elite athletes, one-third of the participants had EIB, whereas only 5.1% had inspiratory stridor. The authors highlighted the role of post-exercise serial spirometry as well as the lack of response to B2 agonist treatment in differentiating vocal fold dysfunction from exercise-induced bronchoconstriction [6].

In summary, asthma, EIA, and EIB are common in athletes. There are many commonalities in the triggers and clinical presentation of these diseases and EILO. A comprehensive history and physical examination are crucial to accurate assessment of patients with respiratory symptoms. Pulmonary function testing and methacholine challenge are useful diagnostic tests but are not always diagnostic.

8.3.2   Psychological Disturbances

Psychological disturbances are not uncommon in athletes. There are numerous studies in the literature indicating that athletes are under significant stress and at risk of developing psychological illnesses. In a study by Powell et al. on paradoxical vocal fold movement disorders in juveniles, 12 of 22 participants had history of social stress [14]. In a study by Chiang et al. of 104 patients with exercise-induced PVFMD, psychiatric disturbances were diagnosed in 26% of cases [11]. Similarly, in a study by Marcinow et al. that included 46 athletes with PVFMD, gastroesophageal reflux disease and psychiatric diseases were among the most common comorbid conditions present in 28% and 15% of cases, respectively [12]. In another study by Husein et al. on the psychological profile of patients with PVFMD, the authors showed elevated scores for hypochondriasis and hysteria, consistent with conversion disorders. Female patients exhibited higher negative stress in comparison to the normal population. The study was conducted on 45 newly diagnosed cases, and the assessment consisted of administering 2 validated questionnaires, the Minnesota Multiphasic Personality inventory and the Life Experiences Survey [39]. A substantial number of stressors can predispose to psychological difficulties in athletes, especially during at the early years through college age. These include a previous history of mental illnesses, the need to impress peers and parents, engagement in highly competitive sports, and prior injuries and/or trauma [67].

In summary, the prevalence of psychological disturbances in athletes is high. The commonly are the result of mental stress, trauma, and prior history of physical injuries. Early recognition of these disturbances is crucial in the diagnosis and management of athletes with EILO.

8.3.3   Gastroesophageal Reflux Disease (GERD)
and Laryngopharyngeal Reflux Disease (LPR)

Gastroesophageal reflux disease is reported frequently in athletes. Its high prevalence is attributed to alteration in esophageal motility and lower esophageal sphincter pressure as discussed in Chap. 5 in the section on the GERD/LPR as a significant voice risk factor. Gastroesophageal reflux disease also is a known comorbid condition in patients with laryngeal dysfunction. In 1996, Loughlin and Koufman described 12 patients with a history of paroxysmal laryngeal spasm that was associated with gastroesophageal reflux disease. The authors showed clinical evidence of gastroesophageal reflux in 92% of cases and abnormal pH meter in 83% of cases. All patients improved on anti-reflux treatment. The authors highlighted the extra-esophageal manifestation of GERD in the etiology of patients with a paroxysm of laryngeal spasm [68]. In a study by Powell et al. on paradoxical vocal fold movement disorders in 22 patients aged 18 years and below, the authors showed evidence of GERD in 19 patients. Arytenoid edema and inter-arytenoid abnormalities were found in 77% and 86% of cases, respectively [14]. In a study of 30 patients with paradoxical vocal fold dysfunction, Patel et al. showed laryngeal signs of LPR in 16 participants and findings suggestive of chronic laryngitis in 4 patients. The authors emphasized the need to diagnose coexisting laryngeal abnormalities in patients with inappropriate vocal fold movement disorders [65]. In the study by Hussein et al. on the psychological profile of patients with PVFD, gastroesophageal reflux disease was diagnosed in 51% of the cases, in addition to other comorbidities [39]. Similarly, the pathogenic role of LPR as a comorbid condition was substantiated by Murry et al. in their study of 16 patients diagnosed with symptoms of LPR, cough, and PVFM. The authors showed an improvement in laryngeal sensory response with a significant decrease in reflux symptom index score [69]. LPR-induced damage to the laryngeal mucosa with subsequent accentuation of the glottic reflex for closure has been suggested. This alteration in the mucosal stimulus threshold is in agreement with the hypersensitivity theory demonstrated in patients with vocal fold dysfunction and irritable laryngeal movement disorders [70].

There is a strong linkage between reflux disease and EILO in athletes. As discussed in the section on "Laryngeal Hypersensitivity: Its Pathogenic Role in EILO in Athletes," alterations in the laryngeal mucosal lining's sensory threshold may lead to abnormal laryngeal behavior and thus jeopardize the airway. Athletes with LPR also may exhibit dysfunctional movement of the true and false vocal folds, secondary to alterations in laryngeal mucosal lining sensitivity.

8.3.4   Neurogenic Laryngeal Movement Disorders

The clinical presentation of EILO may mimic that of patients with neurogenic laryngeal movement disorders. Suspected patients must be investigated thoroughly for the presence of unilateral or bilateral vocal fold paresis or paralysis. Prior history of surgery to the neck, base of skull, and chest should alert the caring physician to the possibility of iatrogenic injury to the recurrent and/or superior laryngeal nerves [71, 72]. Central neurologic disorders such as Parkinson's disease, amyotrophic lateral sclerosis, and multiple sclerosis also should be investigated. [73–77] Abnormal laryngeal movement in the form of impaired vocal fold mobility, tremor, excessive rigidity, and delayed movement onset is a common laryngeal finding in up to 54% of patients with neurologic diseases and no systemic manifestations. For instance, one-third of patients with amyotrophic lateral sclerosis present with bulbar symptoms and narrowing of the glottis aperture [76]. In a study by Forshew and Bromberg, one out of five patients with advanced ALS suffered from laryngeal spasm [77]. Similarly, patients with Parkinson's disease may present with stridor and respiratory distress secondary to bilateral vocal fold paralysis [73–75]. Though these cases are rare, physicians should be aware of the laryngeal hyperkinetic behavior in patients with Parkinson's disease.

8.4 Voice Changes in Athletes with EILO

Voice changes are not uncommon in athletes with EILO. Although EILO affects breathing primarily, thus leading to stridor and shortness of breath, phonatory disturbances also have been reported by numerous authors, with a prevalence up to 60% of cases [10–12]. Marcinow et al., in their study of 46 athletes with VFMD, reported change in voice quality in 15% of cases [12]. Morris et al., in their review of vocal fold dysfunction in athletes, reported dysphonia in 12% of cases [10]. Similarly, Chiang et al. studied 104 patients with EILO and reported dysphonia in 60% of cases. The change in voice quality was described as hoarseness and/or voice breaks [11]. Hence, voice complaints should be sought in patients with EILO.

8.4.1 Why the Voice Changes in Athletes with EILO?

Voice changes in athletes with EILO can be attributed to several factors, the most important of which is phonotrauma. The involuntary contraction of the adductor muscles during inspiration and/or throughout the glottic cycle leads to a forceful glottal approximation with increase in the collision forces between the vocal folds. This increase in the collision forces can lead to an increase in vocal folds' epithelial injury and vascular disruption with bleeding. The impact pressure is mostly accentuated at the mid-membranous portion of the vocal folds [78–80]. The healing process results in remodeling of the lamina propria's constituents sometimes leading to exudative lesions and possible scar formation. This is documented in numerous studies showing the prevalence of nodules, polyps, granuloma, and ulceration in 11–25% of patients with PVFMD [11, 12]. Injury to the vocal fold also may be the result of the increase in airflow velocity between the vocal folds during stridor. The high-speed ventilation and the increase in mean flow rate during an attack of stridor can lead to vocal fold injury. Based on the review by Titze, aerodynamic pressure is a major mechanical stress in phonation related to the subglottal pressure and glottal area (entry and exit), which is markedly reduced in patients with EILO [81].

Similarly, cough, which is a common symptom in patients with EILO, is also a phonotraumatic behavior. Cough is often reported in patients with laryngeal hypersensitivity and shares common pathophysiology with globus, muscle tension dysphonia, and EILO [33]. Based on a review by Altman et al. on the neurologic mechanisms of PVFM, the authors noted PVFM, GERD, and vagal neuropathy as common causes of cough. The authors stressed the intersection between disorders in breathing and other abnormal laryngeal behaviors [82]. This is in agreement with a study by Vertigan and Gibson on cough triggers in 53 patients with refractory cough, which also showed that phonation was a frequent trigger in 71% of cases. The authors alluded to the neuropathic origin of cough and central reflex sensitization [83]. Based on a review by Vertigan et al., the frequency of cough was reported as high as 16.5/h in patients with vocal fold dysfunction [32]. All the above studies support the high prevalence of cough in patients with VFMD and the common pathophysiology between the two. Cough is also a mechanical stress that can affect phonation. The forceful closure of the vocal folds during cough is associated with an increase in the impact force between the vocal folds. The increase in the collision force is attributed to the high-speed velocity before the impact which is reduced to zero during the collision [78, 81]. As cough is a phonotraumatic behavior, it is clear that athletes with EILO who complain of cough are at risk for phonatory disturbances.

Another cause of dysphonia in athletes with EILO is reflux (GERD and LPR). As discussed in the previous sections of this chapter and in Chap. 5 of this book, the prevalence of gastrointestinal symptoms in athletes can reach up to 70% and increases markedly in patients with EILO. In the study by Altman et al. on ten patients with PVFM, 80% had LPR as a coexisting disorder [84]. This high prevalence is in agreement with other studies documenting higher frequency and longer duration of reflux episodes in symptomatic athletes during exercise in comparison with asymptomatic athletes [85]. The high prevalence of reflux disease in these patients may be a cause of disordered phonation. The exposure of the laryngeal mucosa to the acidic and nonacidic reflux material leads to inflammatory changes and mucosal lesions ranging from pachydermia to premalignant and malignant lesions [86, 87]. As a result, patients may suffer from an array of voice and swallowing symptoms. A detailed discussion on reflux disease and voice disorders can be found elsewhere [88]. In addition, dysphonia in athletes with EILO may be secondary to stress. Acute and chronic stress are common in athletes with a prevalence of 45% and 25%, respectively [89, 90]. The prevalence is higher in patients with prior history of physical injuries or sexual assault [91]. The clinical presentation of stress-related disorders varies from intrusion, negative mood/cognition, derealization and decreased emotional response, to hypervigilance and aggressiveness [92]. Stress also is known to affect the phonatory apparatus negatively. Stressed speakers may complain of voice breaks, change in voice pitch, and loudness. Voice-related symptoms commonly described include lump sensation in the throat and muscle tension in the neck [93, 94]. EILO may be associated with all of these symptoms.

8.5   Treatment

The treatment of EILO in athletes requires a multidisciplinary approach that includes a laryngologist, a speech-language pathologist, a psychotherapist, and very often a respiratory therapist, pulmonologist, and allergist. Given the diversity in the clinical presentation and the numerous associated comorbid diseases and etiologies, there is no consensus in the management. The lack of consensus can be ascribed to many factors, among which is the disparity in the terms used to describe exercise-induced airway symptoms in athletes. Other factors contributing to the nonuniformity in treatment are the reduced awareness of EILO among healthcare providers, the limited number of otolaryngologists who have been trained in the management of PVFMD, the limited number of speech-language therapists trained in this disorder, and the limited accessibility to therapeutic resources. Moreover, cross-cultural differences sometimes have precluded sharing with the patient the psychological aspect of EILO [84, 95].

The treatment of EILO in athletes is similar to that in nonathletes. It varies markedly in the literature with no standardization in the approach or follow-up. The treatment modalities most commonly adopted in isolation or combination are voice therapy, cognitive therapy with laryngeal feedback, botulinum toxin therapy, and psychotherapy and hypnosis. The choice of treatment is individualized according to the patient's characteristics [95–98]. In acute cases, when patients present to the emergency room with severe respiratory symptoms, continuous positive airway pressure (CPAP) is used commonly to secure the airway. CPAP acts by delivering intermittent pulses of positive air pressure, resulting in widening of the airway. Alternatively, heliox, a combination of helium and oxygen, can be inhaled. [98] The use of heliox in the treatment of patients with acute attacks of PVCM has been described as early as 1995 by Reisner and Borish [98]. The decrease in air density results in a decrease in flow turbulence, which in turn leads to a decrease in respiratory effort.

In this section, the authors review the most common treatment modalities used. However, we emphasize that in our hands, the most effective approach includes comprehensive evaluation to determine each individual's etiology and then focused treatment for the etiology. In addition to the history, physical and laryngoscopy, we routinely include pulmonary function tests, 24-h pH monitoring with symptom index, and laryngeal EMG.

8.5.1   Voice Therapy and Breathing Exercises

Voice therapy by a trained speech-language pathologist or phoniatric is the treatment modality used most commonly in patients with induced laryngeal obstruction. It starts with the patient's reassurance and education about the patient's condition. Sharing with the patient and family the knowledge that the condition is not life-threatening cannot be overemphasized, although providers should be aware that in extremely rare cases in patients with underlying cardiovascular diseases it can be [95]. Following the patient's education, behavioral modification is initiated with the primary focus being on breathing exercises and the use of abdominal support for controlled inhalation and exhalation. Patients learn how to use diaphragmatic breathing while avoiding unnecessary tension in the larynx and its neighboring structures. Learning what is referred to "rescue breathing" allows the patient to avoid or mitigate an impending attack. Rescue breathing consists mainly of deep nasal inhalation followed by slow exhalation through the mouth with the lips being pursed. [96] The rationale of rescue breathing is similar to that of semiocclusive voice therapy exercises often recommended for the treatment of laryngeal muscle tension dysphonia. The objective is to enhance the glottic aperture by reducing unnecessary tension in the vocal folds and other laryngeal muscles [95, 96]. Exhaling against the resistance of pursed lips also provides positive expiratory pressure that helps hold laryngeal tissues apart. Another breathing technique commonly adopted is the EILO-biphasic inspiratory technique. It modulates the inspiratory and expiratory airflow through the laryngeal inlet using various oropharyngeal maneuvers such as clenching on the teeth. Alternatively, patients are encouraged to produce sounds similar to the word "hoover" to modulate the airflow and increase intra-laryngeal pressure [97].

In summary, voice therapy focused on abdominal breathing, and support is key in the management of athletes with EILO. Increasing patients' education about the nature of their condition is extremely important. This can help avoiding unnecessary medical treatment and at times surgical intervention to secure the airway.

8.5.2   Cognitive Behavioral and Laryngeal Control Therapy

Similar to voice therapy, cognitive behavioral therapy enhances the cognitive skills involved in control of laryngeal muscle during respiration. Laryngeal control therapy with audio and visual biofeedback has gained popularity as the gold standard treatment approach in patients with induced laryngeal obstruction with no treatable organic cause such as LPR or respiratory dystonia [84, 85]. By cultivating laryngeal muscle memory, patients learn how to avoid inappropriate laryngeal movements such as the adduction of the vocal folds during breathing. In a study of 36 adolescents and children, Richards-Mauze et al. showed marked improvement in symptom severity, self-perception of control, and functional disability scores following therapy. The authors stressed the benefits of cognitive-behavioral intervention in enhancing the coping capability of affected patients [99]. Olin et al. described real-time laryngoscopic visualization as a therapeutic means that allows feedback from the patient during the attack. The authors reported the safety, learning value, and effectiveness of this therapeutic technique in 81%, 78%, and 58% of the cases, respectively [100]. In a study by Chiang et al. that included 67 patients with exercise-induced vocal fold movement disorder (EVFMD) who underwent laryngeal control therapy, 48% of those who completed one treatment session improved or had complete regression of symptoms. Approximately 82% of those who completed two therapy sessions noted the resolution of their symptoms. On average, the number of sessions needed for improvement was 2.2 in the EVFMD group [11]. In a study by Marcinow et al., laryngeal control therapy was the most recommended and adopted treatment modality. Approximately 69% of the study group had improvement in symptoms, and the overall success rate, including those lost to follow-up, was 43%. Approximately 50% of patients had two treatment sessions or fewer, and only 7% had four or more treatment sessions. Among those who attended three or more treatment sessions, 92% had complete remission of their symptoms or at least improvement [12].

Cognitive therapy is a viable alternative treatment modality for EILO. Visualization of vocal fold movement during inspiration may help patients learn how to control their laryngeal behavior. Patient collaboration and perseverance are needed for a successful outcome.

8.5.3   Botulinum Toxin Injection

Botulinum toxin (BT) is a potent toxin produced by *Clostridium botulinum*. It acts by inhibiting the release of acetylcholine at the neuromuscular junction leading to chemical denervation and paresis or paralysis at the site of injection. Its clinical use has grown over the last few decades given its therapeutic benefit in the treatment of dystonia and neurologic conditions characterized by sustained and repetitive involuntary muscle contractions [95]. These include cervical dystonia, hemifacial spasm, blepharospasm, essential tremor, rest tremor, and simple motor tics [101, 102]. Many laryngeal movement disorders are treated successfully with BT, among which are laryngeal tremor, spasmodic dysphonia, respiratory dystonia, and ILO [103–106]. Unlike other dystonias such as spasmodic dysphonia, it is common for teenage athletes to "outgrow" respiratory dystonia and become asymptomatic after several months or years of BT injections.

The successful treatment of these conditions has broadened the clinical application of Botox in the management of EILO, particularly in athletes refractory to conventional therapy. In 1991, Blitzer et al. were the first to describe Botox injection for the treatment of respiratory and obstructive laryngeal dystonia [103]. A few years later, Garibaldi et al. described BT injection in a competitive athlete who improved for 2 months following the injection [104]. In a review by Morris et al. in 2006, the authors reported nine cases of paradoxical vocal fold movement disorders treated successfully with BT injection [95]. Maillard et al. described the added value of BT injection in the management of PVFM and in avoiding the need for a tracheotomy. The authors described a 35-year-old man who presented with hypercapnic respiratory failure and who was managed successfully with intra-laryngeal BT injection. Notably, the patient had had previous tracheal intubation (four times) and had been treated in error for asthma [105]. In 2000, Altman et al. reviewed their experience with ten patients with PVFM, five of whom were treated with BT injection. The authors alluded to the viability of Botox injection as an alternative treatment in patients diagnosed with this disorder [84]. Similarly, in their review of 46 athletes with PVFMD, Marcinow et al. reported 2 who were treated with BT injection. The authors emphasized the advantage of this treatment modality in addition to laryngeal control therapy in the management of these patients [12]. Montojo et al. described a 13-year-old child with PVFM who was treated successfully with vocal fold BT injection. The procedure was done in an office setting under local anesthesia using a flexible laryngoscope [106]. In 2019, DeSilva et al. reviewed their case series of 13 patients with refractory paradoxical vocal fold movement disorders who underwent repeated Botox injection at an average of 3.85 injections per patient. During a follow-up period of 5–69 months, the authors reported improvement and complete remission of symptoms in 84.7% and 18.2% of cases, respectively. The dyspnea severity index and resolution of dyspnea symptoms were used as outcome measures [107]. In a recent review of the characteristics of 40 patients with PVFM, Vance et al. reported asthma, LPR, allergy, and psychiatric disorders in 65%, 78%, 48%, and 33% of cases, respectively. The authors reported improvement following voice therapy and LPR treatment in 43% of cases and an improvement in 90% of cases following BT injections. In conclusion, the authors stressed the diverse etiologies of this disorder and the superior benefit of combined treatment in the management of this disorder [108].

In summary, intra-laryngeal BT injection is a viable treatment in patients with laryngeal obstructive symptoms who have respiratory dystonia. Adverse side effects such as change in voice quality can be minimized as BT doses are individualized and adjusted over time.

8.5.4 Hypnosis

Hypnosis is a common therapeutic technique used in the treatment of pain, anxiety, depression, claustrophobia, tinnitus, and many behavioral disorders. The technique focuses on relaxing the mind and allowing control over the function of various systems in the body. According to the American Psychological Association, hypnosis is an effective therapeutic means that can help people change behaviors and manage chronic conditions among which is laryngeal dysfunction or paradoxical vocal fold dysfunction [109]. Caraon and Otoole described a 14-year-old boy who developed inspiratory stridor associated with adduction of the vocal folds on indirect laryngoscopy. Failure to respond to asthma medications made the treating physician suspect a conversion disorder, and the patient was offered hypnosis as an alternative therapy. Following two sessions of hypnotherapy, the patient had full recovery [110]. Similarly, Smith described a 16-year-old athlete who presented with stridor and adduction of the vocal fold throughout the glottic cycle on laryngeal endoscopy. The patient was under a lot of stress and awaiting wrestling competitive games. He was offered hypnosis during which he was asked to visualize his vocal folds opening during inspiration. On follow-up, the patient was asymptomatic with no recurrence of his attacks [111].

Hypnosis is a well-described psychotherapy technique used commonly in the treatment of behavioral disorders. Its application in patients with EILO remains embryonic although few case reports have been published in the literature. Future studies are needed to define appropriate patient selection and to confirm its efficacy in the management of affected patients.

In summary, given the multifaceted etiology of EILO, the management strategy of affected patients should be individualized. The most commonly adopted treatment modalities are voice therapy, cognitive therapy, psychotherapy, and BT injections. The treatment of confounding diseases when present, such as asthma, LPR, allergy, and psychiatric disorders, is equally important in controlling the severity and frequency of the attacks and in avoiding recurrence.

References

1. Patterson RO, Schatz HM. Munchausen's stridor: non-organic laryngeal obstruction. Clin Allergy. 1974;4(3):307–10.
2. Christopher KL, Wood RPII, Eckert RC, Blager FB, Raney RA, Souhadrada JF. Vocal-cord dysfunction presenting as asthma. N Engl J Med. 1983;308:1566–70.
3. Olin JT, Clary MS, Deardorff EH, et al. Inducible laryngeal obstruction during exercise: moving beyond vocal cords with new insights. Phys Sportsmed. 2015;43(1):13–21.
4. Christensen PM, Heimdal JH, Christopher KL, et al. ERS/ELS/ACCP 2013 international consensus conference nomenclature on inducible laryngeal obstructions. Eur Respir Rev. 2015;24(137): 445–50.
5. Lakin RC, Metzger WJ, Haughey BH. Upper airway obstruction presenting as exercise-induced asthma. Chest. 1984;86:499–501.
6. Nielsen EW, Hull JH, Backer V. High prevalence of exercise-induced laryngeal obstruction in athletes. Med Sci Sports Exerc. 2013;45(11):2030–5.
7. Rundell KW, Spiering BA. Inspiratory stridor in elite athletes. Chest. 2003;123(2):468–74.
8. Mikita J, Parker J. High levels of medical utilization by ambulatory patients with vocal cord dysfunction as compared to age- and gender-matched asthmatics. Chest. 2006;129:905–8.
9. Liao KS, Kwak PE, Hewitt H, Hollas S, Ongkasuwan J. Measuring quality of life in pediatric paradoxical vocal fold motion using the SF-36v2. J Voice. 2017;31(4):518.e1–5.
10. Morris MJ, Christopher KL. Diagnostic criteria for the classification of vocal cord dysfunction. Chest. 2010;138:1213–23.
11. Chiang T, Marcinow AM, deSilva BW, Ence BN, Lindsey SE, Forrest LA. Exercise-induced paradoxical vocal fold motion disorder: diagnosis and management. Laryngoscope. 2013;123:727–31.
12. Marcinow AM, Thompson J, Chiang T, Forrest LA, deSilva BW. Paradoxical vocal fold motion disorder in the elite athlete: experience at a large division I university. Laryngoscope. 2014;124(6):1425–30.
13. Al-Alwan A, Kaminsky D. Vocal cord dysfunction in athletes: clinical presentation and review of the literature. Phys Sportsmed. 2012;40:22–7.
14. Powell DM, Karanfilov BI, Beechler KB, Treole K, Trudeau MD, Forrest LA. Paradoxical vocal cord dysfunction in juveniles. Arch Otolaryngol Head Neck Surg. 2000;126(1):29–34.
15. Tervonen H, Niskanen MM, Sovijarvi AR, Hakulinen AS, Vilkman EA, Aaltonen LM. Fiberoptic videolaryngoscopy during bicycle ergometry: a diagnostic tool for exercise-induced vocal cord dysfunction. Laryngoscope. 2009;119:1776–80.

16. Heimdal JH, Roksund OD, Halvorsen T, Skadberg BT, Olofsson J. Continuous laryngoscopy exercise test: a method for visualizing laryngeal dysfunction during exercise. Laryngoscope. 2006;116:52–7.
17. Christensen P, Thomsen SF, Rasmussen N, Backer V. Exercise-induced laryngeal obstructions objectively assessed using EILOMEA. Eur Arch Otorhinolaryngol. 2010;267(3):401–7.
18. Olin JT, Clary MS, Fan EM, et al. Continuous laryngoscopy quantitates laryngeal behaviour in exercise and recovery. Eur Respir J. 2016;48:1192–200.
19. Maat RC, Roksund OD, Halvorsen T, et al. Audiovisual assessment of exercise-induced laryngeal obstruction: reliability and validity of observations. Eur Arch Otorhinolaryngol. 2009;266:1929–36.
20. Walsted ES, Swanton LL, van van Someren K, et al. Laryngoscopy during swimming: a novel diagnostic technique to characterize swimming-induced laryngeal obstruction. Laryngoscope. 2017;127:2298–301.
21. Morris MJ, Grbach VX, Deal LE, Boyd SY, Morgan JA, Johnson JE. Evaluation of exertional dyspnea in the active duty patient: the diagnostic approach and the utility of clinical testing. Mil Med. 2002;167(4):281–8.
22. Morris MJ, Deal LE, Bean DR, Grbach VX, Morgan JA. Vocal cord dysfunction in patients with exertional dyspnea. Chest. 1999;116(6):1676–82.
23. Newman KB, Mason UG 3rd, Schmaling KB. Clinical features of vocal cord dysfunction. Am J Respir Crit Care Med. 1995;152(4):1382–6.
24. Olin JT, Clary MS, Connors D, et al. Glottic configuration in patients with exercise-induced stridor: a new paradigm. Laryngoscope. 2014;124(11):2568–73.
25. Sataloff RT, Mandel S, Heman-Ackah YD, Abaza M. Laryngeal electromyography. 3rd ed. San Diego: Plural Publishing; 2017. p. 1–181.
26. Scherer RC. Laryngeal function during phonation. In: Sataloff RT. Professional voice: the science of art of clinical care, 4th ed. San Diego: Plural Publishing; 2017. p. 281–308.
27. Wysocki J, Kielska E, Orszulak P, Reymond J. Measurements of pre- and postpubertal human larynx: a cadaver study. Surg Radiol Anat. 2008;30:191–9.
28. Hocevar-Boltezar I, Krivec U, Sereg-Bahar M. Laryngeal sensitivity testing in youth with exercise-inducible laryngeal obstruction. Int J Rehabil Res. 2017;40:146–51.
29. Famokunwa B, Walsted ES, Hull JH. Assessing laryngeal function and hypersensitivity. Pulm Pharmacol Ther. 2019;56:108–15.
30. Benninger C, Parsons JP, Mastronarde JG. Vocal cord dysfunction and asthma. Curr Opin Pulmon Med. 2011;17(1):45–9.
31. Kolnes LJ, Stensrud T. Exercise-induced laryngeal obstruction in athletes: contributory factors and treatment implications. Physiother Theory Pract. 2019;35(12):1170–81.
32. Vertigan AE, Kapela SM, Kearney EK, Gibson PG. Laryngeal dysfunction in cough hypersensitivity syndrome: a cross-sectional observational study. J Allergy Clin Immunol Pract. 2018;6(6):2087–95.
33. Vertigan AE, Bone SL, Gibson PG. Laryngeal sensory dysfunction in laryngeal hypersensitivity syndrome. Respirology. 2013;18(6):948–56.
34. Ryan NM, Vertigan AE, Gibson PG. Chronic cough and laryngeal dysfunction improve with specific treatment of cough and paradoxical vocal fold movement. Cough. 2009;5(1):1–8.
35. Wilhelm FH, Gevirtz R, Roth WT. Respiratory dysregulation in anxiety, functional cardiac, and pain disorders: assessment, phenomenology, and treatment. Behav Modif. 2001;25(4):513–45.
36. McFadden ER Jr, Zawadski DK. Vocal cord dysfunction masquerading as exercise-induced asthma. A physiologic cause for "choking" during athletic activities. Am J Respir Crit Care Med. 1996;153:942–7.
37. Powell SA, Nguyen CT, Gaziano J, Lewis V, Lockey RF, Padhya TA. Mass psychogenic illness presenting as acute stridor in an adolescent female cohort. Anna Otol Rhinol Laryngol. 2007;116(7):525–31.

38. Forrest LA, Husein T, Husein O. Paradoxical vocal cord motion: classification and treatment. Laryngoscope. 2012;122(4):844–53.
39. Husein OF, Husein TN, Gardner R, et al. Formal psychological testing in patients with paradoxical vocal fold dysfunction. Laryngoscope. 2008;118(4):740–7.
40. Revill AL, Vann NC, Akins VT, et al. Dbx1 precursor cells are a source of inspiratory XII premotoneurons. elife. 2015;4:e12301.
41. Kottick A, Del Negro CA. Synaptic depression influences inspiratory–expiratory phase transition in Dbx1 interneurons of the preBötzinger complex in neonatal mice. J Neurosci. 2015;35(33):11606–11.
42. Vann NC, Pham FD, Hayes JA, Kottick A, Del Negro CA. Transient suppression of Dbx1 pre-Bötzinger interneurons disrupts breathing in adult mice. PLoS One. 2016;11(9):e0162418.
43. Hisa Y, Bamba H, Koike S, Shogaki K, Tadaki N, Uno T. Neurotransmitters and neuromodulators involved in laryngeal innervation. Ann Otol Rhinol Laryngol Supp. 1999;108:3–14.
44. Ramaswamy S, Shankar SK, Manjunath KY, Devanathan PH, Nityaseelan N. Ultrastructure of the ganglion on human internal laryngeal nerve. Neurosci Res. 1994;18(4):283–90.
45. Ibanez M, Valderrama-Canales FJ, Maranillo E, et al. Human laryngeal ganglia contain both sympathetic and parasympathetic cell types. Clin Anat. 2010;23(6):673–82.
46. Demmink-Geertman L, Dejonckere PH. Neurovegetative symptoms and complaints before and after voice therapy for nonorganic habitual dysphonia. J Voice. 2008;22(3):315–25.
47. Helou LB, Wang W, Ashmore RC, Rosen CA, Abbott KV. Intrinsic laryngeal muscle activity in response to autonomic nervous system activation. Laryngoscope. 2013;123(11):2756–65.
48. Sataloff RT. Clinical anatomy and physiology of the voice. In: Sataloff RT. Professional voice: the science of art of clinical care, 4th ed. San Diego: Plural Publishing; 2017. p. 157–95.
49. Iwarsson J, Sundberg J. Effects of lung volume on vertical larynx position during phonation. J Voice. 1998;12:159–65.
50. Iwarsson J. Effects of inhalatory abdominal wall movement on vertical laryngeal position during phonation. J Voice. 2001;15:384–94.
51. Dempsey JA, McKenzie DC, Haverkamp HC, Eldridge MW. Update in the understanding of respiratory limitations to exercise performance in fit, active adults. Chest. 2008;134(3):613–22.
52. Vertigan AE, Gibson PG, Theodoros DG, Winkworth AL, Borgas T, Reid C. Involuntary glottal closure during inspiration in muscle tension dysphonia. Laryngoscope. 2006;116:643–9.
53. Aaron AJ, Deems DA, Sataloff RT. Spasmodic dysphonia. In: Sataloff RT. Professional voice: the science of art of clinical care, 4th edition. San Diego: Plural Publishing; 2017. p. 1077–100.
54. Boulet LP, Turmel J, Côté A. Asthma and exercise-induced respiratory symptoms in the athlete: new insights. Curr Opin Pulm Med. 2017;23(1):71–7.
55. Lacroix VJ. Exercise-induced asthma. Phys Sportsmed. 1999;27(12):75–92.
56. Kurowski M, Jurczyk J, Krysztofiak H, Kowalski ML. Exercise-induced respiratory symptoms and allergy in elite athletes: allergy and asthma in polish Olympic athletes (a(2)POLO) project within GA(2)LEN initiative. Clin Respir J. 2016;10(2):231–8.
57. Salem L, Dao VA, Shah-Hosseini K, et al. Impaired sports performance of athletes suffering from pollen-induced allergic rhinitis: a cross-sectional, observational survey in German athletes. J Sports Med Phys Fitness. 2018;59(4):686–92.
58. Perrotta F, Simeon V, Bonini M, et al. Evaluation of allergic diseases, symptom control, and relation to infections in a Group of Italian Elite Mountain Bikers. Clin J Sport Med. 2020;30(5):465–9.
59. Christensen PM, Thomsen SF, Rasmussen N, Backer V. Exercise-induced laryngeal obstructions: prevalence and symptoms in the general public. Eur Archi Otorhinolaryngol. 2011;268(9):1313–9.
60. Côté A, Turmel J, Boulet LP. Exercise and asthma. Semin Respir Crit Care Med. 2018;39(1):19–28.
61. Brennan FH Jr, Alent J, Ross MJ. Evaluating the athlete with suspected exercise-induced asthma or bronchospasm. Curr Sports Med Rep. 2018;17(3):85–9.

62. Bonini M, Silvers W. Exercise-induced bronchoconstriction: background, prevalence, and sport considerations. Immunol Allergy Clin N Am. 2018;38(2):205–14.
63. Levai IK, Hull JH, Loosemore M, Greenwell J, Whyte G, Dickinson JW. Environmental influence on the prevalence and pattern of airway dysfunction in elite athletes. Respirology. 2016;21(8):1391–6.
64. Bougault V, Drouard F, Legall F, Dupont G, Wallaert B. Allergies and exercise-induced bronchoconstriction in a youth academy and reserve professional soccer team. Clin J Sport Med. 2017;27(5):450–6.
65. Patel NJ, Jorgensen C, Kuhn J, Merati AL. Concurrent laryngeal abnormalities in patients with paradoxical vocal fold dysfunction. Otolaryngol Head Neck Surg. 2004;130(6):686–9.
66. Hull JH, Godbout K, Boulet LP. Exercise-associated dyspnea and stridor: thinking beyond asthma. J Allergy Clin Immunol Pract. 2020;8(7):2202–8.
67. Sutcliffe JH, Greenberger PA. Identifying psychological difficulties in college athletes. J Allergy Clin Immunol Pract. 2020;8(7):2216–9.
68. Loughlin CJ, Koufman JA. Paroxysmal laryngospasm secondary to gastroesophageal reflux. Laryngoscope. 1996;106(12):1502–5.
69. Murry T, Branski RC, Yu K, Cukier-Blaj S, Duflo S, Aviv JE. Laryngeal sensory deficits in patients with chronic cough and paradoxical vocal fold movement disorder. Laryngoscope. 2010;120(8):1576–81.
70. Andesron JA. Work-associated irritable larynx syndrome. Curr Opin Allergy Clin Immunol. 2015;15(12):150–5.
71. Slomka WS, Abedi E, Sismanis A, Barlascini CO Jr. Paralysis of the recurrent laryngeal nerve by an extracapsular thyroid adenoma. Ear Nose Throat J. 1989;68(11):855–6.
72. Baranyai L, Madarasz G. Recurrent nerve paralysis following lung surgery. J Thorac Cardiovasc Surg. 1963;46(4):531–6.
73. Stelzig Y, Hochhaus W, Gall V, Henneberg A. Laryngeal manifestations in patients with Parkinson disease. Laryngorhinootologie. 1999;78(10):544–51.
74. Plasse HM, Lieberman AN. Bilateral vocal cord paralysis in Parkinson's disease. Arch Otolaryngol. 1981;107(4):252–3.
75. Read D, Young A. Stridor and parkinsonism. Postgrad Med J. 1983;59(694):520–1.
76. Hamdan AL, Sataloff RT, Hawkshaw MJ. Laryngeal manifestations of neurologic disorders. In: Laryngeal manifestations of system diseases. San Diego: Plural Publishing; 2019. p. 87–118.
77. Forshew DA, Bromberg MB. A survey of clinicians' practice in the symptomatic treatment of ALS. Amyotroph Lateral Scler Other Motor Neuron Disord. 2003;4(4):258–63.
78. Jiang JJ, Titze IR. Measurement of vocal fold intraglottal pressure and impact stress. J Voice. 1994;1;8(2):132–44.
79. Primov-Fever A, Lidor R, Meckel Y, Amir O. The effect of physical effort on voice characteristics. Folia Phoniatr Logop. 2013;65(6):288–93.
80. Baken RJ. An overview of laryngeal function of voice production. In: Sataloff RT. Professional voice. The science and art of clinical care. 4th ed. San Diego: Plural Publishing; 2017. p. 259–80.
81. Titze IR. Mechanical stress in phonation. J Voice. 1994;8(2):99–105.
82. Altman KW, Simpson CB, Amin MR, Abaza M, Balkissoon R, Casiano RR. Cough and paradoxical vocal fold motion. Otolaryngol Head Neck Surg. 2002;127(6):501–11.
83. Vertigan AE, Gibson PG. Chronic refractory cough as a sensory neuropathy: evidence from a reinterpretation of cough triggers. J Voice. 2011;25(5):596–601.
84. Altman KW, Mirza N, Ruiz C, Sataloff RT. Paradoxical vocal fold motion: presentation and treatment options. J Voice. 2000;14(1):99–103.
85. van Nieuwenhoven MA, Brouns F, Brummer RJ. Gastrointestinal profile of symptomatic athletes at rest and during physical exercise. Eur J Appl Physiol. 2004;91(4):429–34.

86. Sataloff RT, Castell DO, Katz PO, Sataloff DM, Hawkshaw MJ. Reflux and other gastroenterologic conditions that may affect the voice. In: Sataloff RT. Professional voice: the science and art of clinical care. 4th ed. San Diego: Plural Publishing; 2017. p. 907–98.
87. Lechien JR, Saussez S, Harmegnies B, Finck C, Burns JA. Laryngopharyngeal reflux and voice disorders: a multifactorial model of etiology and pathophysiology. J Voice. 2017;31(6):733–52.
88. Jr Akst LM, Hamdan AL, Schindler A, et al. Evaluation and management of laryngopharyngeal reflux disease: state of the art review. Otolaryngol Head Neck Surg 2019;160(5):762–782.
89. Wismen T, Foster K, Curtis K. Mental health following traumatic physical injury: an integrative literature review. Injury. 2013;44(11):1383–90.
90. Aron CM, Harvey S, Hainline B, Hitchcock ME, Reardon CL. Post-traumatic stress disorder (PTSD) and other trauma-related mental disorders in elite athletes: a narrative review. Br J Sports Med. 2019;53(12):779–84.
91. Timpka T, Spreco A, Dahlstrom O, et al. Suicidal thoughts (ideation) among elite athletics (track and field) athletes: associations with sports participation, psychological resourcefulness and having been a victim of sexual and/or physical abuse. Br J Sports Med. 2021;55:198–205.
92. Regier DA, Kuhl EA, Kupfer DJ. The DSM-5: classification and criteria changes. World Psychiatry. 2013;12(2):92–8.
93. Holmqvist S, Santtila P, Lindström E, Sala E, Simberg S. The association between possible stress markers and vocal symptoms. J Voice. 2013;27(6):787.e1–787.e10.
94. Van Lierde K, Van Heule S, De Ley S, Mertens E, Claeys S. Effect of psychological stress on female vocal quality. Folia Phoniatr Logop. 2009;61(2):105–11.
95. Morris MJ, Allan PF, Perkins PJ. Vocal cord dysfunction: etiologies and treatment. Clin Pulm Med. 2006;13(2):73–86.
96. Sandage MJ, Zelazny SK. Paradoxical vocal fold motion in children and adolescents. Lang Speech Hearing Serv Sch. 2004;35:353–62.
97. Johnston KL, Bradford H, Hodges H, Moore CM, Nauman E, Olin JT. The Olin EILOBI breathing techniques: description and initial case series of novel respiratory retraining strategies for athletes with exercise-induced laryngeal obstruction. J Voice. 2018;32:698–704.
98. Reisner C, Borish L. Heliox therapy for acute vocal cord dysfunction. Chest. 1995;108(05):1477.
99. Richards-Mauzé MM, Banez GA. Vocal cord dysfunction: evaluation of a four-session cognitive–behavioral intervention. Clin Pract Pediatr Psychol. 2014;2(1):27–38.
100. Olin JT, Deardorff EH, Fan EM, et al. Therapeutic laryngoscopy during exercise: a novel non-surgical therapy for refractory EILO. Pediatr Pulmonol. 2017;52(6):813–9.
101. Jabbari B. History of botulinum toxin treatment in movement disorders. Tremor Other Hyperkinet Mov. 2016;6:394.
102. Peckham EL, Lopez G, Shamim EA, et al. Clinical features of patients with blepharospasm: a report of 240 patients. Eur J Neurol. 2011;18:382–6.
103. Brinn MF, Blitzer A, Braun N, Stewart C, Fahn S. Respiratory and obstructive laryngeal dystonia: treatment with botulinum toxin (Botox). Neurology. 1991;41(suppl 1):291.
104. Garibaldi E, LaBlance G, Hibbett A, Wall L. Exercise-induced paradoxical vocal cord dysfunction: diagnosis with videostroboscopic endoscopy and treatment with Clostridium toxin. J Allergy Clin Immunol. 1993;91:200.
105. Maillard I, Schweizer V, Broccard A, Duscher A, Liaudet L, Schaller MD. Use of botulinum toxin type a to avoid tracheal intubation or tracheostomy in severe paradoxical vocal cord movement. Chest. 2000;118(3):874–7.
106. Montojo J, González R, Hernández E, Zafra M, Plaza G. Office-based laryngeal injection of botulinum toxin for paradoxical vocal fold motion in a child. Int J Pediatr Otorhinolaryngol. 2015;79(7):1161–3.
107. deSilva B, Crenshaw D, Matrka L, Forrest LA. Vocal fold botulinum toxin injection for refractory paradoxical vocal fold motion disorder. Laryngoscope. 2019;129(4):808–11.

108. Vance D, Heyd C, Pier M et al. Paradoxical vocal fold movement: a retrospective analysis. J Voice. Published online May 2020.
109. American Psychological Association. Hypnosis. https://www.apa.org/search?query=hypnosis. Published 2008.
110. Caraon P, O'toole C. Vocal cord dysfunction presenting as asthma. Ir Med J. 1991;84(3):98–9.
111. Smith MS. Acute psychogenic stridor in an adolescent athlete treated with hypnosis. Pediatrics. 1983;18:991–4.

Chapter 9
Laryngeal Trauma in Athletes and Its Implication for Voice

9.1 Introduction

Sports activity is common worldwide. In the United States, it is estimated that one out of four adults plays at least one type of sport. The top five sports played by men are golf, basketball, soccer, baseball/softball, and football, whereas those played by women are running or track, baseball/softball, tennis, volleyball, and swimming [1]. A main drive to engage in sports for both genders is the health benefit associated with physical activity. Physical activity is linked strongly to physiologic maturation and development. There is growing evidence supporting the advantageous role of sports activity for daily function. Additional benefits include improvement in psychosocial behavior and alleviation of mental illnesses [2].

The health benefits of sports come at a cost. Strenuous physical activity may cause burnout, eating disorders, hormonal imbalance, and musculoskeletal and head and neck injuries [2, 3]. The site of injury varies with the type of sport, style of competition, level of expertise, and environmental factors. In a review of 208 cases of head and neck trauma in sports activities, the nose, mandible, and zygomatic complexes were the most common sites of injury in 56.25%, 15.86%, and 13.45% of cases, respectively [3]. Laryngeal injury is also substantial risk for those who engage in sports. The associated airway compromise may be life-threatening, and long-term phonatory sequelae can be disabling. Additional burdens associated with laryngeal injury include emotional and psychological disturbances that often are underestimated or underdiagnosed and untreated.

This chapter reviews sports-related injuries to the larynx and their variation with age and gender. Familiarity with their clinical presentations, diagnostic workup, and management strategies is essential for healthcare professionals. Understanding the pathophysiology of dysphonia in affected patients is important for healthcare providers, particularly otolaryngologists and voice therapists. It is also paramount for athletes given the known impact of laryngeal injury on their physical performance, readiness to resume competitive games, and quality of life in general.

© The Author(s), under exclusive license to Springer Nature Switzerland AG 2021
A.-L. Hamdan et al., *Voice Disorders in Athletes, Coaches and other Sports Professionals*, https://doi.org/10.1007/978-3-030-69831-7_9

9.2   Sports-Related Laryngeal Injuries: Variations with Sports Type, Age, and Gender

Laryngeal trauma is not very common. Based on a study that included 21,140 admissions to the trauma center at Boston Medical Center, only 12 patients had laryngeal injuries. This figure represents 0.06% of the trauma visits to a level I trauma center [4]. This concurs with a large review of 30,000 trauma cases by Gussack et al., of whom only 0.04% had injury to the larynx and trachea [5]. The low prevalence of laryngeal trauma, accounting for less than 1% of blunt trauma cases, can be attributed to the protected position of the larynx in the neck with shielding of the larynx by the mandible superiorly, the sternocleidomastoid muscles laterally, and the sternum inferiorly [4–6]. The most common causes of laryngeal trauma are motor vehicle accidents, strangulation, and sports-related injuries. Based on a review of 256 cases of blunt airway trauma by Kiser et al. in 2001, motor vehicle collision accounted for 59% of all cases. The most commonly described offending objects were the steering wheel and dashboard [7]. With advancements in car safety measures over the last two decades, strangulation and sports activity are becoming the main causes of laryngeal trauma.

Sports-related laryngeal injuries vary with the type of sport and rarely occur in isolation. In a review of head and neck trauma by Frenguelli et al., sports-related injuries were reported in 22.7% of the trauma cases presenting to otolaryngologists in a university setting in Italy [3]. The injuries were encountered mostly in soccer games, accounting for 62.5% of the total sports-related trauma. Similarly, in a study by Mendis and Anderson of 28 patients with blunt laryngeal trauma 13 of whom sports related, 50% occurred in ice hockey players (6 out of 13), while the remaining occurred in soccer, rugby, racing, and skiing [8]. The study was a retrospective chart review of patients who presented to head and neck trauma service at Boston University over the course of 10 years. These figures are similar to the high rate of head and neck injuries reported in football and soccer players in the United States [9, 10]. In a review of sports-related neck injuries presenting to the emergency department over the course of 10 years, Delaney and Kashmiri reported the highest rate in American football and soccer (114.706 and 19.341, respectively) [9].

Sports-related laryngeal injuries, similar to other sports-related head and neck injuries, are due mostly to collision among players during aerial challenges. In a review by Fuller of 163 video sequences of head and neck injuries in international football, the use of upper extremities and head accounted for 33% and 30% of the causes of injury, respectively [11]. In another review by Frenguelli et al., collision among soccer players accounted for 159 of 208 total impact-related injuries [3]. Similarly, sports-related laryngeal injuries can be ball related. French and Kelley stressed in their case series of lacrosse-related laryngeal fractures the risk of ball-related injuries in this sport as commonly reported also in hockey players (puck rather than ball). The injury is ascribed partially to the high-speed ball which can exceed 100 miles/h, leading to massive trauma to an unprotected neck. The authors emphasized the need for players and goalkeepers to use throat protective gears [12]. Similarly, Liberman and Mulder argued that pucks in hockey games are a major threat to players. The authors described three cases of laryngeal fractures, two being the result of high-velocity puck injury [13]. In another review of 41 injuries in base-ball players, 2 of whom were diagnosed with tracheal collapse, Boden et al. reported pitcher hit by a batted ball and collision among fielders as the most common causes of injury ($n = 14$ and $n = 9$, respectively) [14]. The high prevalence of ball-related injuries and collision among players has led to development in the safety regula-tions and to vigorous enforcement of preventive measures in the sports industry. Additional preventive measures have included enhancement in sports' technique, improvement in surveillance, increased athletes' education, and strict adherence to permitted game tactics such as blocking and tackling [14].

The prevalence of sports-related laryngeal injuries varies with age. Differences in physical, psychosocial, and somatic development across different age groups need to be considered in the assessment of athletes with laryngeal trauma [15–18]. In a study on age profiles of sport participants, Eime et al. reported two-thirds of their study group (64.1%) to be below the age of 20 years and 27.6% to be between the ages of 10 and 14 years [17]. These results are in agreement with the study by Maia et al. that showed a linear increase in sport participation by 0.7 h/week/year until the age of 16.8 years. After the age of 16.8 years, there was a deceleration at a rate of 0.07 h/week. Note that this was a longitudinal study that included 588 boys aged 13–18 years who were followed for 6 years using a standardized sport participation questionnaire [18]. Despite the above, recent investigations indicate that sports activity is very common in subjects in their six and seventh decades of life. In a study that included 2497 males and 1559 females aged 58–67 years, Cozijnsen et al. showed an increase in sports participation that was attributed par-tially to the high level of education and the decrease in physical health restrictions [19]. This increase in sports' participation with age can explain partially the rela-tively high rate of sports-related laryngeal fractures. The increased risk of laryngeal fractures with age is ascribed to the decreased resilience and increased ossification of the laryngeal cartilages. Numerous studies indicate that ossification of laryngeal cartilages increases with age. The ossification is understood as an adaptive process to vocal loading throughout life [20, 21]. In a radiologic study that included 359 patients, Mupparapu et al. showed that laryngeal ossification starts at the third decade of life and increases with age [20]. In another review by Sataloff et al. on the impact of aging on voice, the authors noted ossification of the laryngeal carti-lages even earlier during adulthood [21]. This may help explain why sports-related serious laryngeal injuries and fractures in young athletes are less common despite their participation in high-velocity and aggressive sports. Young athletes and chil-dren enjoy so-called laryngeal elasticity which allows better tolerance of trauma to the neck. Additional protective factors against laryngeal structures in young ath-letes are the high-positioned larynx and the abundant percutaneous fat in the neck [3].

Sports-related laryngeal injuries vary also with gender. The prevalence of laryngeal trauma is higher in males compared to females, with a ratio of almost 4:1 [22, 23]. This gender difference in the prevalence of laryngeal trauma is attributed mostly to the historic disparity in sports participation between males and females and to the disparity in media public perception of athletes across genders [22]. Despite reform in policies over the last few decades, which aimed to increase females in sports participation, a significant gender difference still is noted across the world. In the United States, participation by men is twice that of women (35% vs. 16%, respectively) [1]. Similar gender disparity in sports participation is observed in European countries. Based on a study by Tuyckom et al., males were more likely than females to participate regularly in sports than females in Belgium, France, Greece, Latvia, Lithuania, Slovakia, Spain, and the United Kingdom, while the opposite was true in Denmark, Finland, Sweden, and the Netherlands [16].

Another important factor that needs to be considered in the understanding of gender difference in laryngeal fractures is sexual dimorphism in the anatomy of the laryngeal skeleton. Men are more prone to laryngeal fractures because of the associated high rate of laryngeal cartilage ossification. In a computerized tomography study by Yeager et al., the extent of thyroid cartilage ossification was found to be greater in men compared to women [24]. In another cephalometric study of 141 men and 218 women aged 10–59 years, the authors showed a higher preponderance of laryngeal cartilage ossification in men compared to women and a greater extent of ossification in thyroid cartilages compared to cricoid cartilages [20]. In a study by Classeen et al. on men and women between the ages of 41 and 60 years, the authors reported significantly higher bone formation in the thyroid cartilages of men in comparison to women [25]. The study was conducted using light microscopic examination and serial X-ray images.

Sports-related laryngeal trauma is a common cause of laryngeal injury in athletes. It is very common in high-velocity sports such as ice hockey, soccer, and rugby. The injury is due mostly to collision among players and/or field-related equipment. Sports-related laryngeal injuries vary with age and gender. Men are affected more than women, and elderly athletes are more prone to laryngeal fractures than young athletes. The disparity in laryngeal injury between genders and across different age groups is attributed largely to differences in laryngeal cartilages calcification.

9.3 Clinical Presentation of Sports-Related Laryngeal Trauma

9.3.1 History and Physical Findings in Sports-Related Laryngeal Trauma

Sports-related laryngeal trauma, like other causes of laryngeal trauma, can lead to dysfunction in phonation, breathing, and deglutition. In the absence of a penetrating injury, the symptoms following trauma are attributed mostly to inability of laryngeal soft tissues to oscillate normally within the cartilaginous laryngeal framework, very similar to brain injury following head trauma [26]. Fractures often occur because of anterior trauma that compresses the larynx posteriorly against the bone of the cervical spine. As in non-sports-related laryngeal trauma, the most commonly reported symptoms aside from neck pain are dysphonia, impairment in breathing, and dysphagia [26–30]. Mendis and Anderson reviewed the clinical presentation of 13 patients with sports-related blunt laryngeal trauma and reported dysphonia and neck pain as the most common symptoms ($n = 13$). These were followed by shortness of breath and/or stridor in 8 of 13 cases [8]. In another review on the diagnosis and management of laryngotracheal trauma, Francis et al. reported dysphonia and respiratory distress in 4 and 6 of 23 patients, respectively [28]. Similarly, in a review of the clinical findings in 22 patients with laryngeal fracture, one of which was attributed to sports injury, Kim et al. reported hoarseness in 18% of cases. The most common presenting symptom was neck pain in 68.1% of cases [29]. Other less commonly reported symptoms in sports-related laryngeal trauma include dysphagia, odynophagia, and hemoptysis. In the aforementioned report by Kim et al., two-thirds of the patients with laryngeal fractures reported odynophagia. In a review of the clinical presentation of 30 patients with external laryngeal trauma, Yen et al. reported dysphagia and hemoptysis in 18 and 11 cases, respectively [30]. When present, these symptoms indicate possible injury to the mucosal lining of the pharynx and/or cervical esophagus, in addition to the larynx. In a review of 51 patients with trauma to the cervical trachea, Reece and Shatney reported esophageal injury in 21% of cases, with hemoptysis being a symptom in 1 out of 5 patients. Dysphonia was reported in 46% of patients with laryngeal injury [31]. Although it is important to note that dysphagia and hemoptysis may be symptoms and signs of esophageal injury, not all patients with these symptoms are affected. In the study by Yen et al., none of the 18 patients with dysphagia and none of the 11 patients with hemoptysis had significant esophageal injury on esophagoscopy [30].

The clinical presentation of sports-related laryngeal trauma can be misleading and does not always reflect the extent of laryngeal injury. The delay in phonatory and airway symptoms of up to 48 or 72 h following trauma may mask the severity of the injury and often lead to underdiagnosis. Haft et al. reported a 33-year defense man for a hockey league team who sustained trauma to the neck by a high-velocity hockey puck. Although the player was stunned after the impact, he was able to resume playing. After a short lapse of time, the patient developed dysphonia and dysphagia which prompted medical assistance. The player had laryngeal injury that was managed successfully using conservative measures [32]. Similarly, Rejali et al. described a 33-year-old patient with mandibular fracture who developed dyspnea and hoarseness 24 h following sports-related trauma to the face. His airway compromise was attributed to progressive supraglottic laryngeal edema that was managed conservatively using steroids [33]. These studies highlight that lack of airway and/or phonatory symptoms at the time of presentation does not exclude substantial laryngeal injury, and hence a thorough physical examination of the head and neck and larynx is mandatory in the evaluation of patients who have sustained laryngeal trauma. The neck examination usually reveals point tenderness at the site of trauma, swelling, and ecchymosis. In a review by Fuhrman et al. that included ten patients with laryngotracheal injuries presenting to level I trauma center, cervical tenderness and anterior neck contusion occurred in nine and four patients, respectively [27]. Less commonly described physical findings in sports-related laryngeal trauma include depressed laryngeal prominence (Adam's apple) and step deformities along the laryngeal skeleton. When cervical landmarks are distorted, laryngeal fractures should be sought. The presence of subcutaneous emphysema and/or crepitus on physical examination should raise the suspicion of laryngeal fractures and/or disruption of the laryngeal mucosal lining. Detachment of the vocal folds' anterior attachment to the thyroid cartilage (Broyles ligament) can lead to laxity of the vocal folds and restriction in its ability to contract or elongate. Severe symptoms such as contracted voice range, loss of volume, loss of low-pitch and high notes, and decreased intensity are reported often.

When laryngeal injury is suspected, laryngeal examination using either a flexible nasopharyngoscope or a rigid telescope (or both) is always recommended. The most common laryngeal findings are edema and submucosal hematoma with or without mucosal lacerations (Figs. 9.1 and 9.2). In the review by Yen et al. which included 30 patients with external laryngeal trauma, the most common laryngeal findings on direct and indirect laryngeal examination were arytenoid swelling, vocal fold injury, and superficial mucosal lacerations in 7, 6, and 5 cases, respectively. Other findings in the study group included mixed injuries in five cases, cricoarytenoid dislocation in four cases, thyroid cartilage fractures in two cases, and epiglottic fracture in one case [30]. The hematoma may be well localized, supraglottic, subglottic, or glottic or may be diffuse and not be confined to one laryngeal site. When present, serial laryngeal examination is recommended, and airway symptoms should be monitored. Less commonly described endoscopic findings include exposed laryngeal cartilages and/or impairment of motion or fixation of the vocal folds. The impairment in vocal fold mobility can be unilateral or bilateral and usually is ascribed to either a large vocal fold hematoma weighing on the vocal fold, to a displaced

Fig. 9.1 A 50-year-old man with history of blunt trauma to the neck presented with dysphonia and difficulty swallowing. The laryngeal examination shows a submucosal hematoma involving the aryepiglottic folds, left arytenoid, and bilateral true vocal folds

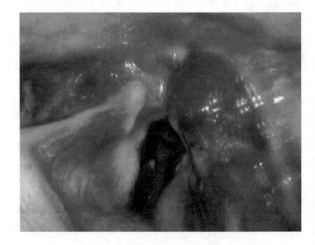

Fig. 9.2 The same patient
as Fig. 9.1, 1 year later.
The patient was managed
conservatively with voice
rest and hydration

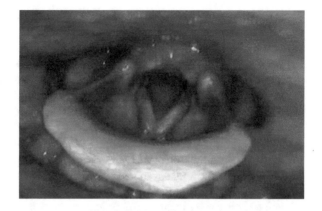

fracture of the thyroid cartilage, and/or to injury to the cricoarytenoid joint, or to the
laryngeal nerves. In a review by Yen et al., 4 patients out of 30 had cricoarytenoid
dislocation [30]. Though impairment in vocal fold mobility is rare and usually
occurs on one side, bilateral vocal fold fixation should not be overlooked in patients
with stridor. Levine et al. reported a case of upper airway obstruction secondary to
impaired bilateral vocal fold mobility in a 26-year-old man who sustained blunt
laryngeal trauma [34]. The patient had a thyroid cartilage fracture and retropharyn-
geal hematoma which obstructed his airway and necessitated an emergency tracheotomy to secure the airway. Another finding that is encountered rarely following
laryngeal trauma is vocal fold/process granuloma. Garret and Lee reported a
20-year-old-female who presented with persistent and progressive airway symptoms and a change in voice quality following conservative management of sports-
related laryngeal trauma. On examination, the patient had a large mass filling the
supraglottis and occluding the airway. The patient underwent awake tracheotomy
and excision of the mass under microlaryngoscopy. The authors highlighted the
need to consider post-trauma pyogenic granuloma in the workup of laryngeal
masses, though traumatic granulomas are encountered more frequently in the oral
cavity [35]. Vocal process avulsion also can occur from external laryngeal trauma,
although that injury is usually caused by intubation.

Strobovideolaryngoscopy (SVL) is recommended in the evaluation of patients
with sports-related laryngeal trauma presenting with dysphonia. SVL provides
valuable information about vocal fold closure and the vibratory behavior of the
vocal folds during phonation. In a review by Remacle on the contribution of videostroboscopy to otolaryngology practice, the author noted its essential usefulness in
68% of cases and its ability to correctly diagnose in 13% of cases [36]. The author
(RTS) and colleagues have found it essential in a substantially higher percentage of
cases [37, 38]. Incomplete vocal fold closure, phase asymmetry, and aperiodicity
need to be considered as signs of possible vocal fold injury or disruption of laryngeal mucosal lining, keeping in mind the discrepancies between telescopic laryngeal examinations and intraoperative findings [39]. In a review by Mendis and
Anderson, 5 of 13 patients with laryngeal trauma had incomplete closure of the

vocal folds. Moderate impairment in mucosal waves was reported in 1–19% of the cases bilaterally and was attributed to mucosal edema and submucosal hematoma [8]. In a study on the usefulness of SVL in the management of 40 patients with acute laryngeal trauma, Kennedy et al. reported phase asymmetry and aperiodicity in all 7 patients who underwent stroboscopic examination. Moreover, five patients had decreased amplitude of vibration, and one patient had impaired mobility of the vocal fold secondary to subluxation of the arytenoid cartilage. The authors stressed the added value of SVL in the assessment and management of patients with laryngeal trauma [40]. SVL also is valuable in the assessment of patients with sports-related, long-term phonatory sequel secondary to vocal fold scarring. In the aforementioned study, all seven patients had improvement in voice quality on long-term follow-up, but laryngeal stroboscopic examination remained abnormal. The clinical and phonatory changes following laryngeal trauma can be attributed to scar and/or atrophic changes of the vocal folds [41]. Decrease in vocal fold pliability is a diagnostic sign of vocal fold structural change following injury. Based on a review of vocal fold scar by Hansen and Thibault, there is an increase in collagen I in the early phase of repair, followed by replacement with thick collagen and a decrease in elastin fibers which become fragmented and disorganized. There is also a decrease in hyaluronic acid in the early phase of wound repair (rabbit model) and its redistribution across the different layers of the lamina propria [42].

9.3.2 Radiologic Imaging in Sports-Related Laryngeal Trauma

Radiologic imaging is key to assessing the extent of laryngeal injury in sports-related laryngeal trauma. The most commonly ordered tests are plain cervical radiography and/or computerized tomography (CT) of the head and neck [8, 28, 43, 44]. Plain radiography of the neck is a standard diagnostic test used in detecting cervical spine injuries and presence of subcutaneous emphysema and in delineating the position and integrity of the hyoid bone which may be altered in patients with laryngotracheal separation. Computerized tomography (CT) of the larynx used to be recommended mostly as an adjuvant diagnostic tool with a high index of reliability, particularly in patients with blunt laryngeal trauma [45, 46]. Now, it is the standard study. In a review by Francis et al., 4 patients out of 12 who had undergone laryngoscopy had missed injuries [28]. CT of the neck helped to identify laryngotracheal injury in 100% of cases who had imaging, whereas laryngoscopy had a diagnostic yield of only 67%. CT scan of the neck is most helpful in identifying fractures of the hyoid bone and thyroid and/or cricoid cartilages, and it may identify cricoarytenoid and thyroarytenoid joint injuries especially in older athletes whose larynges are ossified at least partially (Fig. 9.3). In a study by Mendis and Anderson, the thyroid cartilage was the most common site of fracture in eight of nine patients with laryngeal fractures. Only two patients had concomitant fractures at other laryngeal sites, namely, at the cricoid cartilage and the hyoid bone [8]. In a review of 22 patients with laryngeal fractures, 1 of which was sport related, Kim et al. reported

Fig. 9.3 A 23-year-old
man who sustained blunt
laryngeal trauma by a
tennis racket.
Computerized tomography
of the neck shows a
vertical fracture of the
right thyroid cartilage

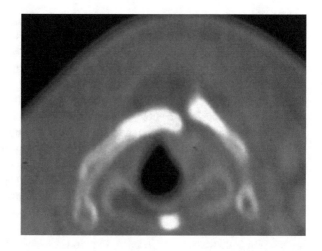

comminuted laryngeal fractures in 4. The most common site of fracture was the
thyroid cartilage ($n = 18$), followed by the cricoid cartilage and arytenoid cartilage
in 3 cases [29]. In addition to its ability to delineate laryngeal fractures, CT scan of
the neck is very useful in detecting laryngeal soft tissue injuries, particularly in
patients with a large, expanding hematoma that impairs the visualization of the
laryngeal lumen. However, CT usually should be obtained only when the airway is
not at risk. Signs of subcutaneous emphysema and perilaryngeal or peripharyngeal
air pockets are indicative of laryngeal and/or pharyngeal mucosal tears. CT scan of
the neck can assist the treating physician in deciding on the need for surgical exploration [8]. In a review of 16 cases of laryngeal injury, Scaglione et al. reported
questionable and non-correct physical examination in 60% of cases and nondiag-
nostic or incorrect laryngoscopic findings in 40% of patients with class II laryngeal
injury based on Schaefer classification which is used commonly in the classification
of laryngeal injury [46]. Class I patients are those with minimal laryngeal mucosal
lacerations or hematoma and minimal compromise of the airway; class II patients
are those with edema and/or hematoma resulting in various degrees of airway compromise; class III patients are those with massive edema, mucosal lacerations with
exposed cartilages, displaced fractures, and/or immobile vocal folds; and class IV
patients are those similar to group II and with unstable laryngeal framework.
Computerized tomography of the neck helped in the management of these cases and
in avoiding surgery in one patient. Computerized tomography of the head and neck
also is useful in ruling out concomitant head and neck vascular and/or neurologic
injuries and in identifying concomitant factures of the maxillofacial skeleton that
often are neglected or missed in patients presenting with airway symptoms. In a
study on sports-related laryngeal trauma by Mendis and Anderson, 1 of 12 cases
with laryngeal fractures had facial fractures. One patient with laryngeal fracture was
also diagnosed with an ankle fracture [8].

   Barium swallow is another radiologic test often requested in patients with symptoms and signs of pharyngeal and/or esophageal injury. In a review of ten cases of

acute laryngotracheal trauma, Mathisen and Grillo reported esophageal transection in one. The authors also noted esophageal injury in 4 cases out of 17 who had delayed treatment and stressed the need for early diagnosis of these injuries in order to avoid potentially fatal complications. There was no mention whether these patients had barium swallow or esophagoscopy [44]. Similarly, Bernat et al. described a case of esophageal injury following blunt trauma to the neck that was associated with laryngotracheal separation. The authors advocated the need for immediate reconstruction of the mucosal injury and restoration of the mucosal lining [47]. In an analysis of 57 patients with penetrating injuries to the laryngotracheal complex, Grewal et al. reported combined airway and digestive tract injuries in 19% of cases. Given that injuries to the upper digestive tract are associated with a high mortality rate, the authors advocated for contrast esophagogram and/or esophagoscopy in patients with suspected injury. Contrast esophagography, with or without fluoroscopy, usually is performed using a dilute barium sulfate paste or a water-soluble contrast agent in order to reduce the risk of mediastinitis in cases of esophageal perforation. It is worth noting that the false-negative rate of esophagography is up to 40%, which emphasizes the need for esophagoscopy, particularly in patients with a high index of suspicion [48]. Signs indicative of possible perforation on esophagoscopy are the presence of bleeding and/or air bubbles within the esophagus. Less commonly ordered radiologic tests include angiography and magnetic resonance imaging (MRI) of the neck. The former is requested to rule out vascular injuries, namely, injury to the carotid artery and its branches, whereas MRI is recommended particularly to rule out cervical spine injury. In a study by Francis et al., 10 out of 23 patients with laryngotracheal trauma had associated mostly vascular and cervical spine injuries [28].

In summary, the importance of a diligent history taking in sports-related laryngeal trauma cannot be overemphasized. Voice and airway symptoms may be delayed and may not be commensurate with the apparent severity of injury. Patients need to undergo laryngeal examination at the time of presentation even in the absence of phonatory and/or airway symptoms. More than one laryngeal examination is warranted in patients with mucosal edema and/or laryngeal hematoma. Radiologic imaging using CT scan of the head and neck is useful mostly in detecting laryngeal fractures or joint dislocation, especially following blunt trauma. The cartilages affected the most are the thyroid and cricoid cartilages. CT also is useful in ruling out maxillofacial and cervical spine injury. A barium swallow is recommended in cases of suspected pharyngeal or esophageal mucosal injury.

9.3.3   Direct Laryngoscopy and Laryngeal Exploration

In patients with severe laryngeal injury, diagnostic evaluation of the larynx under suspension laryngoscopy is indicated. Although flexible laryngeal examination and SVL are important in assessing laryngeal injuries, their diagnostic yield may be suboptimal. In a study by Kennedy et al., the authors emphasized that indirect laryngeal examination is not always a substitute to direct laryngoscopy which allows magnified visualization of laryngeal structures and palpation [40]. In a study by Young et al. on the accuracy of SVL, ten patients had their diagnosis changed on direct laryngoscopy. The authors reported an accuracy of 36% and emphasized the need for a flexible consent form in the operative treatment of affected patients [39]. In a review of laryngotracheal trauma by Heman-Ackah and Sataloff, indications for operative evaluation included airway compromise, expanding hematoma, lacerations of the true vocal folds and/or anterior commissure, injury to the thyroarytenoid muscles, and impaired mobility of one or both vocal folds. Additional indications included herniation of pre-epiglottic fat and destabilized laryngeal fractures [49]. Sataloff also has stressed the importance of cricothyroid joint injuries [50]. They are missed far more often than cricoarytenoid joint injuries but impair the ability to change pitch or project the voice. He described a 38-year-old world-class basketball player who had sustained 12 traumatic laryngeal injuries during his career, mostly caused by elbows striking to his larynx. His dysphonia prevented him from being hired as a coach in the National Basketball Association until unique surgery focusing on his cricothyroid joint improved his volume and quality [50].

9.4 Pathophysiology of Dysphonia in Sports-Related Laryngeal Trauma

Dysphonia is a common complaint in patients with sports-related laryngeal injuries. Despite the suspended position of the larynx in the neck and its ability to deflect trauma in all directions except posteriorly, it remains vulnerable to injuries from collision between players, sports sticks, field instruments, balls, or pucks, or simply from falling [49]. Dysphonia following sports-related trauma can be due to structural vocal fold changes, impairment in vocal fold mobility, alterations in vocal tract resonance, and to impairment in breathing, as reviewed below.

9.4.1 Vocal Fold Structural Changes in Sports-Related Laryngeal Trauma

Sports-related laryngeal trauma may jeopardize all three laryngeal functions, including phonation. Vocal fold structural changes are among the most common causes of dysphonia in these patients even in the absence of laryngeal fractures. Twisting of the larynx and/or compression of the laryngeal framework against the posterior cervical spine can traumatize the glottis and supraglottic soft tissues. Athletes with sports-related laryngeal injury commonly present with submucosal hematoma that may be localized or diffuse, and hematoma may involve one or both vocal folds [51]. When present, the hematoma may disturb the body-cover interface and jeopardize vocal fold vibration. The shearing forces, among other mechanical stresses in phonation, are disturbed [52]. Vocal fold hematoma also can lead to change in voice quality by increasing vocal fold mass and/or changing vocal fold tension and length, two major determinants of voice pitch. If left untreated, it can result in vocal fold scar and increased stiffness. Similar phonatory sequelae may result from vocal fold mucosal lacerations. Scar and tethering of the mucosal cover to the underlying vocal fold ligament can lead to permanent change in voice pitch, loudness, and timber. In a review of 33 cases of laryngeal fractures, one-third of which had been caused by sports injury, Juutilainen et al. reported "fair" subjective voice outcome (altered but still functional as perceived by the patient) and contracted voice range in 13 and 6 patients, respectively. The inability to reach the high notes was attributed to the restricted elasticity or ability of the vocal folds to stretch [53]. Brosch et al., in their review of three cases of laryngeal trauma, emphasized the long-term voice sequelae of submucosal hematoma and reiterated the poor correlation between the extent of laryngeal injury at presentation and the clinical course afterward. One out of the three cases had a localized vocal fold hematoma that progressed to what the authors referred to as "post-traumatic functional dysphonia" [54]. If left untreated, post-traumatic dysphonia may evolve into pressed phonation with symptoms and signs of laryngeal hyperfunction. Early diagnosis and intervention are crucial in order to minimize vocal fold scar and permanent change in voice quality [55].

9.4.2   Vocal Fold Impaired Mobility in Sports-Related Laryngeal Trauma

Another cause of dysphonia following sports-related laryngeal trauma is impairment in vocal fold mobility. The impairment in vocal fold mobility may be secondary to a mass effect of large glottic and supraglottic submucosal hematoma and to subluxation/dislocation of the cricoarytenoid joint, to paresis/paralysis, or to a combination of these conditions. If the vocal fold is fixed in the paramedian or lateral position, glottic insufficiency with incomplete closure of the vocal folds during phonation usually results. Patients complain of breathiness, loss of power, and often aspiration and dysphagia. If the vocal fold is fixed in the midline and the injury is bilateral, patients often have shortness of breath and stridor [56]. In a study by Kennedy on 40 patients with laryngeal trauma, 1 patient had impaired mobility of the vocal fold secondary to arytenoid subluxation [40]. The presence of suspected arytenoid subluxation or dislocation should prompt direct endoscopic exploration and reduction [49]. Vocal fold impaired mobility also may be secondary to displaced thyroid cartilage fractures. Detachment of the anterior commissure attachment can result in laxity and impaired closure of the vocal folds, and fractures of the thyroid may alter vocal fold height or mobility. Trauma also can cause neuropraxia and paresis or paralysis of laryngeal nerves. If left untreated, the long-term sequelae of untreated sports-related laryngeal trauma include permanent change in voice quality.

9.4.3 Alteration in Vocal Tract Resonance in Sports-Related Laryngeal Trauma

Dysphonia may be caused by change in vocal tract resonance. Vocal tract resonant frequencies are determined by the shape and configuration of the vocal tract, as well as the thickness and continuity of its mucosal lining [57]. In a study on vocal tract and surrounding tissue resonance, Hanna et al. showed that vocal tract wall thickness and "non-rigidity" affect the acoustic properties of a speaker. The authors demonstrated that the bandwidths of the acoustic resonance are attenuated partially by the properties of vocal tract wall [58]. Similarly, Sulter et al. reported that the spatial configuration of the vocal tract can be determined acoustically. The study was conducted on a male subject whose vocal tract dimensions were measured using magnetic resonance imaging while he was asked to perform various phonatory tasks [59].

Athletes with sports-related laryngeal trauma may develop changes in the cross-sectional area and volume of their vocal tract. These changes usually lead to alterations in the strength, position, and interspace of the vocal tract harmonics. The presence of mucosal edema, tears, as well as pooling of mucus secondary to impaired laryngeal sensation may exacerbate the phonatory changes. Severe laryngeal trauma also may alter the length of the vocal tract by disturbing its muscular and ligamentous attachments. Dislocated fractures of the hyoid bone and/or comminuted fractures of the thyroid cartilage may either shorten or lengthen the vocal tract. With changes in vocal tract length, there are changes in the position and dispersion of formant frequencies. The acoustic properties may be affected in patients with concomitant oropharyngeal hematoma which can lead to permanent stiffness and/or thickening of the pharyngeal wall, altering the size and pliability of the resonance structures. Changes in the cross-sectional area and volume of the oropharynx and hypopharynx may lead to alteration in formant frequencies, particularly the first and second formants. A detailed review of voice resonance has been provided by Sundberg [57].

9.4.4 Impaired Breathing in Sports-Related Laryngeal Trauma

Dysphonia in patients with sports-related trauma may be due also to impairment in breathing. The impairment in breathing can be secondary to musculoskeletal or neural injuries to the chest, as in cases of rib fractures, or to pulmonary dysfunction secondary to pneumomediastinum and/or pneumothorax [60, 61]. The fundamental role of breathing in phonation is well known. Breathing enables the oscillator by sustaining a pressure gradient across the glottis that sets the vocal folds into oscillation [62]. Impairment in breathing can result in significant changes in voice quality and endurance. Commonly reported symptoms include loss of volume, decreased vocal range, voice fatigue, and inability to project the voice. Breathing also plays an important role in modulating the type of phonation and voice pitch by affecting the position of the larynx and the adductor forces for glottic closure. A high-positioned larynx with a hard glottal attack is commonly observed in patients with low-lung volume [59, 63]. Hence, compensatory laryngeal behavior may develop leading to pressed phonation.

In summary, dysphonia in sports-related laryngeal injuries is due mostly to vocal fold structural change and/or impaired mobility of the vocal folds. Alteration in vocal tract resonance secondary to mucosal edema, hematoma, and/or scar can contribute to the change in voice quality. Impairment in breathing is an important possible etiology especially in patients with pulmonary dysfunction and musculoskeletal injuries.

9.5 Management of Sports-Related Laryngeal Injury in Athletes

9.5.1 Airway Management in Sports-Related Laryngeal Injury

The management of sports-related laryngeal injury in athletes is challenging. Comprehensive workup and early intervention are invaluable, as late diagnosis and treatment may lead to adverse sequelae. Securing the airway and controlling hemorrhage are the first considerations in emergent trauma. Securing the airway starts by proper positioning of the mandible using chin lift or jaw thrust, clearing the oral cavity of secretions, blood and/or foreign bodies, and inserting an oral airway to prevent collapse of the base of tongue against the posterior pharyngeal wall when necessary. Assistance using a bag-valve mask often is needed to ensure ventilation [64]. Failure to sustain oxygenation prompts the need for endotracheal tube insertion and/or a tracheotomy. Alternatively, patients may undergo percutaneous needle cricothyrotomy under local anesthesia [65]. The rationale for either is to bypass the vocal folds and minimize the risk of aspiration. There is extensive debate in the literature on whether the insertion of an endotracheal tube is hazardous and should be avoided or not. Hence, the management of the emergency airway in patients with laryngeal trauma and respiratory symptoms should be individualized. In their report on the acute management of external laryngeal trauma, Schaefer et al. recommended tracheotomy under local anesthesia [46]. The author advocated avoidance of intubation in patients with impeding airway obstruction, particularly those with evidence of mucosal tears and/or exposed laryngeal cartilage. Exempted patients were those with nonsignificant laryngeal injuries and/or normal laryngeal examination [46]. Similarly, Fuhrman et al., in their study which included eight patients with airway emergencies, recommended tracheotomy to secure the airway. The authors emphasized that intolerance of patients with laryngeal trauma to the supine position should guide the treating physician toward performing an immediate tracheotomy [27]. Heman-Ackah and Sataloff, in their review of laryngotracheal trauma, advocated placement of the tracheotomy two rings below the site of injury or at the site of laryngotracheal separation if one is present. The authors also noted that tracheotomy allows exposure of missed or unidentified laryngotracheal injury, an important added value [49]. Gussack et al. argued that endotracheal intubation using a small tube is a safe alternative to tracheotomy, if performed cautiously with minimal manipulation of the pharyngeal and laryngeal lumen [5]. Intubation must be considered with great caution if cervical spine injury has not been ruled out. Notably, flexible laryngoscopic intubation while the patient is awake and the use of the GlideScope (Verathon, Inc., Bothell, Washington, USA) may allow better visualization of the laryngeal lumen during intubation than techniques of intubation used by anesthesiologists routinely (Fig. 9.4). In a study by Bhojani et al., most patients with laryngeal trauma and who needed emergency airway (37 out of 71) were intubated successfully. A higher percentage of patients with blunt trauma required emergency airway procedures in comparison to patients with penetrating trauma (78.9% vs. 46.2%, respectively). The authors stressed the high mortality in patients who undergo tracheotomy and surgical repair. Note that none of the laryngeal trauma cases in that study were sports related [66]. Grewal et al. reviewed the records of 57 patients with penetrating laryngotracheal trauma and reported the need for emergency airway management in 56% of cases. Endotracheal intubation was successful in 14 of 32 patients. The authors advocated intubation in patients with minor to

Fig. 9.4 Picture of a GlideScope (Verathon, Inc., Bothell, Washington, USA)

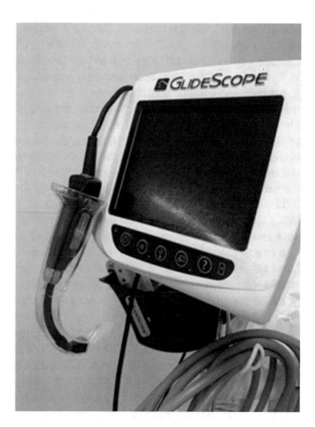

moderate laryngeal injuries and tracheotomy in patients with major laryngeal injuries [48]. In a study by Jewett et al. that included 392 patients with external laryngeal trauma, 139 had tracheotomy. The mortality of those who underwent tracheotomy was higher than that of those who underwent no tracheotomy or surgical repair [67]. Notably, a large percentage of those who underwent tracheotomy had other injuries to the head, chest, and other sites, which may explain the higher mortality rate.

Management of airway obstruction in athletes with sports-related laryngeal trauma is challenging. Cases should be individualized taking into consideration the extent of laryngeal injury, degree of airway compromise, and availability of well-trained care providers. Associated comorbidities should not be missed, including cervical spine injury. Other causes of respiratory distress such as central neurologic disorders, cervical neuromuscular injuries, pneumomediastinum, and/or pneumothorax must be investigated.

9.5.2   Conservative Treatment of Sports-Related Laryngeal Trauma

The management of sports-related laryngeal trauma depends on the severity of injury, the patient's clinical presentation, the availability of medical resources, and the time when athletic activity needs to be resumed. Although there are no studies in the literature on the correlation between symptoms, signs, and treatment outcome in patients who undergo surgical intervention vs. conservative (nonsurgical) treatment, most sports-related laryngeal injuries are managed conservatively. The trend toward conservative management might be ascribed to the fact that most sports-related laryngeal trauma is blunt in nature and mild in severity. In a study by Danic et al. on the prevalence and management of laryngotracheal trauma in peacetime vs. wartime, the authors reported a higher percentage of patients with blunt laryngeal trauma treated conservatively, in comparison to patients with penetrating injuries [68]. Similarly, in a review by Schaefer and Close, patients with mild laryngeal injury with edema, minor mucosal lacerations, and no exposed laryngeal cartilage were treated conservatively. Patients with non-displaced single laryngeal fractures also were managed nonsurgically [46]. In another review of 77 patients with acute laryngeal trauma, Bent et al. advocated conservative treatment of patients with small endolaryngeal hematoma, minor mucosal lacerations, and no displaced laryngeal fractures [69]. While these publications did not address sports-related injuries, the principles of treatment apply.

Conservative management of sports-related laryngeal trauma includes head bed elevation, proper hydration, and close monitoring of the upper airway using serial indirect or flexible laryngeal endoscopy. Administration of humidified air and the use of systemic steroids in cases of severe edema may be helpful. The use of antibiotics is controversial, but many otolaryngologists prescribe them when there is exposed cartilage. In selected patients, maintaining the airway by keeping the endo-tracheal tube in place until there is regression of edema and airway patency is restored may be the only needed treatment [46, 49].

In summary, the clinical signs indicating conservative management include nor-mal or nearly normal laryngeal examination, the presence of only minimal edema, non-expanding hematoma, minor mucosal lacerations, normal mobility of the vocal fold, and single non-displaced laryngeal fracture. Treatment consists of assuring the patency of the airway, hydration, antibiotic or steroid coverage when appropriate, and close observation.

9.5.3 Surgical Treatment of Sports-Related Laryngeal Trauma

The timing of surgical intervention, as well as the type of surgery to be performed, in patients with sports-related laryngeal injury is controversial. In patients with severe laryngeal injury, surgical intervention usually is recommended early in the course of management, i.e., within the first 24 hours. Early surgical repair promotes good outcome and helps avoid extensive scarring, webs, and granulation tissue for-mation [49]. In a study by Bent et al. that included 77 patients with laryngeal trauma who were treated within 48 h, the phonatory outcome was good in 3 of 4 cases with dysphonia. Moreover, 91% of the study group had good airway toward the end of treatment [69]. Similar results were reported in a study by Schaefer on the acute management of laryngeal trauma. The authors advocated early intervention keeping in mind the lack of association between severity of injury and symptoms [46]. Patients with cricoarytenoid joint subluxation and/or dislocation warrant special attention. Early diagnosis and reduction of the subluxation and/or dislocation are important in avoiding long-term joint ankyloses with subsequent impaired mobility of the vocal fold [50, 70]. That being stated, early intervention in patients with severe laryngeal injury appears valuable in preserving good voice quality and air-way patency, whereas delay in treatment may predispose to numerous complica-tions and long-term airway and phonatory sequelae [71].

Surgical intervention may be endoscopic only, external, or combined [49], but this chapter will discuss external surgery. External surgical intervention starts with neck exploration with or without internal laryngeal exposure. Neck exploration allows inspection of the laryngeal framework, control of bleeding in case of expand-ing cervical hematoma, and repair of neurologic injuries. Exposure of the larynx usually is indicated in cases of extensive laryngeal mucosal tears and/or when the laryngeal cartilage is exposed or displaced. Other indications for internal laryngeal exposure include disruption of the anterior commissure, destabilized laryngeal framework secondary to multiple fractures, and/or impaired mobility of the vocal fold [49]. In a study by Mendis and Anderson, two-thirds of patients with laryngeal trauma needed surgical intervention, 54% of whom belonged to class III severity according to Schaefer Fuhrman classification [8]. Similarly, in a review of 120 cases of laryngeal trauma, Schaefer and Close advocated surgical intervention for patients with extensive mucosal lacerations and/or displaced laryngeal fractures. A single displaced thyroid cartilage fracture with intact laryngeal lumen can be reduced and fixed through neck exploration without laryngeal exposure [46]. The author (RTS) has reduced such fractures bimanually with a Hollinger laryngoscope, popping the fracture into position using a technique similar to that used to reduce a nasal fracture.

The internal larynx is exposed usually either through a laryngofissure or thyrotomy, depending on the site of laryngeal fracture and stability of the laryngeal framework. When the larynx is exposed, mucosal tears and muscle lacerations are sutured using absorbable sutures. Mucosal lacerations are closed primarily, and mucosal defects are covered using adjacent local flaps or grafted mucosa. Rotation flaps may be used from the false vocal folds and/or epiglottis. Herniated pre-epiglottic contents are restored to their normal anatomic position, and crushed tissues are debrided. Internal fixation of laryngeal fractures with the aim of stabilizing the laryngeal framework is achieved using either sutures, wires, or mini-plates (Figs. 9.5, 9.6, 9.7, and 9.8). It is important to note that the use of wires in approximating laryngeal fractures allows a two-dimensional repair, whereas the use of mini-plates allows a three-dimensional repair. The use of mini-plates has been recommended highly in cases of multiple displaced fractures, particularly in the presence of surgical defects

Fig. 9.5 Schematic illustration of a paramedian thyroid cartilage fracture crossing the midline

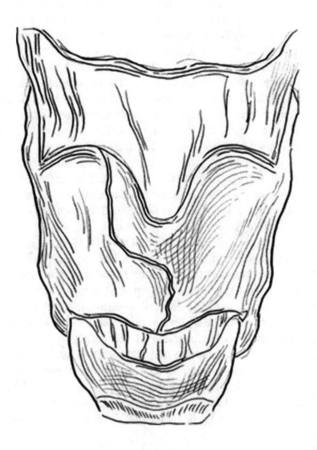

Fig. 9.6 Schematic illustration of paramedian and midline thyroid cartilage fractures stabilized with mini-plates

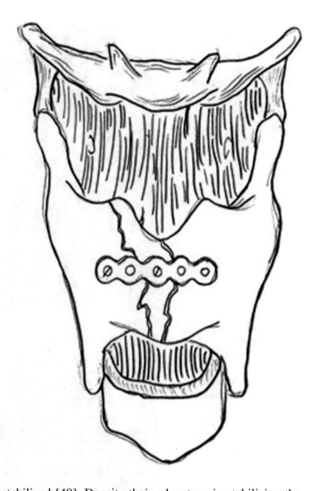

or when the larynx is destabilized [49]. Despite their advantage in stabilizing the laryngeal framework, thus allowing it to stand the stresses of deglutition and phonation, a major drawback is their palpability even years after insertion. This drawback often necessitates their removal at a later stage. Recently described alternatives are the Inion biodegradable plates, made of glycolic and lactic acid polymers. The author (RTS) avoids plating in the vast majority of cases by using figure-of-eight sutures to re-approximate and stabilize cartilage fragments. In areas of severe comminution, cyanoacrylate can be very effective. Tasca et al. reported a 29-year-old rugby player who sustained trauma to his neck that resulted in a displaced vertical thyroid cartilage fracture. The patient complained of neck pain, loss of the high notes, and clicking on palpation of his laryngeal framework. The patient underwent open reduction and internal fixation of his laryngeal fracture 3 weeks after the injury using Inion biodegradable plates. One year following the surgery, the plates were non-palpable on examination [72]. In rare cases, laryngeal stents may be used to stabilize the laryngeal framework. The main indications for use of stents are

Fig. 9.7 Surgical
laryngeal exposure after
the installation of
mini-plates for a lateral
thyroid cartilage fracture

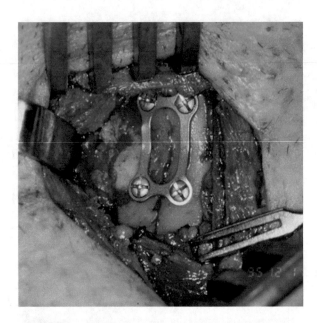

Fig. 9.8 Surgical
laryngeal exposure after
the installation of
mini-plates for a midline
thyroid cartilage fracture

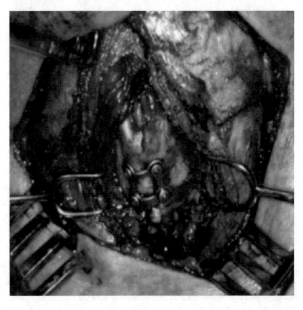

comminuted fractures, extensive mucosal injuries with large denuded surfaces, and
injury to the anterior commissure. Though stents help keep the endolaryngeal lumen
patent and in minimizing web formation, their use decreased markedly over the last
two decades. The reason for the decrease in their popularity is the associated pressure necrosis to surrounding structures and formation of granulation tissue [49].
When stents are needed, these complications usually can be avoided through use of
soft, deformable stent.

Despite all the advances in management of patients with laryngeal trauma, the mortality rate remains substantial. This is due mostly to associated injuries, namely, head trauma, chest trauma, vascular injuries, and esophageal perforation. In a review of 72 patients with laryngeal trauma, Bhojani et al. reported vascular and chest trauma in 8 and 11 cases, respectively. Head trauma and esophageal injuries occurred in six and five patients, respectively [66]. Similarly, in a review by Jewett et al. of 392 patients with external laryngeal trauma, skull base/intracranial injuries, cervical spine, and esophageal/pharyngeal injuries occurred in 13%, 8%, and 3% of cases, respectively [67]. In a study by Grewal et al., 86% of patients with penetrating laryngotracheal injuries had associated injuries. Most common of these were chest injuries ($n = 17$), digestive ($n = 11$), and vascular ($n = 10$). Five patients presented with unstable hemodynamic status, and two had cardiorespiratory arrest. Angiography was recommended for evaluation of vascular injuries. Less common associated injuries were neurologic injuries and injuries to the face and extremities [48].

Surgical intervention is recommended in patients with extensive sports-related laryngeal injury. Common indications include multiple mucosal lacerations, denuded cartilages, thyroarytenoid muscle injury, detached anterior commissure, and displaced laryngeal fractures. Surgery consists primarily of restoring the mucosal lining by suturing the edges and/or using mucosal flaps and reducing and stabilizing the laryngeal fractures using sutures, wires, or mini-plates. Early initiation of voice therapy is invaluable to avoid late and irreversible phoniatric dysfunction. Athletes with laryngeal injury should not resume sport before complete restoration of airway patency and laryngeal framework integrity.

References

1. Datz T. Poll: three in four adults played sports when they were younger, but only one in four still play. Harvard T.H. Chan School of Public Health. https://www.hsph.harvard.edu/news/press-releases/poll-many-adults-played-sports-when-young-but-few-still-play. Updated 15 June 2015. Accessed 25 Aug 2020.
2. Malm C, Jakobsson J, Isaksson A. Physical activity and sports—real health benefits: a review with insight into the public health of Sweden. Sports. 2019;7(5):127.
3. Frenguelli A, Ruscito P, Bicciolo G, Rizzo S, Massarelli M. Head and neck trauma in sporting activities: review of 208 cases. J Craniomaxillofac Surg. 1991;19(4):178–81.
4. Jalisi S, Zoccoli M. Management of laryngeal fractures--a 10-year experience. J Voice. 2011;25(4):473–9.
5. Gussack GS, Jurkovich GJ, Luterman A. Laryngotracheal trauma: a protocol approach to a rare injury. Laryngoscope. 1986;96(6):660–5.
6. Schaefer SD. The acute management of external laryngeal trauma. A 27-year experience. Arch Otolaryngol Head Neck Surg. 1992;118(6):598–604.
7. Kiser AC, O'Brien SM, Detterbeck FC. Blunt tracheobronchial injuries: treatment and outcomes. Ann Thorac Surg. 2001;71(6):2059–65.
8. Mendis D, Anderson JA. Blunt laryngeal trauma secondary to sporting injuries. J Laryngol Otol. 2017;131(8):728–35.

9. Delaney JS, Al-Kashmiri A. Neck injuries presenting to emergency departments in the United States from 1990 to 1999 for ice hockey, soccer, and American football. Br J Sports Med. 2005;39(4):e21.
10. Dec KL, Cole SL, Metivier S. Screening for catastrophic neck injuries in sports. Curr Sports Med Rep. 2007;6(1):16–9.
11. Fuller CW, Junge A, Dvorak J. A six-year prospective study of the incidence and causes of head and neck injuries in international football. Br J Sports Med. 2005;39(1):i3–9.
12. French C, Kelley R. Laryngeal fractures in lacrosse due to high speed ball impact. JAMA Otolaryngol Head Neck Surg. 2013;139(7):735–8.
13. Liberman M, Mulder DS. Airway injuries in the professional ice hockey player. Clin J Sport Med. 2007;17(1):61–7.
14. Boden BP, Tacchetti R, Mueller FO. Catastrophic injuries in high school and college baseball players. Am J Sports Med. 2004;32(5):1189–96.
15. Brown KA, Patel DR, Darmawan D. Participation in sports in relation to adolescent growth and development. Transl Pediatr. 2017;6(3):150–9.
16. Van Tuyckom C, Scheerder J, Bracke P. Gender and age inequalities in regular sports participation: a cross-national study of 25 European countries. J Sports Sci. 2010;28(10):1077–84.
17. Eime RM, Harvey JT, Charity MJ, Casey MM, Westerbeek H, Payne WR. Age profiles of sport participants. BMC Sports Sci Med Rehab. 2016;8(1):6–16.
18. Maia JA, Lefevre J, Claessens AL, Thomis MA, Peeters MW, Beunen GP. A growth curve to model changes in sport participation in adolescent boys. Scand J Med Sci Sports. 2010;20(4):679–85.
19. Cozijnsen R, Stevens N, Van Tilburg TG. The trend in sport participation among Dutch retirees, 1983–2007. Ageing Soc. 2013;33(04):698–719.
20. Mupparapu M, Vuppalapati A. Ossification of laryngeal cartilages on lateral cephalometric radiographs. Angle Orthod. 2005;75(2):196–201.
21. Sataloff RT, Kost KM, Linville SE. The effects of age on the voice. In: Sataloff RT. Professional voice: the science and art of clinical care. 4th ed. San Diego: Plural Publishing; 2017. p. 585–604.
22. Dickson KE. Public perception of male athletes Vs. female athletes in the media. 2015. LSU master's thesis. 3865. https://digitalcommons.lsu.edu/gradschool_theses/3865
23. Scheerder J, Vanreusel B, Taks M. Stratification patterns of active sport involvement among adults: social change and persistence. Int Rev Sociol Sport. 2005;40(2):139–62.
24. Yeager VL, Lawson C, Archer CR. Ossification of the laryngeal cartilages as it relates to computed tomography. Investig Radiol. 1982;17(1):11–9.
25. Claassen H, Schicht M, Sel S, Paulsen F. Special pattern of endochondral ossification in human laryngeal cartilages: X-ray and light-microscopic studies on thyroid cartilage. Clin Anat. 2014;27(3):423–30.
26. Sidle DM, Altman KW. The contralateral injury in blunt laryngeal trauma. Laryngoscope. 2002;112(9):1696–8.
27. Fuhrman GM, Stieg FH 3rd, Buerk CA. Blunt laryngeal trauma: classification and management protocol. J Trauma. 1990;30(1):87–92.
28. Francis S, Gaspard DJ, Rogers N, Stain SC. Diagnosis and management of laryngotracheal trauma. J National Med Assoc. 2002;94(1):21–4.
29. Kim JP, Cho SJ, Son HY, Park JJ, Woo SH. Analysis of clinical feature and management of laryngeal fracture: recent 22 case review. Yonsei Med J. 2012;53(5):992–8.
30. Yen PT, Lee HY, Tsai MH, Chan ST, Huang TS. Clinical analysis of external laryngeal trauma. J Laryngol Otol. 1994;108(3):221–5.
31. Reece GP, Shatney CH. Blunt injuries of the cervical trachea: review of 51 patients. South Med J. 1988;81(12):1542–8.
32. Hanft K, Posternack C, Astor F, Attarian D. Diagnosis and management of laryngeal trauma in sports. South Med J. 1996;89(6):631–3.

33. Rejali SD, Bennett JD, Upile T, Rothera MP. Diagnostic pitfalls in sports related laryngeal injury. Br J Sports Med. 1998;32(2):180–1.
34. Levine RJ, Sanders AB, LaMear WR. Bilateral vocal cord paralysis following blunt trauma to the neck. Ann Emerg Med. 1995;25(2):253–5.
35. Garrett MM, Lee WT. Obstructing pyogenic granuloma as a result of blunt laryngeal trauma. Otolaryngol Head Neck Surg. 2007;136(3):489–90.
36. Remacle M. The contribution of videostroboscopy in daily ENT practice. Acta Otorhinolaryngol Belg. 1996;50(4):265–81.
37. Sataloff RT. Strobovideolaryngoscopy in professional voice users: results in clinical value. Ann Otol Rhinol Laryngol. 1988;1(4):359–64.
38. Romak JJ, Heuer RJ, Hawkshaw MJ, Sataloff RT. The clinical voice laboratory. In: Sataloff RT. Professional voice: the science and art of clinical care. 4th ed. San Diego: Plural Publishing; 2017. p. 405–38.
39. Young WG, Shama L, Petty B, Hoffman MR, Dailey SH. Comparing videostroboscopy and direct microlaryngoscopy: an argument for flexible consent and operative plan. J Voice. 2019;33(2):143–9.
40. Kennedy TL, Gilroy PA, Millman B, Greene JS, Pellitteri PK, Harlor M. Strobovideolaryngoscopy in the management of acute laryngeal trauma. J Voice. 2004;18(1):130–7.
41. Hantzakos A, Dikkers FG, Giovanni A, et al. Vocal fold scars: a common classification proposal by the American laryngological association and European laryngological society. Eur Arch Otorhinolaryngol. 2019;276(8):2289–92.
42. Hansen JK, Thibeault SL. Current understanding and review of the literature: vocal fold scarring. J Voice. 2006;20(1):110–20.
43. Scaglione M, Romano L, Grassi R, Pinto F, Calderazzi A, Pieri L. Diagnostic approach to acute laryngeal trauma: role of computerized tomography. Radiol Med. 1997;93(1–2):67–70.
44. Mathisen DJ, Grillo H. Laryngotracheal trauma. Ann Thorac Surg. 1987;43(3):254–62.
45. Steven DS. The acute management of external laryngeal trauma. Arch Otolaryngol Head Neck Surg. 1992;118(6):598–604.
46. Schaefer SD, Close LD. Acute management of laryngeal trauma. Update. Ann Otol Laryngol. 1989;98(2):98–104.
47. Bernat RA, Zimmerman JM, Keane WM, Pribitkin EA. Combined laryngotracheal separation and esophageal injury following blunt neck trauma. Facial Plast Surg. 2005;21(3):187–90.
48. Grewal H, Rao PM, Mukerji S, Ivatury RR. Management of penetrating laryngotracheal injuries. Head Neck. 1995;17(6):494–502.
49. Heman-Ackah YD, Sataloff RT. Laryngotracheal trauma. In: Sataloff RT. Professional voice: the science and art of clinical care. 4th ed. San Diego: Plural Publishing; 2017. p. 1611–27.
50. Sataloff RT. Cricoarytenoid and Cricothyroid joint injury: evaluation and treatment. In: Sataloff RT. Professional voice: the science and art of clinical care. 4th ed. San Diego: Plural Publishing; 2017. p. 1629–39.
51. Glatterer MS Jr, Toon RS, Ellestad CH, et al. Management of blunt and penetrating external esophageal trauma. J Trauma. 1985;25(8):784–92.
52. Titze IR. Mechanical stress in phonation. J Voice. 1994;8(2):99–105.
53. Juutilainen M, Vintturi J, Robinson S, Bäck L, Lehtonen H, Mäkitie AA. Laryngeal fractures: clinical findings and considerations on suboptimal outcome. Acta Otolaryngol. 2008;128(2):213–8.
54. Brosch S, Johannsen HS. Clinical course of acute laryngeal trauma and associated effects on phonation. J Laryngol Otol. 1999;113(1):58–61.
55. Sataloof RT, Hawkshaw MJ. Vocal fold scar. In: Sataloff RT. Professional voice: the science and art of clinical care. 4th ed. San Diego: Plural Publishing; 2017. p. 1587–603.
56. Sataloff RT. Vocal fold paresis and paralysis. In: Sataloff RT. Professional voice: the science and art of clinical care. 4th ed. San Diego: Plural Publishing; 2017. p. 1059–76.

57. Sundberg J. Vocal tract resonance. In: Sataloff RT. Professional voice: the science and art of clinical care. 4th ed. San Diego: Plural Publishing; 2017. p. 309–28.
58. Hanna N, Smith J, Wolfe J. Frequencies, bandwidths and magnitudes of vocal tract and surrounding tissue resonances, measured through the lips during phonation. J Acoust Soc Am. 2016;139(5):2924.
59. Sulter AM, Miller DG, Wolf RF, Schutte HK, Wit HP, Mooyaart EL. On the relation between the dimensions and resonance characteristics of the vocal tract: a study with MRI. Magn Reson Imaging. 1992;10(3):365–73.
60. Putukian M. Pneumothorax and pneumomediastinum. Clin Sports Med. 2004;23(3):443–54.
61. Mihos P, Potaris K, Gakidis I, Mazaris E, Sarras E, Kontos Z. Sports-related spontaneous pneumomediastinum. Ann Thorac Surg. 2004;78(3):983–6.
62. Sataloff RT. Clinical anatomy and physiology of the voice. In: Sataloff RT. Professional voice: the science and art of clinical care. 4th ed. San Diego: Plural Publishing; 2017. p. 157–95.
63. Iwarsson J, Sundberg J. Effects of lung volume on vertical larynx position during phonation. J Voice. 1998;12(2):159–65.
64. Norris RL, Peterson J. Airway management for the sports physician: part 1: basic techniques. Phys Sportsmed. 2001;29(10):23–9.
65. Norris RL, Peterson J. Airway management for the sports physician: part 2: advanced techniques. Phys Sportsmed. 2001;29(11):15–28.
66. Bhojani RA, Rosenbaum DH, Dikmen E, et al. Contemporary assessment of laryngotracheal trauma. J Thorac Cardiovascular Surg. 2005;130(2):426–32.
67. Jewett BS, Shockley WW, Rutledge R. External laryngeal trauma analysis of 392 patients. Arch Otolaryngol Head Neck Surg. 1999;125(8):877–80.
68. Danic D, Prgomet D, Sekelj A, Jakovina K, Danic A. External laryngotracheal trauma. Eur Arch Otorhinolaryngol. 2006;263(3):228–32.
69. Bent JP 3rd, Silver JR, Porubsky ES. Acute laryngeal trauma: a review of 77 patients. Otolaryngol Head Neck Surg. 1993;109(3):441–9.
70. Rubin AD, Hawkshaw MJ, Moyer CA, Dean CM, Sataloff RT. Arytenoid cartilage dislocation: a 20-year experience. J Voice. 2005;19(4):687–701.
71. Corner BT, Gal TJ. Recognition and management of the spectrum of acute laryngeal trauma. Case Report J Emerg Med. 2012;43(5):e289–93.
72. Tasca RA, Sherman IW, Wood GD. Thyroid cartilage fracture: treatment with biodegradable plates. Br J Oral and Maxillofac. 2008;46(2):159–60.

Chapter 10
Sex Hormone Disturbances in Athletes: Implications for Voice

10.1 Introduction

Body function is hormone dependent. Growth and sex hormones have a hypertrophic effect on body organs leading to marked structural and functional development. At puberty, there is differentiation of secondary sex characteristics with marked alteration of the genitourinary system under the influence of estrogen, progesterone, and testosterone. Hormones in turn are under the control of the hypothalamic-pituitary axis and the release of follicle-stimulating hormones (FSH) and luteinizing hormones (LH) [1, 2]. In parallel with the differentiation in primary and secondary sex characteristics, there are marked musculoskeletal, hemodynamic, and psychological changes. These include muscle hypertrophy, an increase in hemoglobin concentration, and alteration in mental drive. These changes are particularly important in athletes. The hormone-induced myogenic effect, improvement in oxygen concentration, increase in mental drive, and sense of competition all improve athletic performance and exercise tolerance [3–5].

This chapter reviews hormonal effects in athletes with emphasis on the prevalence and etiology of hormonal disturbances in this population. Endogenous causes of hyperandrogenism such as polycystic ovaries and disorders in sexual development, as well as exogenous causes such as intake of anabolic steroids, are stressed. Healthcare providers and sports professionals should be familiar with the impact of hyperandrogenism on voice and the pathophysiology of the androgenic voice in female athletes.

A.-L. Hamdan et al., *Voice Disorders in Athletes, Coaches and other Sports Professionals*, https://doi.org/10.1007/978-3-030-69831-7_10

10.2   Hormone Variations in Athletes

10.2.1   Hormone-Induced Effects in Athletic Performance: Gender Dichotomy

Testosterone has a significant effect on musculoskeletal structures [6–10]. It enhances osteoblast differentiation and bone mineralization leading to an increase in bone marrow density. The osteogenic effect is enhanced further in athletes by mechanical loading and training [7]. Testosterone also has an anabolic effect on skeletal muscles leading to an increase in muscle mass and subsequently strength. It acts by promoting preferential differentiation of mesenchymal pluripotent cells into the myogenic lineage. In parallel, testosterone leads to a decrease in the modulation of these cells into adipogenesis, thus decreasing fat concentration and mass. Testosterone-induced growth effect on musculoskeletal structures is facilitated by growth factors and cytokines. The effect is exerted directly and indirectly via its 5-alpha reduction to dihydrotestosterone and its aromatization to estradiol [8]. In an animal study by Manttari et al., testosterone injection was similar to training in inducing an increase in myoglobin concentration, although the effect varied among different muscle groups. The administration of testosterone increased the concentration of myoglobin in the plantaris muscles, whereas training caused an increase in myoglobin concentration in both plantaris and gastrocnemius muscles [9].

The relationship between testosterone level, bone formation, and muscle strength/ mass is dose dependent. With an increase in testosterone level, there is an increase in bone mineralization, as well as an increase in protein metabolism and myogenic activity. As testosterone level is 15 times higher in men compared to women [5], it is clear that there is a dichotomy in athletic performance across genders. The dose-response relation between athletic performance and testosterone level is present also within the same gender. Based on a review by Bermon, hyperandrogenic females have a competitive benefit of 2–5% in comparison to those with a normal androgen level. The authors attributed this competitive edge to the known androgen-enhancing effect on musculoskeletal structures [11]. Similarly, in a study on the correlation between serum androgen levels and performance in track and field, Bermon and Garnier showed that female athletes with the highest levels of free testosterone had significantly better performance in 400 m and 800 m runs in comparison to female athletes with lower free testosterone level. Moreover, male sprinters had higher values of free testosterone in comparison to other male athletes [12]. Similarly, Cook et al. showed that elite athletes had free testosterone concentrations that were double those of non-elite athletes [13], and Bermon et al. stressed the need for establishing normative serum androgen levels in the stratification process between elite female athletes and non-elite female athletes [14].

In summary, there is a strong link between athletic performance and testosterone level. The difference in testosterone across genders has led to a dichotomy in athletic performance between men and women. Moreover, athletic women with hyperandrogenism are considered to have an advantage over those with a normal androgen level.

10.2.2   Hormone Disturbances in Athletes

Hormone disturbances are common in athletes due to dysfunction in the hypothalamic-pituitary axis [15, 16]. As a result, athletes may suffer from amenorrhea, menstrual irregularities, and other signs and symptoms of hyperandrogenism. This can be due to either endogenous or exogenous causes. The most common causes of endogenous hyperandrogenism are PCOS and disorders in sex differentiation (DSD), whereas the most common causes of exogenous hyperandrogenism are the intake of oral contraceptives and/or anabolic-androgenic steroids, as discussed below.

10.2.2.1   Athletic Amenorrhea

Based on the *American College of Sports Medicine*, amenorrhea is one component of the "female athlete triad" often reported as a result of excessive physical activity and/or decrease in energy intake [17]. The reduction in the release of gonadotropin-releasing hormone (GRH) leads to suppression in LH and FSH secretion, with subsequent attenuation in the production of sex steroids by the ovaries. As a result, there is a marked decrease in the concentration of progesterone, estradiol, and testosterone. This drop in sex steroid levels leads to "athletic amenorrhea," or loss of menstruation, a clinical entity encountered commonly in female athletes who exercise intensively [15, 18–20]. Based on a study by Sheid et al., the prevalence of functional hypothalamic amenorrhea and oligo-amenorrhea in female athletes can reach up to 40%, a figure that is markedly higher than that reported in nonathletic women [21]. Two hypotheses are suggested in the literature to explain menstrual irregularities and/or delay in the onset of puberty in female athletes. One is the "critical fat" hypothesis which states that a minimal amount of fat is needed to sensitize the hypothalamic-pituitary-ovarian axis (HPO), and the second is the "metabolic fuel" hypothesis which attributes the HPO axis suppression to a negative energy balance [22–25]. Both hypotheses stress that fertility is linked to abundance in energy in order to assure that reproduction occurs only in favorable conditions.

10.2.2.2   Polycystic Ovary Syndrome in Athletes

Polycystic ovary syndrome (PCOS) is a clinical entity suspected in athletes with irregular menstrual cycles and/or androgenic signs such as hirsutism, acne, or male pattern baldness. Based on the Rotterdam consensus, PCOS is syndrome characterized primarily by features of hyperandrogenism and evidence of polycystic ovaries on imaging [26]. The diversity in clinical presentation and the distribution of patient care among healthcare providers of various specialties have led to underdiagnosis of this condition despite its known adverse effects [27]. In a large review of 873 patients investigated for hyperandrogenism, PCOS was among the most common causes, accounting for 82% of the cases [28]. In a study by Lowe et al. on polycystic ovaries in Australian women, the authors reported a prevalence of 23%. The study was conducted on 100 women who had undergone transvaginal ultrasound as part of the workup of their husband's sterility [29]. In another study by Hagmar et al. on reproductive system dysfunction in female Olympic athletes, one out of four had menstrual dysfunction, and PCOS was the most common cause [30]. Similarly, in their study on polycystic ovary-like syndrome in competitive swimmers, Coste et al. reported a prevalence of 50% among those with hyperandrogenism [31].

The hyperandrogenic state in female athletes with PCOS is no doubt advantageous for athletic performance as discussed in the section on hormonal dichotomy [11–14, 32]. For further corroboration, in a study by Guzelce et al., women with PCOS were found to have a higher average power of lower limb extension and flexion in comparison to controls matched by age and body mass index (BMI). Muscle mechanical function measured using isokinetic dynamometry correlated with bioavailable testosterone level [33]. Given the hypertrophic myogenic effect of androgen, PCOS must be investigated in female athletes with signs and symptoms of hyperandrogenism. Other causes must be excluded as well.

10.2.2.3 Disorders in Sex Differentiation

Disorder in sexual development (DSD) is an uncommon condition characterized by atypical gonadal and chromosomal development with the presence of ambiguous genitalia. Women with DSD have increased production of testosterone from their undescended testes, which leads to signs and symptoms of hyperandrogenism that markedly affect their psychosexual well-being [14, 34–37]. The clinical evaluation of these patients entails biochemical and psychosocial assessment as well as genetic evaluation [34]. Given the known role of androgen in gender difference and its enhancing effect on physical performance, exercise resistance, and training, identification of women with DSD is extremely important particularly in athletes [35, 36]. Although rare, DSD must be excluded in female athletes with signs of hyperandrogenism. In a study that included 849 elite female athletes, 5 cases of DSD were identified. The prevalence of hyperandrogenic 46, XY DSD in athletes was 7/1000, which is 140 times higher than the normal population. The prevalence of 46, XY DSD in the normal population is 1 in 20,000 [37].

10.2.2.4 The Use of Oral Contraceptives in Female Athletes

Oral contraceptives (OC) consist of a combination of estrogen, usually ethinyl estradiol, and often progesterone. The composition and dosage of each component vary across the different generations of oral contraceptives. Ethinyl estradiol concentration, for instance, ranges between 0.02 and 0.05 mg/d in monophasic pills, whereas in triphasic pills it does not exceed 0.04 mg/d. Similarly, progesterone derivatives are available in eight different forms and different concentrations. Despite the variations in the concentration of its constituents, OC act primarily by suppressing the mid-cycle surge of gonadotropins, thus reducing the endogenous production of progesterone and estrogen responsible for pregnancy [38, 39]. Because of their success, the prescription of OC has increased markedly over the last decades, particularly in athletes. In a study by Brynhildsen et al. of 716 female elite athletes in different types of sports, the authors reported use of OC in almost half the cases [40]. In a study of 430 elite female athletes, Martin et al. reported the use of hormonal contraceptive in 49.5% of cases and their usage at some point in time in 69.8% of cases. The authors stressed the need to balance the benefits and side effects of these medications, keeping in mind individual variations [41]. Similarly, Rechichi et al., in their review on athletic performance, quoted an OC use of up to 83% in elite athletes with a mean age of 25 years [42].

The upsurge in the intake of OC came at a cost. Depending on the concentration of estrogen and progesterone, and on their relative binding affinity to estrogen, progesterone, and androgenic receptors, several cardiorespiratory and metabolic side effects of OC have been described. The synthetic products in OC have been shown to alter hormone responses to exercise [43, 44], triglyceride mobilization and metabolic cost [45, 46], carbohydrate metabolism [47], glucose variations, and oxidation rate [48]. In athletes, the focus has been primarily on the impact of these metabolic changes on aerobic and anaerobic exercise and on athletic performance. In a study by Casazza et al. on six eumenorrheic women (moderately active), the authors showed that the intake of exogenous steroids causes a decrease in peak exercise capacity. The testing was performed before and after the intake of OC during the luteal and follicular phases [49]. In another study on 12 women, 6 of whom were randomly assigned oral contraceptives, there was a decrease in those using OC in functional aerobic capacity, although there were no significant hemostatic changes and/or changes in lipid-lipoprotein metabolism [50]. Oral contraceptive use also has been associated with a reduction in peak oxygen uptake (VO2) and increased oxygen consumption. A double-blind placebo-controlled study by Lebrun et al. showed a decrease in maximal aerobic capacity (VO2/max) by 4.7% in the oral contraceptive group in comparison to the placebo group [51]. Similarly, Giacomoni et al. reported lower submaximal oxygen consumption by 3–5.8% with the intake of OC during submaximal exercise. The study conducted on ten women who were asked to run continuously for 12 min at different submaximal intensities and on three occasions (during menstruation, i.e., off OC use, and early and late on OC use) showed that pill ingestion improved "running economy" as stated by the authors [52]. These results are in agreement with known hormone-induced changes in respiratory drive and alveolar PCO2 (partial pressure of carbon dioxide in the blood) during a menstrual cycle, which also impact exercise performance and tolerance [53–55]. In a study of 10 females who had their end-tidal PCO2 and base excess measured throughout 16 menstrual cycles, England and Farhi reported a decrease in these variables during the luteal phase. The authors highlighted the consequent decrease in body CO_2 and its metabolic effect [53].

10.2.2.5   The Use of Anabolic-Androgenic Steroids (AAS) in Athletes

The medical use of anabolic steroids has increased markedly over the last few decades particularly in women. The main indication is treatment of medical conditions such as endometriosis, menorrhagia, decreased libido after menopause, and osteoporosis [56–65]. The improvement in postmenopausal symptoms is attributed to elevation in the level of testosterone which decreases markedly at menopause and/or following oophorectomy [63–65]. The use of testosterone replacement also has been on the rise in men diagnosed with andropause, also referred to as late-onset hypogonadism. This term is derived from Greek words "andras" meaning "human male" and the word "pause" meaning "cessation." Based on a European male aging study in 2012 by Tajar et al., late-onset hypogonadism (LOH) is diagnosed by the presence of a decrease in libido and development of impotence, a total testosterone level less than 11 nmol/L, and free testosterone level less than 220 nmol/L. [66] The prevalence rate of LOH is low. In a study by Araujo et al. that included 1475 men between the ages of 30 and 79 years, the prevalence was 5.6%, and it increased with age [67]. Note that this prevalence rate refers to symptomatic androgen deficiency, whereas 11% had free testosterone level less than 5 n/dl. Although the prevalence of symptomatic androgen deficiency ranged between 3.1% and 7.0%, it did not rise in a dose-response fashion with age, probably because of the small sample size in the age brackets. However, in subjects between the ages of 70 and 79 years, the prevalence of symptomatic androgen deficiency reached 18%.

Another indication for the use of anabolic steroids in both men and women is improvement in body image and physical performance [68]. Anabolic-androgenic steroids (AAS) are the most commonly prescribed pharmacologic drugs in the category of appearance and performance-enhancing drugs (APEDS), which also includes growth hormones, insulin, and stimulant diuretics, among others [69]. AAS are a subclass of testosterone derivatives thought to enhance muscle performance and body image. These can be administered in several forms, transdermal gel, oral, and injectable [70]. The overall number of Americans using AAS is on the rise, with late age of onset. According to a study by Pope et al. in 2014, 3–4 million Americans between the age of 13 and 50 years use AAS, and almost one million become dependent [71]. The upsurge in its usage is due partially to social and economic factors in which body image has become a social marker of prestige, authority, and well-being [72]. The ergogenic effect of AAS has been proven in men and women, with ample historical data. AAS act by binding initially to the cytoplasmic androgenic receptors, following which the androgen-receptor complex triggers DNA sequencing and the transcription of mRNA that is responsible for the synthesis of actin and myosin. AAS also act by inhibiting muscle catabolism secondary to a stress-induced surge in glucocorticoid. After the increase in muscle metabolism and decrease in muscle catabolism, there is an increase in muscle mass. In a review of the effect of androgenic-anabolic steroids in athletes, Hartgens and Kuipers reported an increase in bodyweight by 2–5 kg in addition to the gain in strength. The authors attributed the body changes to an increase in lean body mass and a decrease in fat mass [73]. AAS-induced myotrophic effects are very often associated with side effects that include the reproductive, cardiovascular, and endocrine systems, among others. Indirect markers commonly used for detection of anabolic steroid in athletes and for control of their abuse, include signs of hypertension, aggressive behavior, skin changes, and gynecomastia [74, 75].

In summary, sex disturbances are very common in athletes, and the most common is hyperandrogenism. This is due to the increased prevalence of PCOS and the high intake of AAS. Female athletes with hyperandrogenism have a competitive advantage over athletic females with normal androgen level. With increased androgen levels, there is improvement in physical strength and exercise endurance/tolerance. The enhanced muscular performance comes at a cost. Female athletes with hyperandrogenism often suffer from amenorrhea, menstrual irregularities, and other symptoms and signs of excess androgen. The associated hormonal fluctuations also can lead to alterations in respiratory drive that varies with the type of exercise, intensity, duration, and fitness level of the athlete but which could affect athletic performance adversely.

10.3   The Impact of Hormone Disturbances on Voice in Athletes

Sex hormones have major effects on laryngeal structures. These effects are mediated via hormone receptors in soft and cartilaginous structures of the larynx [76–79]. Estrogen, progesterone, and androgen receptors have been demonstrated in various laryngeal tissues, particularly in the cytoplasm and nuclei of the vocal folds [76, 77]. These receptors help explain the differential growth of laryngeal structures at puberty and the role of hormone therapy in patients with laryngeal cancer [78, 79]. Estrogen induces hypertrophic effects on the vocal fold's mucosal lining with marked proliferation of laryngeal glandular secretions. The estrogen-induced increase in submucosal capillary permeability, and the increased polymerization of the lamina propria ground substance, leads to thickening of the vocal folds. Progesterone, however, induces a decrease in glandular secretions with subsequent desquamation and dryness of the mucosal lining [79]. Testosterone enhances the growth of laryngeal muscles and cartilages with widening of the thyroid cartilage angle and development of a thyroid cartilage prominence (Adam's apple) (Fig. 10.1). Subsequently, there is hypertrophy of the thyroarytenoid muscle in all of its dimensions leading to increase in its bulk and lengthening of the vocal folds.

Fig. 10.1 A 30-year-old woman with history of deepening of her voice following the use of androgenic anabolic steroids. Note the prominence of Adam's apple on lateral view

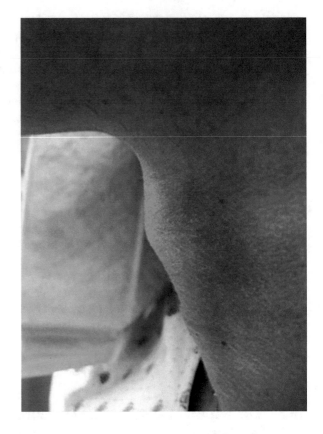

The above facts help explain the hormone-induced voice dimorphism that occurs at puberty. The differential growth of the thyroarytenoid muscles and the descent of the larynx lead to lowering of the fundamental frequency and vocal tract resonance frequencies [80]. As a result, there is deepening of the voice by about one octave in men and one-third octave in women. Vuorenkoski et al. reported a drop in the speaking fundamental frequency in boys from 247–250 Hz at the ages of 8–10 years to 90–100 Hz at puberty. There was also a drop in the speaking fundamental frequency in girls from 253 Hz at the ages of 8–10 years to 180–213 Hz at puberty [81]. Harries et al. performed a longitudinal study on voice characteristics of 26 boys and showed a correlation between the Tanner staging of puberty (Stage 1, no hair; Stage 2, downy hair; Stage 3, scant terminal hair; Stage 4, terminal hair filling the pubic triangle; Stage 5, terminal hair extending beyond the thigh crease [82]) and the Cooksey classification of voice [83]. Cooksey classification is a six-stage classification of the pubertal voice that is based on the singing voice (C staging) and tessitura. It includes the unchanged voice, Midvoice I, Midvoice II, Midvoice IIA (at the climax of the change), the new voice, and emerging adult. Similarly, Pederson et al. reported a significant negative correlation between testosterone level and fundamental frequency ($r = -0.73$) and serum binding globulin ($r = 0.75$). The authors also reported a significant correlation between the fundamental frequency and secondary sex characteristics (pubic hair and testes volume). The study was conducted using 2000 consecutive electrographic cycles [84]. As expected from the information above, a decrease in testosterone secretion (at puberty) results in failure of voice to mature. This is best exemplified by the "castrati" who exhibit a high-pitch voice and small laryngeal structures [85]. In a study by Akcam et al., patients with isolated hypogonadotropic hypogonadism classified as stage I and II (Tanner classification) had significantly higher mean fundamental frequency in comparison to normal males (229.33 Hz vs. 150.40 Hz, respectively). Androgen therapy has been shown to change the fundamental frequency to near normal. This is important to note especially in singers whose voice range and stability are crucial while performing [86]. However, it is important also in athletes and coach instructors who have great vocal demands and whose voice quality is important in projecting credibility. For example, fair or not, a male soprano (due to hypogonadism) is going to have a hard time securing a job as a professional football coach.

In this section the authors review the impact of hyperandrogenism on voice. Given the scarcity of studies on voice changes in athletes with hyperandrogenism, most of the review is on nonathletes with extrapolation to athletes. The information below can be used as material for future research on phonatory changes in athletes with exogenous or endogenous hyperandrogenism.

10.3.1   Effect of PCOS on Voice

The current literature lacks any study on voice changes in athletes with PCOS in comparison to athletes without PCOS. However, there is abundant information on voice changes in patients with PCOS, which can be used reasonably to understand voice changes in female athletes with PCOS. In a study by Hannoun et al. on the prevalence of voice symptoms in patients diagnosed with PCOS, the authors reported loss of voice and deepening of voice in 47.6% and 35.3% of cases, respectively. There was also a significantly higher prevalence of throat clearing and lump sensation in the study group compared to controls. On laryngeal examination, 3 patients out of 17 had vocal fold edema [87]. In a study by Gugatschka et al., the authors reported a nonsignificantly lower fundamental frequency in 24 women with PCOS in comparison to the control group [88]. Similarly, Aydin et al. studied the voice characteristics of 30 patients with PCOS and reported vocal fold structural change and abnormal muscle tension in 56.7% and 36.6% of cases, respectively. However, there was no significant difference in any of the acoustic parameters between the study group and the control group nor in the prevalence of voice complaints between the two groups [89].

In summary, women with PCOS are more likely to have voice symptoms such as deepening in voice and throat clearing in comparison to women without PCOS. These are attributed to structural and functional laryngeal changes. Female athletes with PCOS are also prone to these phonatory symptoms. Given the high prevalence of

PCOS in female athletes in comparison to the normal population, voice care providers should be alerted to the high risk of dysphonia in affected patients. Female athletes complaining of deepening in voice should be investigated for PCOS.

## 10.3.2	Effect of OCP Use on Voice

The effect of OCP use on the female voice is controversial [68, 90–96]. The lack of consensus can be attributed to the disparity in the type of OCP used, to the differences in patient selection, and to differences in the voice outcome measures used. In 2009, Lã et al. conducted a study on the effect of modern (as of 2009) OCP on voice using electrographic measures and reported no effect in 20 professional voice users [90]. The authors advocated the safety of these medications. In another study, they also investigated the impact of oral contraceptives that contain drospirenone on voice in female classical singers and showed a decrease in vocal fold vibratory irregularity, i.e., OCP had a beneficial effect on voice [91]. Similarly, Van Lierde et al. reported no significant difference in any of the measured acoustic parameters in women on OCP vs. controls. The study was conducted on 24 professional voice users who were assessed during the first 3 days of menses and between the 10th and 17th day of pill intake [92]. However, Meurer et al., in their cross-sectional study on the phono-articulatory changes associated with the intake of low-dose OCP, reported better voice acuity in those not on OCP compared to those on OCP. The sustained vowels were recorded in the mid-follicular and mid-luteal phases of the menstrual cycle [93]. Similarly, the same authors 2 years later reported an adverse effect of OCP on voice range. The study was conducted on 72 women (48 of whom were on OCP who were asked to read a sentence in 6 different variations [94]. In a study by Gorham-Rowan and Fowler, the authors showed an increase in peak alternating flow rates and higher F0 in women on OCP vs. those not on OCP. The study was conducted on 16 subjects, and the aerodynamic measures were taken while the vowel /α/ was sustained three times at day 7 and day 14 of the menstrual cycle [95]. Notably, after removal of the outliers in the OCP group, there were no significant differences between those on triphasic OCP and those not on OCP. In 2016, Rodney and Sataloff reviewed the literature on OCP and voice comprehensively [96]. They concluded that unlike early generation OCP which produced adverse voice changes in about 5% of women, modern OCPs do not appear to impact voice adversely and actually may improve it.

In summary, there is confusion in the literature on the effect of OCP use on voice. The lack of consensus is ascribed to differences in patients' selections, generation of OCP studied, and study design. However, recent evidence suggests that the latest-generation OCP usually does not cause dysphonia. Although there are no studies on voice characteristics of athletes using OCP, female athletes complaining of dysphonia should be investigated thoroughly for potential drug-induced adverse effect. Diligent history taking and examination for symptoms and signs of hyperandrogenism in athletes on OCP are warranted. It is also important to read the label of the

OCP. There are OCPs available outside the United States that use androgens instead of progestins. These are not latest-generation OCPs and can cause undesirable voice effects, as can early generation OCPs which also are still available in some countries.

10.3.3   Effect of Anabolic Steroids Intake on Voice

Change in voice quality described as deepening of voice or lowering in pitch is reported commonly as a side effect of anabolic steroid use. Most of the current literature on anabolic steroid-induced dysphonia is derived from studies on treatment of medical conditions such as endometriosis and menopausal syndrome. In a review of 100 patients diagnosed with endometriosis and treated with danazol (West-Coast Pharmaceutical Works LTD, US) 800 mg per day for a mean period of 17.3 weeks, Barbieri et al. reported deepening of voice in 8 patients. Other reported androgenic side effects included weight gain, decrease in breast size, hirsutism, and acne [62]. In a preliminary report by Nordenskjold and Fex on the effect of danazol therapy on voice in 23 women diagnosed with endometriosis, the authors reported change in the mean frequency at 6 months (212 Hz before treatment vs. 202 Hz after treatment) although no significant subjective voice changes were noted except in 1 patient [97]. Wollina et al. reported five cases of adverse effect of topical AAS, among whom was a 44-year-old woman who developed deepening of her voice 6 months following initiation of 2.5% androstanolone gel for the treatment of inner thigh cellulite [98]. Although the laryngeal stroboscopic examination was normal, the voice was described as rough, with a mean speaking frequency of 170 Hz. The patient was treated with voice therapy which led to improvement in her voice quality and to an increase in the mean speaking level by 15 Hz. One of the five reported cases was a bodybuilder who developed acne and striae distensae as side effects of AAS, but there was no mention of change in voice quality. Wardle and Whitehead reported a 27-year-old woman who developed voice changes 7 months following treatment of endometriosis with danazol. The voice became husky, squeaky, and weak with loss of pitch control. The laryngeal examination was not diagnostic. One and half year later, after discontinuing the medication, the voice had not improved [99]. Similarly, in 1990, Boothroyd and Lepre reported a 20-year-old woman diagnosed with endometriosis who suffered permanent deepening of her voice after 3–4 months of treatment with danazol 800 mg per day. Despite cessation of therapy, the change in voice quality was irreversible [61].

Dysphonia also has been reported as an adverse effect of testosterone replacement in menopausal women. In a prospective study by Gerritsma et al. on postmenopausal women with osteoporosis on cyclical hormone therapy, the authors reported significant voice changes in the study group ($n = 22$) in comparison to the control group ($n = 17$). The number of patients with voice complaints increased after 1 year of therapy from 18% to 64%. Loss of high frequencies and lowering of habitual fundamental frequency also increased from 24% to 86% and from 14% to 62%, respectively. There was also a drop in the mean frequency during speech from

213 Hz to 195 Hz and a drop in the highest frequency from 613 Hz to 505 Hz [57]. Similarly, in a study by Huang et al. on the effect of testosterone administration on voice in 46 women status post-hysterectomy with or without oophorectomy, the authors found a significant decrease in average pitch in those receiving 12.5 and 25 mg doses. However, there were no dose-dependent changes in voice using self-reported VHI [100]. The intake of anabolic steroids also has been shown to have adverse effect on voice in female athletes. In a study by Strauss et al. on ten athletic women using anabolic steroids, the authors reported that most subjects noted deepening of the voice in addition to other virilizing signs such as increase in facial hair and hypertrophy of the clitoris [101].

In summary, dysphonia is a common side effect of anabolic steroid use in women. It is often dose dependent and described as deepening of the voice and decrease in pitch. Although most of the studies in the literature are on nonathletes, the same side effects reported in nonathletes may occur in athletes. A change in voice quality in a female athlete taking anabolic steroids should alert the physician to possible laryngeal structural changes. Prompt cessation of these supplements is key in avoiding further irreversible voice changes, especially permanent deepening of the voice. This adverse effect of anabolic steroids is well recognized and has long been used therapeutically to change permanently the voices of female-to-male transgender patients. Once the voice mutation has occurred, it cannot be reversed.

The adverse effect of anabolic steroid on the vocal folds is not limited to women. Men with hypogonadism also may suffer from phonatory adverse events following the intake of anabolic steroids. King et al. reported a 22-year-old tenor, diagnosed with hypogonadism, who, following testosterone replacement, developed marked changes in his voice, described as voice breaks and instability. On acoustic analysis, there was a drop in his F0 from 277.9 Hz to 120.6 Hz, with an increase in cycle-to-cycle variation in pitch and cycle-to-cycle variation in intensity [86]. In 2004, Tinur Ackam et al. investigated voice changes following androgen therapy in 24 patients with isolated hypogonadotropic hypogonadism and reported a drop in the mean fundamental frequency from 229 ± 41 Hz to 173 Hz ± 30 Hz. The decrease in pitch was commensurate with the increase in serum testosterone levels, although these did not reach normal levels [86]. In another study, Ray et al. reported a 47-year old man with history of smoking and regular intake of anabolic steroids, who presented with severe hoarseness associated with dyspnea and shortness of breath. On laryngeal examination, he had severe swelling of the supraglottic and glottic structures resulting in significant narrowing of the airway. Computerized tomography of the neck showed laryngeal muscular hypertrophy with obliteration of the paraglottic space. The patient underwent tracheotomy followed by laryngeal biopsies which confirmed the presence of parakeratosis and epithelial hyperplasia. The laryngeal edematous changes were not commensurate with the commonly observed laryngeal findings in chronic smokers and were believed to be related to steroid use [102].

In summary, voice changes are rare side effects of anabolic steroids in men. Although most of the common literature is on nonathlete men with hypogonadism, the same phonatory side effects may be observed in male athletes who suffer from hypogonadism and in men who use anabolic steroids to enhance athletic performance or body appearance. Affected patients may complain of a constellation of vocal symptoms that include deepening of voice, voice breaks, and voice instability.

10.4 Pathogenesis of Dysphonia in Athletes with Hyperandrogenism

The pathogenesis of voice hyperandrogenism in adults remains a topic of investigation. Several theories have been suggested. These include structural changes in the vocal folds, increase in muscle tissue vs. connective tissue ratio, muscle incoordination, and proprioceptive dysfunction with impairment in muscle memory [56, 57]. This latter is particularly noticeable in singers on virilizing hormone therapy who experience difficulties in placing notes [56]. Among these hypothesizes, laryngeal structural change with an increase in muscle mass is the most popular. Several authors have investigated laryngeal muscle changes following testosterone injections and shown marked histologic changes. Tobias et al. studied the sexually dimorphic effect of androgen on laryngeal muscle fibers of *Xenopus laevis* and demonstrated that androgen injection (dihydrotestosterone) resulted in muscle fiber hypertrophy and conversion of muscle fibers from mixed slow to fast. The effect was not dependent on the state of innervation of these muscles. Androgen injection has helped also reduce laryngeal muscle fiber loss in males and has helped increase muscle fiber number in females [103]. Sassoon et al., in their study on sexual dimorphism of laryngeal structures, stressed the chondrogenic and myogenic effects of testosterone. The study was conducted on clawed frogs, and cell proliferation was measured using electron microscopy/autoradiography [104]. Similarly, Talaat et al. studied the histologic and histochemical effects of anabolic steroids on the female larynx of albino mice and reported thyroarytenoid muscle hypertrophy in addition to epithelial changes. These included hyperplasia and parakeratosis, with vascular congestion and predominance of mucin [105]. In another study, Beckford et al. investigated the effect of androgen stimulation in a sheep model and showed androgen-induced changes in most laryngeal dimensions. There was dose-dependent growth in the laryngeal anteroposterior diameter, thyroid cartilage width, and superior thyroid horn heights, in addition to changes in the thyroid-cartilage angle [106]. Griggs et al. investigated the effect of testosterone injection in nine human subjects and showed an increase in muscle mass and muscle protein synthesis by a mean of 20% and 27%, respectively. Notably, there was no significant increase in whole-body protein synthesis and no increase in muscle fiber diameter. The muscle mass was estimated by measuring creatinine exertion, and nonoxidative flux was used to estimate whole-body protein synthesis [107]. Similarly, Bhasin et al. reported an increase in muscle size (arms, triceps, legs) in men who received testosterone (600 mg weekly for 10 weeks) and had no exercise in comparison to those who did not receive testosterone and had no exercise. Among those who were assigned to exercise, the intake of testosterone also resulted in an increase in muscle size and fat-free mass in comparison to those who did not exercise. Moreover, the intake of supraphysiologic testosterone doses increased muscle strength in all subgroups treated [108].

In summary, voice changes in patients with hyperandrogenism are due mostly to vocal fold structural changes. There is increase in muscle mass and alteration in muscle fiber composition. These histologic changes can explain the decrease in voice pitch observed in patients with high androgen levels.

10.5   Treatment of Androgenic Voice in Female Athletes

Dysphonia is defined as an adverse change in voice quality, pitch or loudness, or as an increase in phonatory effort that impairs communication [109]. Female athletes with a decrease in voice pitch may suffer incongruence between their gender identification and voice quality. Their voice pitch becomes a misleading acoustic cue to who they are, thus often affecting their performance and quality of life. In a recent study by Steward et al. entitled "My Voice Is My Identity: The Role of Voice for Transwomen's Participation in Sport," the authors highlighted the importance of voice and psychosocial moderators of voice in a sports environment. Being identified as a woman was crucial for participation in a sport setting [110]. Similar to transgender patients, female athletes with an androgenic voice initially are offered behavioral therapy to help raise the voice pitch. In a review on the management of the transgender voice, which is analogous in some ways to the androgen-altered voice, McNeill advocated the importance of voice therapy in improving communication behavior [111]. Similarly, in a systematic review of transgender voice feminization that included 212 studies, Nolan et al. reported satisfactory results following voice therapy in the majority of patients. The authors also reiterated the role of voice therapy as an adjunct treatment after pitch alteration surgery [112]. While similar techniques may be used for female athletes with voice masculinization caused by steroids, there are substantial differences in the treatments need for such athletes who are biological females compared with transgender women. So transgender literature must be translated to the athlete female with caution.

In patients who fail voice therapy or who are still unsatisfied with their voice quality, pitch alteration surgery is an option. Pitch alteration surgery focuses on one or more of the known physiologic determinants of pitch, namely, length, tension, and mass. The surgeries performed are cricothyroid approximation or fusion, glottoplasty, and reduction glottoplasty. Other less common surgeries are scarring of the vocal folds to induce stiffening, advancement of the anterior commissure with or without placement of a splint as reported by Guice et al. in 1983 [113] and by Tucker in 1985 [114], and feminization laryngoplasty as described by Thomas and Macmillan [115]. The authors studied the impact of feminization laryngoplasty in a group of 76 patients and reported an increase in the average comfortable speaking pitch, lowest attainable pitch, and highest attainable pitch by 6, 7, and 2 semitones, respectively. Notably, there was no increase in the upper limit of the voice range.

Cricothyroid approximation and glottoplasty remain the most commonly performed pitch-raising procedures. In a systematic review and meta-analysis of transgender phonosurgery that included 13 studies, Song and Jiang reported that shortening of the vocal fold achieved the greatest increase in pitch. The most common surgical techniques used in that review were cricothyroid approximation and glottoplasty [116]. Cricothyroid approximation aims to increase vocal fold tension. Kitajami and colleagues reported a nonlinear relationship between cricothyroid approximation and voice and noted that a 1 mm approximation results in 0.15–0.19 increase in semitones. The study was conducted on excised human larynges to which force was applied to shorten the cricothyroid distance [117]. Yang et al. reported an increase in the fundamental frequency by half an octave and an increase of the lower and upper frequencies of the voice range by 4 semitones following cricothyroid approximation. The study was done on 20 patients who were followed up for 22 months, and the majority of whom were satisfied [118]. Cricothyroid approximation has been criticized for its tendency to fail over time. This problem was eliminated by Sataloff who introduced cricothyroid fusion which is reviewed elsewhere along with therapy and surgery techniques for transgender patients [119], some of which may be applicable to selected athletes. Neumann and Welzel et al. advocated the use of miniplates in cricothyroid approximation. Their study included 67 female patients who were assessed before surgery, after surgery, and 1 year later using laryngoscopy and computer-assisted tomography. The authors reported an increase in the fundamental frequency by one-fourth, and almost one-third of the participants had a feminine voice postoperatively [120]. Glottoplasty is another pitch-raising procedure that is based on denuding the anterior one-third or half the vocal fold (removing its epithelial lining) and then suturing the musculomembranous vocal folds together. The surgery can be performed either endoscopically or through an open approach, but usually it is performed endoscopically. Anderson conducted a study on the outcome of endoscopic web formation assisted with injection augmentation in ten male-to-female transgender individuals and showed an increase in the mean fundamental frequency by 110 Hz postoperatively with no alteration in any of the perturbation parameters or voice range [121]. Donald et al. performed the procedure thru a laryngofissure in three transgender patients who sought a more female voice quality [122]. Similarly, Kunachak et al. reduced the size of the vocal folds by removing part of the thyroid lamina anteriorly, thus creating a new anterior commissure. The surgery performed on six male-to-female transgender patients resulted in an increase in pitch from 147 Hz to 315 Hz [123]. Reduction glottoplasty is also an alternative pitch-raising procedure, whereby part of the thyroarytenoid muscle is removed. With an inverse relationship between mass and pitch, partial resection of the thyroarytenoid muscle results in an increase in voice pitch. The reduction in muscle mass can be performed either endoscopically using could steel instruments or laser or thru an open approach [124, 125]. Alternatively, the thyroarytenoid muscle may be injected with steroids which induce atrophic changes with time (Fig. 10.2).

Fig. 10.2 An endoscopic view of a 30-year-old woman with drug-induced androphonia, which shows percutaneous injection of corticosteroids into the left vocal fold. The patient underwent serial bilateral corticosteroid injection into the thyroarytenoid muscles that resulted in an increase in voice pitch

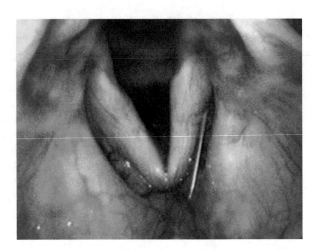

In summary, speech-language pathologists, voice therapists, phoniatrists, and otolaryngologists play important collaborative roles in the management of female athletes with deepening of their voices. When the results of voice and behavioral therapy are not satisfactory, patients may be offered pitch-raising surgery. Although all the above reports are on transgender patients, the same surgical principles and results may be applied to female athletes with androphonia. Nevertheless, it is important to note that not all otolaryngologists are well trained in gender-reassignment surgery. In a cross-sectional survey in the United States that included 22 programs, less than one-third of otolaryngologists had been exposed to transgender patient care and education, only half of whom had been exposed to pitch alteration surgery [124, 126]. The importance of a multidisciplinary approach in the management of these patients cannot be overemphasized, and care by an expert voice team is especially important for female athletes with androphonia for whom subtle and sophisticated judgments must be made to select treatments that address voice concerns without compromising the airway (as happens with planned webbing) to a degree that might affect elite athletic performance.

References

1. Sataloff RT. Endocrine function. In: Sataloff RT. Professional voice. The science and art of clinical care. 4th ed. San Diego: Plural Publishing; 2017. p. 655–69.
2. West JB. Best and Taylor's physiological basis of medical practice, 12th edition. Baltimore: Williams & Wilkins;1991.
3. Hirschberg AL. Female hyperandrogenism and elite sport. Endocr Connect. 2020;9(4):R81–92.
4. Davis SR, Wahlin-Jacobsen S. Testosterone in women—the clinical significance. Lancet Diabetes Endocrinol. 2015;3(12):980–92.
5. Handelsman DJ, Hirschberg AL, Bermon S. Circulating testosterone as the hormonal basis of sex differences in athletic performance. Endocr Rev. 2018;39(5):803–29.

6. Mooradian AD, Morley JE, Korenman SG. Biological actions of androgens. Endocr Rev. 1987;8(1):1–28.
7. Notelovitz M. Androgen effects on bone and muscle. Fertil Steril. 2002;77:34–41.
8. Herbst KL, Bhasin S. Testosterone action on skeletal muscle. Curr Opin Clin Nutr Metab Care. 2004;7(3):271–7.
9. Mänttäri S, Anttila K, Järvilehto M. Testosterone stimulates myoglobin expression in different muscles of the mouse. J Comp Physiol B. 2008;178(7):899–907.
10. Almeida M, Laurent MR, Dubois V, et al. Estrogens and androgens in skeletal physiology and pathophysiology. Physiol Rev. 2017;97(1):135–87.
11. Bermon S. Androgens and athletic performance of elite female athletes. Curr Opin Endocrinol Diabetes Obes. 2017;24(3):246–51.
12. Bermon S, Garnier PY. Serum androgen levels and their relation to performance in track and field: mass spectrometry results from 2127 observations in male and female elite athletes. Br J Sports Med. 2017;51(17):1309–14.
13. Cook CJ, Crewther BT, Smith AA. Comparison of baseline free testosterone and cortisol concentrations between elite and non-elite female athletes. Am J Hum Biol. 2012;24(6):856–8.
14. Bermon S, Garnier PY, Hirschberg AL, et al. Serum androgen levels in elite female athletes. J Clin Endocrinol Metab. 2014;99(11):4328–35.
15. Loucks AB, Mortola JF, Girton L, Yen SS. Alterations in the hypothalamic-pituitary-ovarian and the hypothalamic-pituitary-adrenal axes in athletic women. J Clin Endocrinol Metab. 1989;68(2):402–11.
16. Laughlin GA, Yen SS. Nutritional and endocrine-metabolic aberrations in amenorrheic athletes. J Clin Endocrinol Metab. 1996;81(12):4301–9.
17. Orio F, Muscogiuri G, Ascione A, et al. Effects of physical exercise on the female reproductive system. Minerva Endocrinol. 2013;38(3):305–19.
18. Hirschberg AL. Sport and menses. In: Huhtaniemi L, Martini I, editors. Encyclopedia of endocrine diseases, vol. 2. 2nd ed. Oxford, UK: Academic Press; 2019. p. 461–70.
19. Loucks AB, Verdun M, Heath EM. Low energy availability, not stress of exercise, alters LH pulsatility in exercising women. J Appl Physiol. 1998;84:37–46.
20. Hagmar M, Hirschberg AL, Berglund L, Berglund B. Special attention to the weight control strategies employed by Olympic athletes striving for leanness is required. Clin J Sport Med. 2008;18:5–9.
21. Sheid JL, De Souza MJ. Menstrual irregularities and energy deficiency in physically active women: the role of ghrelin, PYY and adipocytokines. Med Sport Sci. 2010;55:82–102.
22. Mircea CN, Lujan ME, Pierson RA. Metabolic fuel and clinical implications for female reproduction. J Obstet Gynaecol Can. 2007;29:887–902.
23. Loucks AB, Thuma JR. Luteinizing hormone pulsatility is disrupted at a threshold of energy availability in regularly menstruating women. J Clin Endocrinol Metab. 2003;88:297–311.
24. Javed A, Kashyap R, An L. Hyperandrogenism in female athletes with functional hypothalamic amenorrhea: a distinct phenotype. Int J Womens Health. 2015;7:103.
25. Reed JL, De Souza MJ, Mallison RJ, et al. Energy availability discriminates clinical menstrual status in exercising women. J Int Soc Sports Nutr. 2015;12:11.
26. Rotterdam ESHRE/ASRM-Sponsored PCOS Consensus Workshop Group. Revised 2003 consensus on diagnostic criteria and long-term health risks related to polycystic ovary syndrome. Fertil Steril. 2004;81:19–25.
27. Dokras A, Witchel SF. Are young adult women with polycystic ovary syndrome slipping through the healthcare cracks? J Clin Endocrinol Metab. 2014;99(5):1583–5.
28. Azziz R, Sanchez LA, Knochenhauer ES, et al. Androgen excess in women: experience with over 1000 consecutive patients. J Clin Endocrinol Metab. 2004;89(2):453–62.
29. Lowe P, Kovacs G, Howlett D. Incidence of polycystic ovaries and polycystic ovary syndrome amongst women in Melbourne, Australia. Aust N Z J Obstet Gynaecol. 2005;45:17–9.
30. Hagmar M, Berglund B, Brismar K, Hirschberg A. Hyperandrogenism may explain reproductive dysfunction in olympic athletes. Med Sci Sports Exerc. 2009;41(6):1241–8.

31. Coste O, Paris F, Galtier F, Letois F, Maïmoun L, Sultan C. Polycystic ovary-like syndrome in adolescent competitive swimmers. Fertil Steril. 2011;96:1037–42.
32. Burger HG. Androgen production in women. Fertil Steril. 2002;77:3–5.
33. Guzelce EC, Eyupoglu D, Torgutalp S, et al. Is muscle mechanical function altered in polycystic ovary syndrome? Arch Gynecol Obstet. 2019;300(3):771–6.
34. Lee PA, Nordenström A, Houk CP, et al. Global disorders of sex development update since 2006: perceptions, approach and care. Horm Res Paediatr. 2016;85(3):158–80.
35. Linden-Hirschberg A. The role of androgens for body composition and physical performance in women. In: Berga S, Genazzani A, Naftolin F, Petraglia F, editors. Menstrual cycle related disorders. ISGE series. Cham: Springer; 2019. https://doi.org/10.1007/987-3-030-14358-9_4.
36. Vingren JL, Kraemer WJ, Ratamess NA, Anderson JM, Volek JS, Maresh CM. Testosterone physiology in resistance exercise and training. Sports Med. 2010;40(12):1037–53.
37. Croson R, Gneezy U. Gender differences in preferences. J Econ Litererat. 2009;47(2):448–74.
38. Greer JB, Modugno F, Allen GO, Ness RB. Androgenic progestins in oral contraceptives and the risk of epithelial ovarian cancer. Obstet Gynecol. 2005;105:731–40.
39. Fotherby K. Bioavailability of orally administered sex steroids used in oral contraception and hormone replacement therapy. Contraception. 1996;54:59–69.
40. Brynhildsen J, Lennartsson H, Klemetz M, Dahlquist P, Hedin B, Hammar M. Oral contraceptive use among female elite athletes and age-matched controls and its relation to low back pain. Acta Obstet Gynecol Scand. 1997;76(9):873–8.
41. Martin D, Sale C, Cooper SB, Eliott-Sale KJ. Period prevalence and perceived side effects of hormonal contraceptive use and the menstrual cycle in elite athletes. Int J Sports Physiol Perform. 2018;13(7):926–32.
42. Rechichi C, Dawson B, Goodman C. Athletic performance and the oral contraceptive. Int J Sports Physiol Perform. 2009;4(2):151–62.
43. Bonen A, Haynes FW, Graham TE. Substrate and hormonal responses to exercise in women using oral contraceptives. J Appl Physiol. 1991;70(5):1917–27.
44. Bemben DA, Boileau RA, Bahr JM, Nelson RA, Misner JE. Effects of oral contraceptives on hormonal and metabolic responses during exercise. Med Sci Sports Exerc. 1992;24(4):434–41.
45. Casazza GA, Jacobs KA, Suh SH, Miller BF, Horning MA, Brooks GA. Menstrual cycle phase and oral contraceptive effects on triglyceride mobilization during exercise. J Appl Physiol. 2004;97:302–9.
46. McNeill AW, Mozingo E. Changes in the metabolic cost of standardized work associated with the use of an oral contraceptive. J Sports Med Phys Fitness. 1981;21(3):238–44.
47. Spellacy WN. Carbohydrate metabolism during treatment with estrogen, progestogen, and low-dose oral contraceptives. Am J Obstet Gynecol. 1982;142(6):732–4.
48. Suh SH, Casazza GA, Horning MA, Miller BF, Brooks GA. Effects of oral contraceptives on glucose flux and substrate oxidation rates during rest and exercise. J Appl Physiol. 2003;94(1):285–94.
49. Casazza GA, Suh SH, Miller BF, Navazio FM, Brooks GA. Effects of oral contraceptives on peak exercise capacity. J Appl Physiol. 2002;93(5):1698–702.
50. Notelovitz M, Zauner C, McKenzie L, Suggs Y, Fields C, Kitchens C. The effect of low-dose oral contraceptives on cardiorespiratory function, coagulation, and lipids in exercising young women: a preliminary report. Am J Obstet Gynecol. 1987;156(3):591–8.
51. Lebrun CM, Petit MA, McKenzie DC, Taunton JE, Prior JC. Decreased maximal aerobic capacity with use of a triphasic oral contraceptive in highly active women: a randomised controlled trial. Br J Sports Med. 2003;37(4):315–20.
52. Giacomoni M, Falgairette G. Decreased submaximal oxygen uptake during short duration oral contraceptive use: a randomized cross-over trial in premenopausal women. Ergonomics. 2000;43(10):1559–70.
53. England SE, Fahri LE. Fluctuations in alveolar CO_2 and in base excess during the menstrual cycle. Respir Physiol. 1976;26:157–61.
54. Reilly T, Whitley H. Effects of menstrual cycle phase and oral contraceptive use on endurance exercise. J Sports Sci. 1994;2:150.

55. Bryner RW, Toffle RC, Ullrich IH, Yeater RA. Effect of low dose oral contraceptives on exercise performance. Br J Sports Med. 1996;30:36–40.
56. Baker J. A report on alterations to the speaking and singing voices of four women following hormonal therapy with virilizing agents. J Voice. 1999;13:496–507.
57. Gerritsma EJ, Brocaar MP, Hakkesteegt MM, Birkenhager JC. Virilization of the voice in postmenopausal women due to the anabolic steroid nandrolone decanoate (Deca-Durabolin). The effects of medication for one year. Clin Otolaryngol. 1994;19:79–84.
58. Spooner JB. Classification of side effects to danazol therapy. J Int Med Res. 1997;5:15–7.
59. Hardt W. Clinically relevant side effects of danazol. Orynakol Prax. 1987;11:457–70.
60. Dmowski WP. Endocrine properties and clinical application of danazol. Fertil Steril. 1979;31(3):237.
61. Boothroyd CV, Lepre F. Permanent voice change resulting from danazol therapy. Aus N Z J Obstet Gynaecol. 1990;30:275–6.
62. Barbieri RL, Evans S, Kistner RW. Danazol in the treatment of endometriosis: analysis of 100 cases with a 4-year follow-up. Fertil Steril. 1982;37:737–46.
63. Achilli C, Pundir J, Ramanathan P, Sabatini L, Hamoda H, Panay N. Efficacy and safety of transdermal testosterone in postmenopausal women with hypoactive sexual desire disorder: a systematic review and meta-analysis. Fertil Steril. 2017;107(2):475–82.
64. Cappola AR, Ratcliffe SJ, Bhasin S, et al. Determinants of serum total and free testosterone levels in women over the age of 65 years. J Clin Endocrinol Metab. 2007;92(2):509–16.
65. Laughlin GA, Barrett-Connor E, Kritz-Silverstein D, von Mühlen D. Hysterectomy, oophorectomy, and endogenous sex hormone levels in older women: the Rancho Bernardo Study. J Clin Endocrinol Metab. 2000;85(2):645–51.
66. Tajar A, Huhtaniemi IT, O'Neill TW, et al. Characteristics of androgen deficiency in late-onset hypogonadism: results from the European Male Aging Study (EMAS). J Clin Endocrinol Metab. 2012;97(5):1508–16.
67. Araujo AB, Esche GR, Kupelian V, et al. Prevalence of symptomatic androgen deficiency in men. J Clin Endocrinol Metab. 2007;92(11):4241–7.
68. Hamdan AL, Sataloff RT, Hawkshaw MJ. Laryngeal manifestations of endocrine disorders. In: Hamdan AL, Sataloff RT, Hawkshaw MJ. Laryngeal manifestations of systemic diseases. San Diego: Plural Publishing; 2018. p. 313–40.
69. Albertson TE, Chenoweth JA, Colby DK, Sutter ME. The changing drug culture: use and misuse of appearance- and performance-enhancing drugs. FP Essent. 2016;441:30–43.
70. Barceloux DG, Palmer RB. Anabolic-androgenic steroids. Dis Mon. 2013;59:226–48.
71. Pope HG Jr, Kanayama G, Athey A, Ryan E, Hudson JI, Baggish A. The lifetime prevalence of anabolic-androgenic steroid use and dependence in Americans: current best estimates. Am J Addict. 2014;23(4):371–7.
72. Monaghan L. Creating "The perfect body": a variable project. Body Soc. 1999;5:267–90.
73. Hartgens F, Kuipers H. Effects of androgenic-anabolic steroids in athletes. Sports Med. 2004;34(8):513–54.
74. Christou GA, Chtristou MA, Ziberna L, Christou KA. Indirect clinical markers for the direction of anabolic steroid abuse beyond the conventional doping control in athletes. Eur J Sport Sci. 2019;19(9):1276–86.
75. Kersey RD, Elliot DL, Goldberg L, et al. National Athletic Trainers' association. National Athletic Trainers' association position statement: anabolic-androgenic steroids. J Athl Train. 2012;47:567–88.
76. Newman SR, Butler J, Hammond EH, et al. Preliminary report on hormone receptors in the human vocal fold. J Voice. 2000;14:72–81.
77. Voelter C, Kleinsasser N, Joa P, Nowack I, Martinez R, Hagen R, Voelker HU. Detection of hormone receptors in the human vocal fold. Eur Arch Otorhinolaryngol. 2008;265:1239–44.
78. Verma A, Schwartz N, Cohen DJ, Boyan BD, Schwartz Z. Estrogen signaling and estrogen receptors as prognostic indicators in laryngeal cancer. Steroids. 2019;152:108498.
79. Abitbol J, Abitbol P, Abitbol B. Sex hormones and the female voice. J Voice. 1999;13(3):424–46.

80. Shoffel-Havakuk H, Carmel-Neiderman NN, Halperin D, et al. Menstrual cycle, vocal performance, and laryngeal vascular appearance: an observational study on 17 subjects. J Voice. 2018;32(2):226–33.
81. Vuorenkoski V, Lenko HL, Tjernlund PE, Vuorenkoski L, Perheentupa J. Fundamental voice frequency during normal and abnormal growth, and after androgen treatment. Arch Dis Child. 1978;53(3):201–9.
82. Emmanuel M, Bokor BR. Tanner stages. In: StatPearls. Treasure Island: StatPearls Publishing; 2020. Available from: https://www.ncbi.nlm.nih.gov/books/NBK470280/. Updated 22 Aug 2020. Accessed 15 Nov 2020.
83. Harries ML, Walker JM, Williams DM, Hawkins S, Hughes IA. Changes in the male voice at puberty. Arch Dis Child. 1997;77(5):445–7.
84. Pedersen MF, Møller S, Krabbe S, Bennett P. Fundamental voice frequency measured by electroglottography during continuous speech. A new exact secondary sex characteristic in boys in puberty. Int J Pediatr Otorhinolaryngol. 1986;11(1):21–7.
85. Akcam T, Bolu E, Merati AL, Durmus C, Gerek M, Ozkaptan Y. Voice changes after androgen therapy for hypogonadotrophic hypogonadism. Laryngoscope. 2004;114(9):1587–91.
86. King A, Ashby J, Nelson C. Effects of testosterone replacement on a male professional singer. J Voice. 2001;15(4):553–7.
87. Hannoun A, Zreik T, Husseini ST, Mahfoud L, Sibai A, Hamdan AL. Vocal changes in patients with polycystic ovary syndrome. J Voice. 2011;25(4):501–4.
88. Gugatschka M, Lichtenwagner S, Schwetz V, et al. Subjective and objective vocal parameters in women with polycystic ovary syndrome. J Voice. 2013;27(1):98–100.
89. Aydin K, Akbulut S, Demir MG, et al. Voice characteristics associated with polycystic ovary syndrome. Laryngoscope. 2016;126(9):2067–72.
90. Lã FM, Howard DM, Ledger W, Davidson JW, Jones G. Oral contraceptive pill containing drospirenone and the professional voice: an electrolaryngographic analysis. Logoped Phoniatr Vocol. 2009;34(1):11–9.
91. Lã FM, Ledger WL, Davidson JW, Howard DM, Jones GL. The effects of a third generation combined oral contraceptive pill on the classical singing voice. J Voice. 2007;21(6):754–61.
92. Van Lierde KM, Claeys S, De Bodt M, Van Cauwenberge P. Response of the female vocal quality and resonance in professional voice users taking oral contraceptive pills: a multiparameter approach. Laryngoscope. 2006;116(10):1894–8.
93. Meurer EM, Fontoura GV, von Eye Corleta H, Capp E. Speech articulation of low-dose oral contraceptive users. J Voice. 2015;29(6):743–50.
94. Meurer EM, Moura AD, Rechenberg L, von Eye Corleta H, Capp E. Vocal range in the speech of users of low-dose oral contraceptives. J Voice. 2017;31(3):390–e17.
95. Gorham-Rowan M, Fowler L. Aerodynamic assessment of young women's voices as a function of oral contraceptive use. Folia Phoniatr Logop. 2008;60(1):20–4.
96. Rodney JP, Sataloff RT. The effects of hormonal contraception on the voice: history of its evolution in the literature. J Voice. 2016;30:726–30.
97. Nordenskjöld F, Fex S. Vocal effects of danazol therapy: a preliminary report. Acta Obstet Gynecol Scand Suppl. 1984;123:131–2.
98. Wollina U, Pabst F, Schönlebe J, Abdel-Naser MB, et al. Side-effects of topical androgenic and anabolic substances and steroids. A short review. Acta Dermatovenerol Alp Panonica Adriat. 2007;16(3):117–22.
99. Wardle PG, Whitehead MI, Mills RP. Non-reversible and wide ranging voice changes after treatment with danazol. Br Med J (Clin Res Ed). 1983;287(6397):946.
100. Huang G, Pencina KM, Coady JA, Beleva YM, Bhasin S, Basaria S. Functional voice testing detects early changes in vocal pitch in women during testosterone administration. J Clin Endocrinol Metab. 2015;100(6):2254–60.
101. Strauss RH, Liggett MT, Lanese RR. Anabolic steroid use and perceived effects in ten weight-trained women athletes. JAMA. 1985;253(19):2871–3.
102. Ray S, Masood A, Pickles J, Moumoulidis I. Severe laryngitis following chronic anabolic steroid abuse. J Laryngol Otol. 2008;122(3):230–2.

103. Tobias ML, Marin ML, Kelley DB. The roles of sex, innervation, and androgen in laryngeal muscle of Xenopus laevis. J Neurosci. 1993;13(1):324–33.
104. Sassoon D, Segil N, Kelley D. Androgen-induced myogenesis and chondrogenesis in the larynx of Xenopus laevis. Dev Biol. 1986;113(1):135–40.
105. Talaat M, Angelo A, Talaat AM, Elwany S, Kelada I, Thabet H. Histologic and histochemical study of effects of anabolic steroids on the female larynx. Ann Otol Rhinol Laryngol. 1987;96(4):468–71.
106. Beckford NS, Schaid D, Rood SR, Schanbacher B. Androgen stimulation and laryngeal development. Ann Otol Rhinol Laryngol. 1985;94(6):634–40.
107. Griggs RC, Kingston WI, Jozefowicz RF, Herr BE, Forbes GI, Halliday DA. Effect of testosterone on muscle mass and muscle protein synthesis. J Appl Physiol. 1989;66(1):498–503.
108. Bhasin S, Storer TW, Berman N, Callegari C, Clevenger B, Phillips J, Bunnell TJ, Tricker R, Shirazi A, Casaburi R. The effects of supraphysiologic doses of testosterone on muscle size and strength in normal men. N Engl J Med. 1996;335(1):1–7.
109. Stinnett S, Chmielewska M, Akst LM. Update on management of hoarseness. Med Clin North Am. 2018;102(6):1027–40.
110. Stewart L, Oates J, O'Halloran P. "My voice is my identity": the role of voice for trans women's participation in sport. J Voice. 2020;34(1):78–87.
111. McNeill EJ. Management of the transgender voice. J Laryngol Otol. 2006;120(7):521–3.
112. Nolan IT, Morrison SD, Arowojolu O, Crowe CS, Massie JP, Adler RK, Chaiet SR, Francis DO. The role of voice therapy and phonosurgery in transgender vocal feminization. J Craniofac Surg. 2019;30(5):1368–75.
113. Guice CE, LeJeune FE, Samuels PM. Early experiences with vocal ligament tightening. Ann Otol Rhinol Laryngol. 1983;92(5):475–7.
114. Tucker HM. Anterior commissure laryngoplasty for adjustment of vocal fold tension. Ann Otol Rhinol Laryngol. 1985;94(6):547–9.
115. Thomas JP, MacMillan C. Feminization laryngoplasty: assessment of surgical pitch elevation. Eur Arch Otorhinolaryngol. 2013;270(10):2695–700.
116. Song TE, Jiang N. Transgender phonosurgery: a systematic review and meta-analysis. Otolaryngol Head Neck Surg. 2017;156(5):803–8.
117. Kitajima K, Tanabe M, Isshiki N. Cricothyroid distance and vocal pitch: experimental surgical study to elevate the vocal pitch. Ann Otol Rhinol Laryngol. 1979;88(1):52–5.
118. Yang CY, Palmer AD, Meltzer TR, Murray KD, Cohen JI. Cricothyroid approximation to elevate vocal pitch in male-to-female transsexuals: results of surgery. Ann Otol Rhinol Laryngol. 2002;111(6):477–85.
119. Heuer RJ, Baroody MM, Sataloff RT. Management of gender reassignment patients. In: Sataloff RT. Professional voice: the science and art of clinical care. 4th ed. San Diego: Plural Publication; 2017. p. 1649–57.
120. Neumann K, Welzel C. The importance of the voice in male-to-female transsexualism. J Voice. 2004;18(1):153–67.
121. Anderson JA. Pitch elevation in trangendered patients: anterior glottic web formation assisted by temporary injection augmentation. J Voice. 2014;28(6):816–21.
122. Donald PJ. Voice change surgery in the transsexual. Head Neck Surg. 1982;4(5):433–7.
123. Kunachak S, Prakunhungsit S, Sujjalak K. Thyroid cartilage and vocal fold reduction: a new phonosurgical method for male-to-female transsexuals. Ann Otol Rhinol Laryngol. 2000;109(11):1082–6.
124. Spiegel JH. Phonosurgery for pitch alteration: feminization and masculinization of the voice. Otolaryngol Clin North Am. 2006;39(1):77–86.
125. Gross M. Pitch-raising surgery in male-to-female transsexuals. J Voice. 1999;13(2):246–50.
126. Massenburg BB, Morrison SD, Rashidi V, et al. Educational exposure to transgender patient care in otolaryngology training. J Craniofac Surg. 2018;29(5):1252–7.

Chapter 11
Voice Health Management in Sports Occupational Voice Users

11.1 Introduction

The estimated prevalence of voice disorders in the general population varies between 0.65% and 15% [1, 2]. Demographic, socioeconomic, and sociocultural factors are important determinants of lifetime occurrence of these disorders. Sports occupational voice users (SOVU), similar to other professional voice users with high voice demands, are at a higher risk of developing dysphonia in comparison to the normal population [3]. Coaches, fitness instructors, and athletes often engage in phonatory tasks while performing strenuous exercise. The need to project their voice during training and competitive events increases vocal load, compromises voice ergonomics, and imposes high stress on their phonatory apparatus. This body kinetic-induced burden is often compounded by comorbid conditions such as asthma and laryngopharyngeal reflux disease, which predispose further voice disorders [4, 5]. Equally important to these individual-related voice risk factors are environmental factors. Exposure to indoor and outdoor allergens and irritants is a significant threat to all components of the phonatory system [6]. Similarly, poor environment acoustics, reverberation, and noise are voice risk factors. Seidman et al. reported an increase in wind noise up to 120 dB when cycling speed reaches 60 mph [7], and Masullo et al. highlighted noise as a significant risk factor in basketball referees who are exposed to high-peak sound pressure level from whistles [8]. Moreover, the high background noise generated by spectators and others forces coaches and athletes to exert excessive effort in order to be heard. The increase in vocal effort is associated with an increase in mechanical stresses of phonation, thus leading to functional and structural voice disorders as discussed in Chap. 5 of this book.

Because of the factors discussed above, SOVU are at substantial risk of having voice symptoms. Long et al. investigated voice problems in aerobic instructors and reported a prevalence of 44% during or after instructing. The authors highlighted the limited knowledge participants had regarding vocal hygiene and education [9].

© The Author(s), under exclusive license to Springer Nature Switzerland AG 2021
A.-L. Hamdan et al., *Voice Disorders in Athletes, Coaches and other Sports Professionals*, https://doi.org/10.1007/978-3-030-69831-7_11

Similarly, Heidel and Torgerson reported that aerobic instructors were more likely to experience hoarseness and/or loss of voice in comparison to aerobic participants. The authors noted water intake, smoking, and sleeping habits in their evaluation of voice and voice-related risk factors [10]. Similarly, in their study of 320 sports and fitness instructors, Fontan et al. described voice difficulties in 55% of the cases. Only one-third of the participants had been informed about vocal hygiene and phonotrauma, although the majority had expressed their interest in learning about preventive voice care measures [11]. Rumbach et al. also reported chronic hoarseness in 39% of 361 group fitness instructors. The authors used a 65-item self-completion questionnaire and highlighted loud speaking as a significant voice risk factor [12]. Similarly, in the investigation of 109 male soccer coaches by Fellman and Simberg, at least 2 voice symptoms occurred in 28.4% of the study group. The authors stressed the need to increase voice awareness in a vocally demanding profession such as soccer [13].

OVU with dysphonia, similar to teachers, singers, and other professional voice users who suffer from voice symptoms, need special attention. With the emergence of multidisciplinary approaches in the management of patients with voice disorders, nonsurgical "conservative" voice management has gained popularity as a primary treatment modality, with fair results in adults and children [14–16]. Given the scarcity of studies on the impact of conservative voice therapy in SOVU, this chapter reviews briefly the management strategies adopted in the nonsurgical treatment of singers, teachers, and other professional voice users. These include mainly vocal hygiene therapy (VHT), vocal function exercises (VFE), and voice amplification (VA). The educational material and therapies presented in this review apply also to SOVU with dysphonia given the similarity in ergonomic voice risk factors and vocal fold pathology in SOVU and other professional voice users. This material is important for primary care physicians, sports physicians, coaches, fitness instructors, and otolaryngologists involved in the voice care of SOVU with voice disorders or at high risk of having voice disorders. It is also useful for SOVU interested in preventing or improving their voice quality by adopting changes in their lifestyle and behavior.

11.2   Vocal Hygiene Therapy, Vocal Function Exercises, and Voice Amplification: Impact on Voice

11.2.1   Vocal Hygiene Therapy

Vocal hygiene therapy (VHT) is a multifaceted management strategy that is used commonly in patients with functional and structural voice disorders. It also is advocated as adjunctive treatment before and after phono-microsurgery, particularly in patients at high risk for having recurrent dysphonia. Vocal hygiene therapy includes educational and behavioral remedies that aim at optimizing voice production and increasing its efficiency. In a review on vocal hygiene for the voice professional by Behlau and Oliveira, the authors described vocal hygiene as a comprehensive program that encompasses education on the anatomy/physiology of phonation and the means to avoid phonotrauma and improve voice health. By learning about the physiology of phonation, patients recognize the critical role of breathing in voice production and the need for adequate breath support in order to project voice with minimal effort. Similarly, patients also learn how to avoid traumatic vocal behavior secondary to voice abuse as in screaming, coughing or throat clearing, voice overuse as in prolonged phonation, and voice misuse as in speaking or singing out of one's comfortable pitch/intensity range. The authors also stress the role of voice health in phonation. Adequate local and systemic hydration, healthy lifestyle, and control of associated morbidities such as asthma and laryngopharyngeal reflux are emphasized [17]. Patients undergoing VHT are encouraged to engage in behavioral modification with respect to their sleeping habits, alcohol consumption, smoking, and the intake of recreational drugs such as androgenic anabolic steroids. Abstention from caffeinated products and the intake of medications with dehydrating effects also are encouraged. A more detailed description of vocal hygiene and other voice therapy techniques can be found in various chapters of the book *Professional Voice: The Science and Art of Clinical Care, 4th Edition* [18].

There are many reports in the literature that support the clinical application of VHT in the management of dysphonia and its value in voice enhancement. In a Cochrane review by Ruotsalainen et al. on the effectiveness of interventions in treating functional voice disorders, the authors commented on the usefulness of both direct and indirect therapy. There was evidence in three out of six studies that combination therapy had a positive effect on self-reported vocal functioning, observer-rated vocal functioning, and objective voice measures [19]. Similarly, Timmermans et al. reviewed the outcome of vocal hygiene in singers and confirmed its positive role in the management of dysphonia. The authors also stressed the need for careful examination and detection of even minor vocal fold structural abnormalities [20]. In a study by Zuim et al. on the association between education and perceived singing voice function, the authors found that those with greater education in voice heath sang more easily. Other factors associated with higher Evaluation of the Ability to Sing Easily (EASE) score included years of training, having a college degree, and singing classical music [21]. In another study by Yiu et al. of 20 amateur singers who were asked to perform various phonatory tasks, the authors showed that those with better vocal hygiene, i.e., who drank adequate quantities of water and rested their voice at regular intervals, were able to sing longer than those who did not [22]. These reports are in agreement with many studies asserting the strong association between hydration, phonation threshold pressure, and laryngeal function [23, 24].

Although the above reports support the role of VHT in professional voice users with and without dysphonia, it is important to note that VHT has its limitations; namely, the high rate of patient attrition attributed to the duration of treatment and its limited impact on patient behavior in some cases [18, 25, 26]. Timmermans et al., in their study on training outcome in future professional voice users, noted that lecturing about vocal hygiene had no effect on "voice-conserving habits" [25].

Another study by the same authors conducted on 23 professional voice users also showed that lecturing about vocal hygiene did not change the daily habits of the participants with regard to smoking, eating, and phonatory behavior [26].

In summary, VHT is an effective therapeutic strategy in singers and teachers with and without voice complaints. Although there are no studies on VHT in SOVU, there is substantial anecdotal experience confirming that this population, similar to other professional voice users, can benefit from this multifaceted treatment. The limited knowledge about voice health and education in the sports industry emphasizes the substantial need for increased education and VHT in SOVU. Future investigation on how VHT can help mitigate individual and environment-related voice risk factors is needed.

11.2.2   Vocal Function Exercises

Voice training and vocal function exercises (VFE), unlike vocal hygiene, are not limited to lecturing and voice education but include active training of various techniques used in the treatment of functional and organic voice disorders. The main target is to restore voice efficiency by decreasing laryngeal muscle tension and imbalance and by improving the coordination between the activity of respiratory and laryngeal muscles and use of the resonance system. By balancing the airflow and glottal aperture, and by enhancing the resonant voice, voice production becomes more efficient and less tiring. For optimal results, VFE need to be individualized and tailored according to the patient's needs and provided by trained, expert voice care professionals [27, 28].

There are many reports in the literature supporting the role of VFE in the management of the speaking and professional voice [29–37]. In a systematic search on the impact of voice training on voice quality, Hazlett et al. reported improvement in at least one voice-related measure in nine out of the ten studies reviewed [29]. In another study of 37 primary school teachers undergoing VFE, Pasa et al. reported improvement in voice symptoms as well as aerodynamic and acoustic measures [30]. Similarly, Meerschman et al. investigated the short-term effect of resonant voice training and straw phonation (a therapeutic technique that involves phonation against gentle resistance) and reported improvement in voice quality and capacity following 6 weeks of therapy. Straw phonation therapy has helped extend the intensity range, whereas resonant therapy has improved the dysphonia severity index [31]. In a randomized, controlled study that included patients with muscle tension dysphonia, Watts et al. showed that those who were treated with voice therapy (stretch-and-flow voice therapy) had better improvement in self-reported rating and acoustic measures in comparison with those who received voice education alone [32]. In another prospective randomized study of 58 teachers with voice disorders, Roy et al. reported more improvement in voice quality and clarity in the subgroup who underwent a 6-week vocal functional exercises program in comparison with those who underwent vocal hygiene therapy alone. The authors advocated VFE as a better treatment alternative than vocal hygiene therapy in the management of dysphonia patients [33], although most voice care professionals use both. Meerschman et al. investigated the effect of three semi-occluded voice therapy (such as straw phonation) programs in 35 patients with dysphonia and reported improvement 3 weeks after treatment. Patients treated with lip trill and straw phonation had a decrease in their dysphonia severity index. Psychosocial improvement also was noted in those who underwent water resistance therapy [34].

The improvement in voice quality following VFE can be attributed to enhancement in aerodynamic function, in addition to improvement in muscle balance and function. Stemple et al. studied the efficacy of VFE in 35 adults randomly assigned to either therapy or placebo or control and reported a decrease in the flow rate and an increase in maximum phonation time in the therapy group [35]. Similarly, Sabol et al. investigated the value of VFE in 20 singers and also noted the same improvement in aerodynamic measures in the experimental group after 4 weeks of treatment [36].

In summary, VFE is an effective treatment strategy for patients with functional and structural voice disorders. Following treatment, patients experience improvement in both subjective and objective voice measures. The improvement in voice quality is accomplished through reduction in vocal dose and an increase in vocal economy. SOVU with dysphonia can also benefit from VFE. The techniques and approaches used in other professional voice users, such as lip trill, straw phonation, and water-resistant therapy, also are applicable in SOVU with dysphonia. Furthermore, this approach is intuitive for athletes who have been trained to accomplish their sports activity by minimizing excess/unnecessary muscle effort and optimizing efficiency for their athletic tasks whether they involve running, swinging a racket, or any other endeavor. The principle of performance economy in athletic activity is the same as that used to optimize voice. Future studies in that field are needed.

11.2.3 Voice Amplification (VA) Strategy

Voice amplification is an alternative treatment strategy in professional voice users with or without dysphonia. It is a conservative approach that aims at reducing vocal dose by amplifying voice, thereby reducing the effort needed to be heard. The voice amplifiers can be either stationary as in a sound-field FM system or portable. Using a sound-field FM system, the spoken voice is detected and then transformed into an electrical signal that is amplified via a speaker. Usually, the speaker is well located in a given place. Alternatively, a portable voice amplification system is carried. This approach allows increasing voice loudness to a level judged to be comfortable for communication [38]. It is important to note that although voice amplification reduces the stress on the vocal folds, it does not target the phonatory behavior, unlike VHT and VFE. That being stated, VA may be a complementary treatment strategy to VHT and VFE in patients with voice disorders [38–43].

Numerous studies concur that vocal dose is reduced in speakers who use VA. In a study by Texiera and Behlau that included 162 teachers with behavioral dysphonia, and who were randomly allocated to either VFE, VA, or as controls, the authors reported improvement in the auditory-perceptual assessment in the VFE and VA subgroups. Moreover, there was significant improvement in glottic closure and size of vocal fold lesions in 11 out of 54 of the VA subgroup [38]. Gaskill et al. investigated the effect of voice amplification on vocal dose in two elementary school teachers and showed reduction in voice intensity, more so in the teacher with voice problems. Notably, the effect persisted for 1 week after the use of the amplifier was discontinued [39]. Masson and Araujo investigated the effect of VA on 53 teachers, half of whom were assigned VA for 4 weeks and whose voice function was assessed before and after. The authors reported a decrease in sound pressure level (SPL) and acoustic irregularities. The authors reiterated the role of VA as a protective strategy against dysphonia [40]. Morrow and Connor investigated the effect of VA in music teachers and reported a significant decrease in voice intensity, cycle dose, and mean phonation time. The authors concurred that VA is effective in reducing phonotrauma [41]. Similarly, Bovo et al. reported a decrease in symptoms of voice fatigue and improvement in voice handicap index (VHI) score, following the use of VA. The study was conducted on 40 female teachers who had grade 1 dysphonia, and half of whom were asked to carry a portable amplifier for 12 weeks [42]. In a randomized clinical trial, Roy et al. showed that the use of voice amplification yielded better subjective treatment outcome than vocal hygiene or no treatment at all. The study included 44 teachers with voice disorders who were assigned either a vocal hygiene therapy program, the use of voice amplification, or no treatment. The outcome measures included VHI, the voice severity self-rating scale, and acoustic measures. However, it is important to note that both treatment subgroups had significant improvement in comparison to the control subgroup and that there was no significant difference between the vocal hygiene and voice amplification subgroups except for self-rating of clarity of voice and ease of projection, which were greater in the VA subgroup [43].

In summary, VA is an alternative therapy to VHT and VFE. Although it does not address directly laryngeal behavior and phonatory habits, speakers who use VA enjoy a reduction in voice intensity and improvement in self-rating of their voice quality. The reduction in loudness undoubtedly decreases the mechanical stress on the vocal folds, thus reducing phonotrauma. It can be used in conjunction with VHT and VFE. SOVU, similar to other professional voice users, may benefit from VA as either a preventive or therapeutic treatment modality.

11.3 Safety Measures in Sports-Related Laryngeal Trauma

Sports-related laryngeal trauma, although rare, has been reported widely in SOVU. Its prevalence varies with the type of sport, age, and gender. High-velocity sports, older age, and male gender are significant predisposing factors [44]. Sports-related laryngeal injuries can be life-threatening and can have long-term phonatory and airway sequelae. Despite the improvement in safety equipment, sport environment remains a threat to vocal health. Pucks, balls, sticks, and bats are a few examples of objects that can cause laryngeal injury. Resultant trauma may cause substantial cervical soft tissue injuries and laryngeal fractures if the neck is left unprotected. Trinidade et al. reported a 23-year-old lacrosse player who sustained laryngeal injury secondary to a direct blow to the neck by a lacrosse ball [45]. Similarly, French and Kelley reported three cases of laryngeal fracture following a ball trauma in lacrosse games. The authors emphasized the need for all players to wear neck protective gears, not just the goalies [46]. Using helmets, neck guards, face masks, and head gear helps secure protection to the head and neck. Based on the baby boomer sports injury report, wearing head helmets in 69% of children and 43% of baby boomers has markedly reduced the seriousness of head injuries [47]. Although protective to the head and neck region, wearing a helmet may still be hazardous to laryngeal structures. Ostby et al. reported three cases of laryngeal fractures following bicycle or motorcycle accidents. The authors attributed the injuries to the position of the helmet buckle in the neck [48].

In addition to wearing the necessary protective sports gear, proper implementation of athletic regulations and rules is important in preventing sports-related laryngeal trauma. Concerns are not only field related but also collision between players. Trauma to the neck by elbow or other body parts can injure the larynx. Based on the 26th annual report of catastrophic sports injuries, several recommendations were made to reduce the number of injuries and fatalities in sports. These included proper education and training of coaches and sports instructors, periodic inspection of sports equipment and tools, and continued research in athletic rules and facilities for further improvement. Some of the recommendations were sports specific such as anchoring of soccer goals in soccer games and ensuring flat surfaces in the field [49]. Otolaryngologists, speech-language pathologists, and other voice care professionals should collaborate with sports medicine physicians, trainers, coaches, athletes, and other interested parties to help develop the most effective, least intrusive approaches to protecting the larynx and voice.

References

1. Morley DE. A ten-year survey of speech disorders among university students. J Speech Hear Disord. 1952;17(1):25–31.
2. Laguaite JK. Adult voice screening. J Speech Hear Disord. 1972;37(2):147–51.

3. Williams NR. Occupational groups at risk of voice disorders: a review of the literature. Occup Med. 2003;53:456–60.
4. Lennelöv E, Irewall T, Naumburg E, Lindberg A, Stenfors N. The prevalence of asthma and respiratory symptoms among cross-country skiers in early adolescence. Can Respir J. 2019;2019:1514353.
5. Waterman JJ, Kapur R. Upper gastrointestinal issues in athletes. Curr Sports Med Rep. 2012;11(2):99–104.
6. Del Giacco SR, Carlsen KH, Du Toit G. Allergy and sports in children. Pediatr Allergy Immunol. 2012;23(1):11–20.
7. Seidman MD, Wertz AG, Smith MM, Jacob S, Ahsan SF. Evaluation of noise exposure secondary to wind noise in cyclists. Otolaryngol Head Neck Surg. 2017;157(5):848–52.
8. Masullo M, Lenzuni P, Maffei L, et al. Assessment of noise exposure for basketball sports referees. J Occup Environ Hyg. 2016;13(6):464–75.
9. Long J, Williford HN, Olson MS, Wolfe V. Voice problems and risk factors among aerobics instructors. J Voice. 1998;12(2):197–207.
10. Heidel SE, Torgerson JK. Vocal problems among aerobic instructors and aerobic participants. J Commun Disord. 1993;26(3):179–91.
11. Fontan L, Fraval M, Michon A, Déjean S, Welby-Gieusse M. Vocal problems in sports and fitness instructors: a study of prevalence, risk factors, and need for prevention in France. J Voice. 2017;31(2):261.e33–8.
12. Rumbach A, Khan A, Brown M, Eloff K, Poetschke A. Voice problems in the fitness industry: factors associated with chronic hoarseness. Int J Speech Lang Pathol. 2015;17(5):441–50.
13. Fellman D, Simberg S. Prevalence and risk factors for voice problems among soccer coaches. J Voice. 2017;31(1):121-e9–15.
14. Rendon MD, Ermakova T, Freymann ML, Ruschin A, Nawka T, Caffier PP. Efficacy of phonosurgery, logopedic voice treatment and vocal pedagogy in common voice problems of singers. Adv Ther. 2018;35(7):1069–86.
15. Hartnick C, Ballif C, De Guzman V, et al. Indirect vs direct voice therapy for children with vocal nodules: a randomized clinical trial. JAMA Otolaryngol Head Neck Surg. 2018;144(2):156–63.
16. Chhetri SS, Gautam R. Acoustic analysis before and after voice therapy for laryngeal pathology. Kathmandu Univ Med J. 2015;13(4):323–7.
17. Behlau M, Oliveira G. Vocal hygiene for the voice professional. Curr Opin Otolaryngol Head Neck Surg. 2009;17(3):149–54.
18. Sataloff RT. Professional voice: the science and art of clinical care. 4th ed. San Diego: Plural Publishing; 2017. p. 1163–324.
19. Ruotsalainen JH, Sellman J, Lehto L, Jauhiainen M, Verbeek JH. Interventions for treating functional dysphonia in adults. Cochrane Database Syst Rev. 2007;(3):CD006373.
20. Timmermans B, Vanderwegen J, De Bodt MS. Outcome of vocal hygiene in singers. Curr Opin Otolaryngol Head Neck Surg. 2005;13(3):138–42.
21. Zuim AF, Lloyd AT, Gerhard J, Rosow D, Lundy D. Associations of education and training with perceived singing voice function among professional singers. J Voice. 2019;S0892–1997(19)30313–3.
22. Yiu EM, Chan RM. Effect of hydration and vocal rest on the vocal fatigue in amateur karaoke singers. J Voice. 2003;17(2):216–27.
23. Verdolini-Marston K, Sandage M, Titze I. Effect of hydration treatment on laryngeal nodules and polyps and related voice measures. J Voice. 1994;8:30–47.
24. Solomon NP, DiMattia MS. Effects of a vocally fatiguing task and systemic hydration on phonation threshold pressure. J Voice. 2000;14(3):341–62.
25. Timmermans B, De Bodt MS, Wuyts FL, Van de Heyning PH. Training outcome in future professional voice users after 18 months of voice training. Folia Phoniatr Logop. 2004;56(2):120–9.
26. Timmermans B, De Bodt MS, Wuyts FL, Van de Heyning PH. Analysis and evaluation of a voice-training program in future professional voice users. J Voice. 2005;19(2):202–10.

27. Sataloff RT. Introduction to treating voice abuse. In: Satalof RT. Professional voice: the science and art of clinical care. 4th ed. San Diego: Plural Publishing; 2017. p. 1163–6.
28. Rose B, Horman M, Sataloff RT. Voice therapy. In: Satalof RT. Professional voice: the science and art of clinical care. 4th ed. San Diego: Plural Publishing; 2017. p. 1171–94.
29. Hazlett D, Duffy OM, Moorhead SA. Review of the impact of voice training on the vocal quality of professional voice users: implications for vocal health and recommendations for further research. J Voice. 2011;25(2):181–91.
30. Pasa G, Oates J, Dacakis G. The relative effectiveness of vocal hygiene training and vocal function exercises in preventing voice disorders in primary school teachers. Logoped Phoniatr Vocol. 2007;32(3):128–40.
31. Meerschman I, Van Lierde K, Peeters K, Meersman E, Claeys S, D'haeseleer E. Short-term effect of two semi-occluded vocal tract training programs on the vocal quality of future occupational voice users: "resonant voice training using nasal consonants" versus "straw phonation". J Speech Lang Hear. 2017;60(9):2519–36.
32. Watts CR, Hamilton A, Toles L, Childs L, Mau T. A randomized controlled trial of stretch-and-flow voice therapy for muscle tension dysphonia. Laryngoscope. 2015;125(6):1420–5.
33. Roy N, Gray SD, Simon M, Dove H, Corbin-Lewis K, Stemple JC. An evaluation of the effects of two treatment approaches for teachers with voice disorders: a prospective randomized clinical trial. J Speech Lang Hear Res. 2001;44(2):286–96.
34. Meerschman I, Van Lierde K, Ketels J, Coppieters C, Claeys S, D'haeseleer E. Effect of three semi-occluded vocal tract therapy programmes on the phonation of patients with dysphonia: lip trill, water-resistance therapy and straw phonation. Int J Lang Commun Disord. 2019;54(1):50–61.
35. Stemple JC, Lee L, D'Amico B. Efficacy of vocal function exercise as a method of improving voice production. J Voice. 1994;8(3):271–8.
36. Sabol JW, Lee L, Stemple JC. The value of vocal function exercises in the practice regimen of singers. J Voice. 1995;9(1):27–36.
37. Calvache C, Guman M, Bobadilla M, Bortnem C. Variation on vocal economy after different semioccluded vocal tract exercises in subjects with normal voice and dysphonia. J Voice. 2020;34(4):582–9.
38. Teixeira LC, Behlau M. Comparison between vocal function exercises and voice amplification. J Voice. 2015;29(6):718–26.
39. Gaskill CS, O'Brien SG, Tinter SR. The effect of voice amplification on occupational vocal dose in elementary school teachers. J Voice. 2012;26(5):667.e19–27.
40. Masson MLV, de Araújo TM. Protective strategies against dysphonia in teachers: preliminary results comparing voice amplification and 0.9% NaCl nebulization. J Voice. 2018;32(2):257.e1–257.e10.
41. Morrow SL, Connor NP. Voice amplification as a means of reducing vocal load for elementary music teachers. J Voice. 2011;25(4):441–6.
42. Bovo R, Trevisi P, Emanuelli E, Martini A. Voice amplification for primary school teachers with voice disorders: a randomized clinical trial. Int J Occup Med Environ Health. 2013;26(3):363–72.
43. Roy N, Weinreich B, Gray SD, et al. Voice amplification versus vocal hygiene instruction for teachers with voice disorders: a treatment outcomes study. J Speech Lang Hear. 2002;45:625–38.
44. Paluska SA, Lansford CD. Laryngeal trauma in sport. Curr Sports Med Rep. 2008;7(1):16–21.
45. Trinidade A, Shakeel M, Stickle B, Ah-See KW. Laryngeal fracture caused by a lacrosse ball. J Coll Physicians Surg Pak. 2015;25(11):843–4.
46. French C, Kelly R. Laryngeal fractures in lacrosse due to high speed ball impact. JAMA Otolaryngol Head Neck Surg. 2013;139(7):735–8.
47. US Consumer Product Safety Commission. Baby boomer sports injuries. April 2000. https://www.cpsc.gov/s3fs-public/pdfs/boomer.pdf. Accessed 20 Nov 2020.

48. Ostby ET, Crawley BK. Helmet clasp cracks larynx? A case series and literature review. Ann Otol Rhinol Laryngol. 2018;127(4):282–4.
49. Mueller FO, Cantu RC. Twenty-sixth annual report fall 1982- Spring 2008. UNC-Chapel Hill website. http://nccsir.unc.edu/files/2014/05/AllSport.pdf. Published 2008. Accessed 20 Nov 2020.

Index

Printed in the United States
by Baker & Taylor Publisher Services